Ralph T. Manktelow

Microvascular Reconstruction

Anatomy, Applications and Surgical Technique

With Section on Paediatrics
by Ronald M. Zuker

Foreword by G. Ian Taylor

Illustrated by Ken Finch

With 288 Figures

Springer-Verlag
Berlin Heidelberg New York Tokyo

Ralph T. Manktelow, M.D., F.R.C.S. (C)
Associate Professor of Surgery,
University of Toronto Faculty of Medicine;
Head, Division of Plastic Surgery,
Toronto General Hospital,
200 Elizabeth Street,
Toronto, Ontario, Canada
M5G 2C4

ISBN-13:978-3-642-70331-7 e-ISBN-13:978-3-642-70329-4
DOI: 10.1007/978-3-642-70329-4

Library of Congress Cataloging-in-Publication Data
Manktelow, Ralph T. Microvascular reconstruction.
Includes bibliographies and index.
1. Blood - vessels -- Surgery. 2. Microsurgery. 3. Flaps (Surgery)
I. Title. [DNLM: 1. Microsurgery--methods. 2. Surgical Flaps.
WO 512 M278m]
RD594. 2. M36 1986 617'.413 85-30323
ISBN-13:978-3-642-70331-7 (U.S.)

2124/3145-543210

To Marg, Blair, Greg, Jennifer and Scott

Foreword

Reconstructive microvascular surgery is now in its teens. At first many thought this new child was a whim and would fail to thrive. Some were uncertain, others with vision either supported or became actively involved in this new area of surgical endeavour. Although initial interest was focused on the replantation of amputated parts, it has been the one stage free transfer of living tissue to a distant site which has launched microsurgery into the surgical spotlight.

From its humble beginnings we have witnessed a revolution in this branch of plastic surgery; many of the long established methods of reconstruction have, like barricades, fallen before the advances made in this field. In its infancy there were relatively few procedures available. There was a tendency to make the patient's problem fit the operation, rather than the reverse, and this frequently led to an inferior result. The then known flaps, such as the groin flap and the deltopectoral flap, were employed. Unfortunately they were sites which posed many technical problems; namely those of vascular anomaly, a short pedicle and vessels of small calibre. Long operations were the norm, and vascular thrombosis was not uncommon. Hospital routine often was disrupted and there was a danger that these new techniques would fall into disrepute.

Over the last decade this state of affairs has changed dramatically. There has been an explosion in the number of free flaps available to the microsurgeon, which offer both versatility and reliability. Many of these have been developed as a result of intensive investigations in the post mortem disecting room. Numerous fresh cadaver dissection and injection studies have defined the vascular architecture of various tissues and combinations of tissues. In our department at The Royal Melbourne Hospital for example over 2,000 such studies have been performed. What is most important is that many of these techniques have evolved to match the patient's needs.

With the introduction of a new flap, there is an initial wave of enthusiasm which must receed through the channels of peer appraisal, ultimately to assume as Ian McGregor has succinctly stated, "its correct pecking order". Many flaps have their champions, so it is appropriate that a book such as this be written by an ardent consumer who has no axe to grind. Ralph Manktelow is such a person and I am honoured by his request to write the foreward to this important work.

Dr. Manktelow has been more than an umpire. He is one of the second generation of surgeons who has helped refine the works of the pioneers. His enquiring mind and considerable clinical experience has offered much to the literature on this subject. In particular his refinements of the free gracilis muscle as a functional unit for reconstruction of the crippled upper limb and the paralysed face are unsurpassed.

Choosing the most appropriate flap to solve a specific reconstructive problem requires the careful analysis of many factors. What tissues do we need, from where can they be best spared, and how can we minimise patient discomfort and cost to the community? The final choice should be based on sensible planning and experience. One after all does not expect a professional golfer to ask his caddy to pass him from the bag, a putter to drive down the fairway, nor a driver to use on the green. We now have at our disposal flaps that can get us out of the rough far more readily than in bygone days. Even the "hole in one" is easier with the development of such procedures as the vascularised osteomyocutaneous flap.

This book does not pretend to cover every aspect of free flap surgery, nor does it assume to be a definitive work on the subject - for reconstructive microvascular surgery is still a rapidly expanding art. The book does however define the problem areas where, at this stage, free flap surgery has the most to offer. From the long list of described flaps Ralph Manktelow and his co-workers have selected a nucleus of reliable and versatile procedures to solve the majority of these reconstructive problems.

The description of the planning and execution of these operations is practical and informative. The illustrations are of a high standard and are designed to aid the surgeon. The book is undoubtably a valuable contribution to the literature on reconstructive surgery.

February, 1986 G. Ian Taylor

Preface

This book is designed to be a 'how to do it' text of microvascular reconstructive surgery. It discusses the selection, anatomy and surgical technique of a spectrum of free tissue transfers. It is written primarily by one surgeon, and is purposely dogmatic in the hope that it will provide useful solutions to patients' problems.

The book is divided into two sections. The first section covers the surgical anatomy and technique involved in elevating each of the free tissue transfers. The second section discusses the applications of these transfers to reconstruction in three specific areas. These areas are the three anatomical regions in which reconstructive microsurgery has made its major contributions: the head and neck, the upper extremity and the lower extremity. The only digression from this plan has been with toe and jejunum transfers. As they are used exclusively in hand, and head and neck respectively, these transfers are described in the second section. Since most of the free tissue transfers are used in all three anatomic regions, rather than repeat their description in each region of application, I have described each transfer once and grouped these descriptions at the front of the book to form Section One.

Each surgeon doing reconstructive microsurgery should have a repertoire of reliable transfers. I believe that the patient will be served best if the surgeon has expertise in a selected group of transfers and does not dabble in every new transfer that is described. The surgeon's inventory of free tissue transfers will include skin flaps, muscle flaps, bone transfers and composite transfers, such as the toe, and jejunum. With this premise in mind, I have elected to describe what are, for me, the most frequently used transfers in each of the tissue types. There are many transfers which have not been included because I do not have extensive experience in their use and feel that the transfers here described will solve the majority of reconstructive problems. There are also a number of recently described and promising flaps which have not been included in this book as their value can only be gauged by the passage of time and broad application.

This book is not designed to be read through from cover to cover. Rather, it is designed to be a reference book which the trainee and the surgeon with experience in reconstructive microsurgery will use to assist them in the management of patients with specific problems. When using this book, the reader will likely turn first to Section II for the appropriate chapter which describes the patient's problem. Then, after reviewing the surgical options, will turn back to Section I for the chapter which describes the most appropriate free tissue transfer.

When I began, in 1973, there were only a few surgeons using microvascular techniques. Now, 12 years later, in almost every country of the world, there are surgeons practicing reconstructive microsurgery. It is for these surgeons, with their varying levels of expertise and training, that this 'what, when and how to' book is written.

Toronto, February 1986 Ralph T. Manktelow

Topographical Index by Region of Application

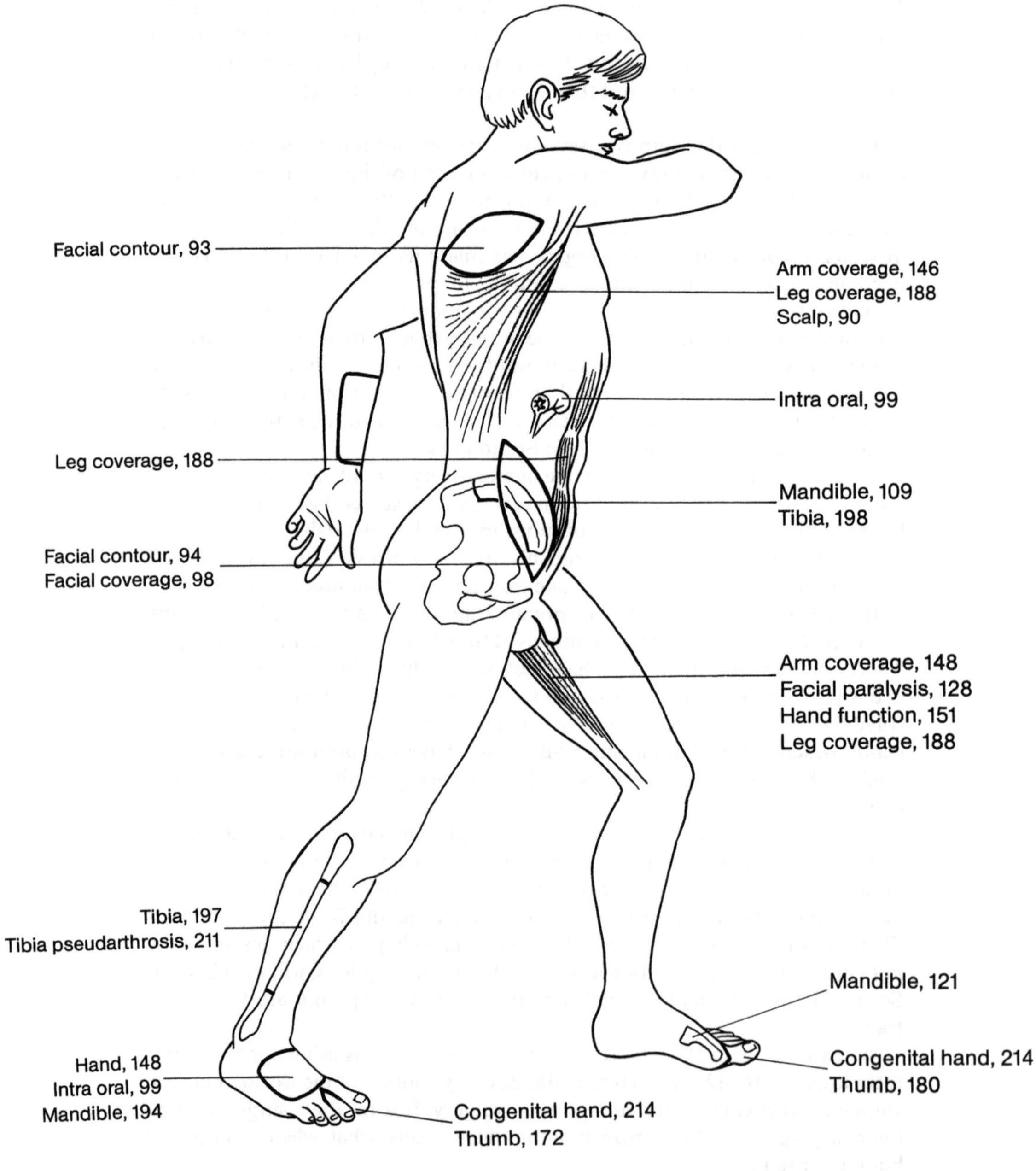

Table of Contents

Acknowledgements

The development of my microsurgical practice was stimulated by exposure to Harry Buncke, John Cobbett, Bob Acland, Bernie O'Brien, Ian Taylor, Chen Zhong-wei, Kiyonori Harii, Alain Gilbert and Harold Kleinert. These surgeons are some of the early giants in reconstructive microsurgery and to them I am most grateful for their teaching and encouragement.

In Toronto, I have had the special pleasure of taking part in the training of other surgeons, and having some of them join me as colleagues. In this manner, Drs. Nancy McKee, Ron Zuker, Jim Mahoney and Brian Boyd and I have developed a group who operate together, form a post graduate teaching service and share in research investigations. The experience of this group has been broadly based with a major microsurgical activity in all three areas of reconstructive microsurgery - the head and neck, the upper extremity and the lower extremity. Included in this book are many of the principles and prejudices developed by these surgeons. I appreciate their contribution.

I am particularly fortunate to have worked with Dr. Ron Zuker as a friend and co-surgeon on most of our difficult cases. Not only does he provide the hands of a skilled microsurgeon, but for these cases, brings an almost intuitive sense of what will work best. From this close co-operation, there have been many benefits to the patient, to the development of the field of reconstructive microsurgery, and to our trainees. As Dr. Zuker has a special interest in children's surgery, he has written the chapter on Paediatric Microsurgery.

Our experience in microsurgery involves over 300 replantations and over 300 free tissue transfers. With these cases, our Fellows and Residents have provided an intellectual stimulus and an untiring support for the heavy demands of the service, and to them I give my sincere thanks.

This book was written with the assistance of my wife, Marg, who provided an incisive editorial pen. For this help and her patience during the preparation of the manuscript, I am most appreciative.

I am particularly grateful for the perseverence of my secretary, Elizabeth Atkinson, who has shepherded this book through its multiple revisions and reorganizations. She accepted the manuscript's preparation with the same good humor, skill and enthusiasm which she puts into the management of my surgical practice.

The realization of this book was possible to a large extent because of the efforts of Ken Finch. His illustrations illuminate the techniques and concepts which are the message of this book. The clarity of his illustrations reflect his understanding of the operative procedures and desire for logical communication.

Chapter 1. Preamble

There are many good texts and manuals which describe the techniques of microvascular anastomoses. It is not the intention of this book to duplicate these descriptions, as it is assumed that the surgeon who uses this book will be skilled in these techniques. The microvascular trainee will quickly appreciate that the microvascular anastomosis, although critical to flap survival, is often the easiest part of a free tissue transfer. More difficult and requiring a broad training and experience in reconstructive surgery is the decision making which goes into each procedure. The success of each reconstruction is as much related to the thoroughness of the preoperative planning as it is to the execution of the operative procedure.

The surgeon wishing to do reconstructive microsurgery will require post graduate training in a centre which specializes in a large volume of reconstructive microsurgery. Before coming to the operating room, the surgeon will have worked in the laboratory and mastered end to end arterial and venous anastomoses, end to side repairs, and the repair of grafts between dissimilar sized vessels. When these skills are developed, he or she is then ready for training in the application of these anastomotic skills to reconstructive techniques.

Free tissue transfers for coverage, although still a valuable application of microsurgical techniques, lead the way to more complex and technically demanding procedures. These are the osteocutaneous reconstructions of the extremities and mandible, toe and partial toe transfers and the functioning muscle reconstructions of the face and extremities. The need to conceptualize, in three dimensions, a reconstruction which includes different but attached tissues, such as skin, muscle and bone, has placed increasing demands upon the reconstructive surgeon.

The development of new free tissue transfers has required an improved understanding of vascular anatomy. Considerable effort has been spent investigating the vascular territories which are supplied by various arteries, and determining the amount of tissue which the artery will support. In developing new transfers, surgeons have had to understand anatomical details which have never previously had an application to reconstructive surgery.

Preoperative Planning

Preoperative planning begins with an assessment of the patient's functional and anatomic deficit. The complete armamentarium of reconstructive techniques should then be reviewed and the technique which provides the best solution with the least difficulty should be used.

If a microsurgical reconstruction is selected, in addition to analyzing the three dimensional size and shape of the defect, the surgeon must assess the available recipient vessels. This assessment is done by clinical, doppler and angiographic examination. The surgeon then reviews the available donor sites which provide the tissue required and selects the most appropriate.

Often the surgeon is faced with a defect which is different from anything he or she has previously reconstructed. In this situation, it is particularly useful to use models and patterns, or go to the anatomy department, create the defect and do the operative procedure in the cadaver. If a careful step by step planning has been carried out, the surgical team can move briskly through the operating procedure with minimal delay.

The Team Approach

For the planning and execution of new and complex cases, a second surgeon is often a great asset. Complex procedures are done most effectively with two teams. One team prepares the recipient area while the other team prepares the tissue for transfer. During the transplantation, the second team is available for a back up should a major problem be encountered. With this approach, there is less surgeon fatigue and often better solutions to the reconstructive problem. Many of the problems which occur in reconstructive microsurgery are decision related and likely to occur at the end of a long procedure when a surgeon is fatigued. If there is a vascular complication after 10 hours of surgery, and a change of operative plan is required, a fatigued surgeon is not as likely to make as good a decision as one who is relatively fresh.

Pedicle Preparation

Although the technique of microvascular anastomosis is well established and frequently described, there has been little emphasis on the technique of preparing the pedicle itself.

Eye loop magnification with high resolution optics of 2.5–4.5 power and high intensity lighting is necessary for adequate visualization of the pedicle.

In each free tissue transfer and each recipient site, there is often a preferred location for identification of the pedicle. The surgeon should begin at this location and then work proximally and distally, separating the pedicle from its surroundings.

Extremity vessels do not normally become obstructed with movements of the extremity because they are surrounded and supported by fatty connective tissue. If the pedicle is dissected with a layer of fat and the venae comitantes left on the artery, the pedicle is less likely to obstruct by kinking and twisting in the recipient site. A skeletonized vessel, particularly a vein, is prone to obstruction through twisting or folding. However, leaving fatty connective tissue on the pedicle may make it more difficult to trace the vessel.

There are a number of ways of managing pedicle side branches. Hemoclips may be applied and are particularly fast and useful. However, if not applied carefully, they will come off or cut the side branch and unwanted bleeding will occur following the transfer. The alternate to clips is the more time consuming ligation with 6-0 to 8-0 sutures. For small branches, a bipolar cautery with jeweller's forceps is the preferred technique. For any of these techniques, the side branch should be divided just beyond its attachment to the main artery, but not so far removed that a blind pouch is created. Great care must be taken that the side branches of the venae comitantes are not inadvertently avulsed, producing an obstructing interstitial hematoma. If a tear is placed in a fragile vena comitans, it should be repaired with micro sutures.

Following the anastomosis, the management of the pedicle is most important. If the pedicle is obstructed by a tight skin closure, by being twisted, or by being draped over a hard object such as a tendon or bone, slowing of flow leading to anastomosis thrombosis is likely to occur. Correct pedicle length is often difficult to determine. A pedicle tends to appear shorter than it really is until the anastomosis is completed and distended by blood. The pedicle should be sufficiently long that it does not have to be stretched to reach the anastomosis. However, excessive pedicle length will produce kinking.

Anaesthetic Considerations

Anaesthesia should be administered in a manner which maintains a normal blood pressure and a good peripheral perfusion. In most non-microvascular procedures, a short period of hypotension is well tolerated by the patient and is not destructive to the operation. However, in the patient with microvascular anastomoses, uninterrupted perfusion with a normal blood pressure is necessary or anastomosis thrombosis will likely occur. Therefore, the fluid volumes must be managed carefully with a tendency to over-transfusion. Blood loss in a long procedure can be deceptively large, as it occurs gradually, slowly and persistently, without any dramatic sudden loss. Monitoring with arterial and central venous lines, hourly urine output and intermittent blood gas and hematocrit evaluations are necessary. If the patient becomes hypothermic, particularly if a transfer to the leg or arm is being done, reactive vasospasm in the extremity will decrease blood flow and may result in anastomosis thrombosis. In order to maintain body temperature, the patient should be placed on a heating blanket, given warmed IV solutions and ventilated with heated and humidified inspired gases. Room temperature control should be maintained at a level which is warm but tolerable for the operating personnel. The patient must be kept in a warm condition in the recovery room as post operative shivering may cause vasoconstriction and shunt blood away from the periphery. To prevent pressure sore problems, a double operating room mattress is used and a sheepskin is placed between the patient and the heating blanket.

The anaesthetic may be general or regional. Regional anaesthetics have the benefit of a vasodilatory effect, but the nature of the procedure or the duration of it may limit its applicability in the individual patient. For a general anaesthetic, the agents should be selected by the anaesthetist on the basis of agents which will not be harmful with a prolonged duration of use, which will not produce cardiac depression, and which allow a prompt reversal of anaesthesia and a quiet return to the awake condition. An agent which produces peripheral vasodilation and subsequent hypotension is not wise, as it will produce vasodilation in all of the patient's vessels except those upon which the surgeon is working. Vessels which have been dissected and are subject to intermittent surgical stimulation have a tendency to vasospasm which will overcome the vasodilating effect of the anaesthetic. These vessels require a good perfusion pressure which occurs only if the patient is normotensive.

Postoperative Monitoring

The most consistently reliable means of monitoring the circulation to a free tissue transfer is by visual observation of the clinical parameters of circulation. Although there has been an extensive effort in the last decade to develop monitoring devices which can evaluate flap circulation, none, except for temperature monitoring, has enjoyed general acceptance. Temperature monitoring of digital replantations and toe to thumb transfers is a reliable way of assessing the volume of blood flow. Because the digit or toe is surrounded by cooling room air, if circulation slows or stops, there will be a prompt drop in the surface temperature. Transfers which are partially buried or lie on a large warm surface area do not show the same temperature response to circulatory changes and so temperature monitoring in skin flaps is not a reliable indicator of circulatory impairment.

For free skin flaps, the color, capillary return, and tissue turgor are the most reliable clinical signs. It is important that the nursing staff be trained to note subtle changes in these clinical signs and record the signs on a flow sheet. At the first sign that there is a change in one of the clinical signs, surgical staff should be notified in order that they can assess the problem. Frequently, a decrease in perfusion is caused by compression from a hematoma, tissue swelling or a tight dressing. Systemic factors such as a drop in the patient's temperature or blood pressure may also decrease flow. With prompt recognition, these factors can often be reversed to prevent the continued decrease in circulation which may lead to thrombosis of the anastomosis.

Microsurgical Instrumentation

There is a plethora of microsurgical instruments available for preparing vascular pedicles and doing microanastomoses. The surgeon should use the ones with which he or she is most comfortable. The microsurgical tray should have a minimum of different types of instrumentation. A complex setup which has a half dozen different types of jeweller's forceps, all of which look alike to the nurse, will frustrate the surgeon and nurse alike. However, there should be at least two types of fine forceps available: a pair of fine tipped jeweller's forceps which are used for the anastomosis, and a pair of heavier forceps, with micro teeth, serrations or other pickup shape on the tips, for the coarser handling of the pedicle. Two needle drivers should be available, one for heavy needles and one, with fine tips, reserved for very fine needles. With experience, each surgeon will develop a preference for a particular style and size of needle driver. Micro scissors, both spring and regular configuration, and a range of vascular clamps should be available. Most surgeons find a double vascular clamp on a bar to be a useful means of holding two vessel ends in proper approximation when initiating the vascular repair.

Part I
Tissue Transfers

Skin Flaps

The ability to transfer tissue based on microvascular anastomoses has created a revolution in reconstructive surgery. The microvascular transfer of a skin flap is the prototype for all other free tissue transfers. The publications of Daniel, Taylor, Harii and O'Brien introduced the concept of a 'free skin flap' based on microvascular anastomoses. After the initial enthusiasm for cutaneous free tissue transfers, interest shifted to the transfer of muscles with or without their accompanying cutaneous flaps. It became apparent that muscle transfers often had a more vigorous blood supply and a longer, larger vascular pedicle than cutaneous flaps. In many situations, this muscle with attached skin flap, the musculocutaneous flap, is preferred to the cutaneous flap.

The advantages of cutaneous flaps are that they are soft and durable and provide a good cosmetic reconstruction. The final size of the flap is predictable, susceptible only to generalized weight gain or loss, whereas a muscle flap undergoes significant atrophy in the first year. The skin flap tolerates ischemia better than muscle, is more likely to recover after re-exploration of an anastomosis thrombosis, and develops more reliable vascular connections with its bed. However, when a skin flap with its thick bed of poorly-vascularized fat is transferred to an area which contains significant bacterial contamination, it may not resist infection as well as a muscle transfer.

The limiting factor in selecting a skin transfer is the availability of donor sites. A donor site for a skin flap is suitable if it contains a reliable pedicle which perfuses the area and if removal of the flap is functionally and cosmetically acceptable. The ideal donor site is one that can be closed directly and leaves a scar which is well hidden during most social activities. The closure of the groin flap is an exellent example of a flap site which leaves a scar that can be well hidden even under a bathing suit. On the other hand, when the donor site requires a split thickness skin graft for closure in a visible area, as occurs with the radial arm flap, the donor site becomes less desirable.

A skin flap may contain an axial cutaneous artery, as found in the groin and scapular flaps, or it may be supplied by a vessel which does not run in the flap but supplies branches to the overlying skin, as in the dorsal foot and radial arm transfers. These cutaneous branches may lie within a loosely defined connective tissue or within a fascial septum.

I have chosen four different skin flaps for inclusion in the book. They are the groin, scapula, dorsal foot and forearm flaps. The groin flap is little used except for buried contour reconstruction but has an important historical place in the development of skin flaps. The scapular flap will provide the answer to many if not most skin coverage problems. However, when a particularly thin or innervated skin flap is required, the dorsal foot and forearm flaps will provide the solution. There are other skin flaps which are available and not described in this book. They include the scalp, delto-pectoral, lateral thoracic, medial and lateral arm, saphenous, thigh and hemi-pulp flaps.

References

1. Daniel RK, Taylor GI (1973) Distant transfer of an island flap by microvascular anastomoses. Plast Reconstr Surg 52: 111
2. Harii K, Ohmori K, Ohmori S (1974) Successful clinical transfer of ten free flaps by microvascular anastomoses. Plast Reconstr Surg 53: 259
3. O'Brien BMcB, McLeod AM, Hayhurst JW, Morrison WA (1973) Successful transfer of a large island flap from the groin to the foot by microvascular anastomosis. Plast Reconstr Surg 52: 271
4. Harii K, Ohmori K, Ohmori S (1974) Free deltopectoral skin flaps. Br J Plast Surg 27: 231
5. Harii K, Ohmori K, Sekigguchi J (1978) The free lateral thoracic flap. Plast Reconstr Surg 62: 212
6. Harii K, Ohmori K, Ohmori S (1974) Hair transplantation with free scalp flaps. Plast Reconstr Surg 53: 410
7. Acland RD, Schusterman M, Godina M, Eder E, Taylor GI, Carlisle I (1981) The saphenous neurovascular free flap. Plast Reconstr Surg 67: 763
8. Buncke HJ, Rose EH (1979) Free toe-to-fingertip neurovascular flaps. Plast Reconstr Surg 63: 607
9. Song YG, Chen GZ, Song YL (1984) The free thigh flap: a new free flap concept based on the septocutaneous artery. Br J Plast Surg 37: 149

Chapter 2. Groin Flap

After McGregor and Jackson introduced the groin flap in 1972, surgeons became more aware of the benefit of including a specific artery within the tissue being transferred. As a pedicled flap, it became the work horse for coverage of upper extremity soft tissue defects, and as a free tissue transfer, it broke new ground in reconstructive surgery [2].

The groin flap provides a large piece of skin and subcutaneous fat. The size of flap available depends upon the patient's build. A number of authors have reported flaps surviving that were over 30 cm in length and 15 cm in width. The donor site scar is excellent as it can usually be closed directly by undermining the abdominal skin and flexing the hip. This procedure may produce a spread scar but it will be well hidden under the bathing suit area. However, the disadvantages of this flap are many. It is particularly bulky in its medial half and not suitable in a fat person. The pedicle is small and short and there are many anatomical variations to the vascular supply. The color of the flap is pale and yellowish when applied to the face and will carry pubic hair on its medial aspect.

Its present day applications include coverage of soft tissue defects and contour reconstruction as a buried flap, particularly in the face. In many areas of the body, other flaps are preferred for soft tissue coverage. Often, a myocutaneous flap will be favoured because it is easier to elevate and has a longer, more reliable pedicle than the groin flap.

Vascular Anatomy

The vascular pedicle for this flap employs one of two possible arteries and one of four possible veins. The flap may be based on the superficial circumflex iliac artery (SCIA) or the superficial epigastric artery (SEA). The variations in the origin, route and distribution of these two arteries may confuse the surgeon. In Harii's clinical experience with 87 groin flaps, there was a common arterial trunk of the SCIA and SEA 29% of the time and, in the remainder of cases, they had separate origins. Harii recommends using the common trunk, if available, or using the SCIA as the pedicle unless the SEA is larger (20%) and then he would use the latter (Fig. 2-1 c) [3, 5, 7].

The SCIA usually takes origin from the anterolateral aspect of the femoral artery, 2–3 cm below the inguinal ligament (Fig. 2-1 A). It runs laterally superficial to the iliacus fascia in the fatty lymphatic tissue found in the femoral triangle. In passing laterally, it runs in a line towards, away from, or parallel to the inguinal ligament [6]. At the medial border of the sartorius muscle, it usually divides into two branches, either of which may be dominant. The superficial branch remains above the sartorius fascia and continues laterally, supplying skin up to and beyond the anterior superior iliac spine. The deep branch pierces the sartorius fascia at its medial border and passes on the deep surface of this fascia to the lateral border of the muscle (Fig. 2-1 b) [1, 3]. Here it exits the fascia 1–4 cm below the ASIS and runs laterally superficial to the fascia lata, supplying skin in the region of the ASIS and laterally. The deep branch also gives off muscle branches to the sartorius. If a long groin flap is required, it is necessary to include the deep branch in the pedicle. In one fifth of cases, the SCIA originates from a branch of the femoral artery, such as the deep circumflex iliac, medial circumflex femoral, or deep or superficial pudenal arteries. Taylor, in 100 dissections, found the SCIA to be present and 1 mm or larger in diameter 98% of the time [9].

The superficial epigastric artery (SEA) usually arises from a location similar to that of the SCIA. It passes superiorly and laterally, superficial to the inguinal ligament, and remains medial to the anterior superior iliac spine, to supply an area of skin above the territory of the SCIA. In view of the dissections and clinical experience of Harii and Taylor & Daniels, it is apparent that the territories of these vessels overlap and the most dependable approach to taking a flap from this area is to plan the flap axis through the centre of both vessels' territories. The largest artery to be found at surgical dissection is

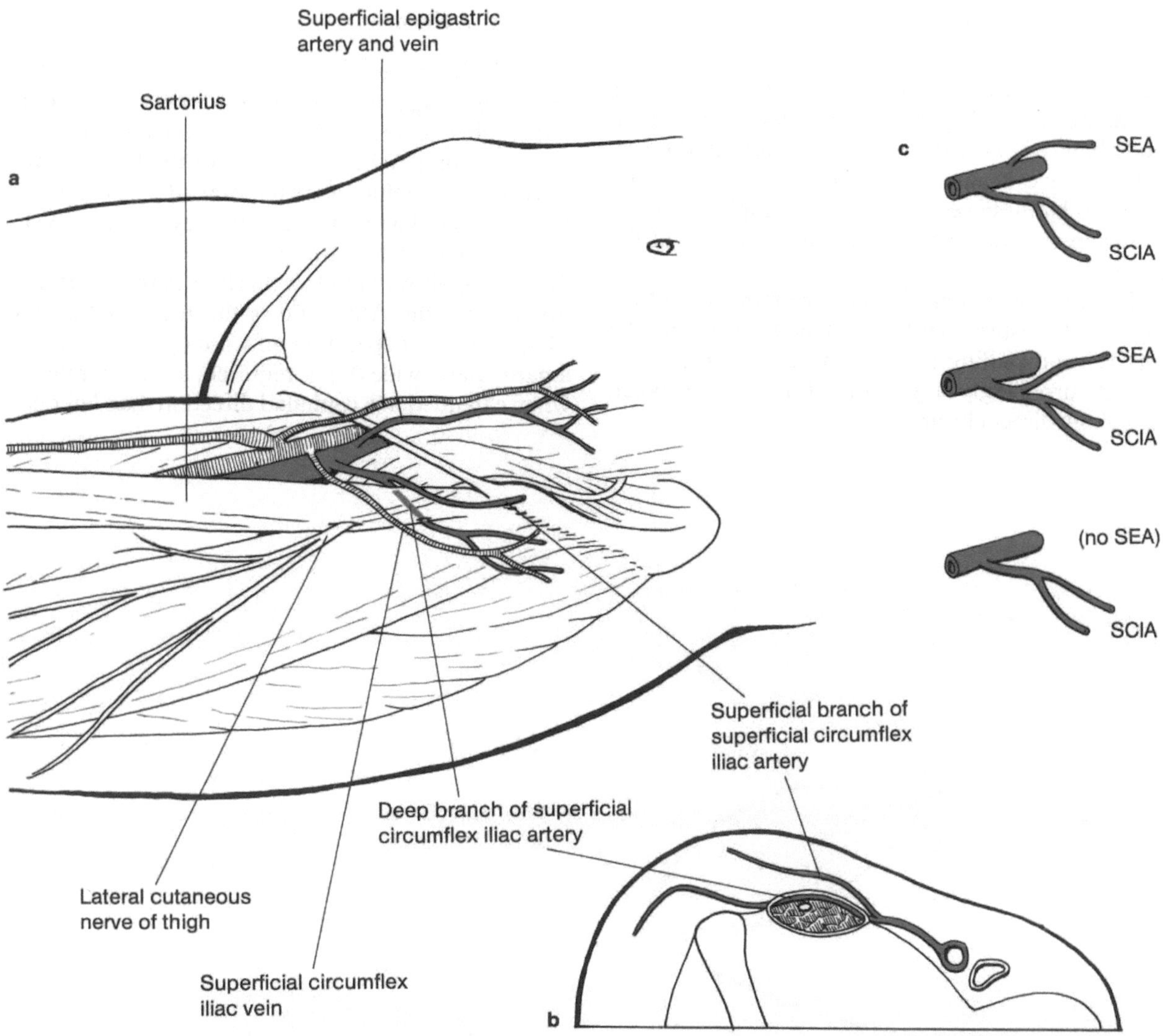

Fig. 2-1. **a** Vascular anatomy of the groin flap. Either the SCIA or SEA may be used as the pedicle for the flap. Although there are venae comitantes with each of these arteries, they are seldom large enough for flap transfer. **b** Cross section of the thigh parallel to and below the inguinal ligament, illustrating the course of the superficial and deep branches of the SCIA in relation to the sartorius muscle. The deep branch passes under the sartorius fascia, entering at the muscle's medial border and leaving at the lateral border to supply the lateral skin of the flap. **c** The SEA and SCIA may have a common or a separate origin, or the SEA may be absent

used as the pedicle. At their origin, these arteries are from 0.8 to 1.8 mm in diameter.

The venous pattern may be equally confusing. The groin area is drained by the superficial epigastric vein (SEV) and superficial circumflex iliac vein (SCIV) and by the venae comitantes of the named arteries. All veins drain into the femoral vein or saphenous bulb. The venae comitantes are small and used infrequently for groin transfer. The SEV and SCIV lie superficial to their respective arteries and usually superficial to scarpa's fascia. In 60% of Harii's cases, they joined to form a common trunk measuring 2 mm or more. This is the preferred vein for anastomoses [4]. In any individual case, of the four veins available, the largest should be used for the transfer.

Elevating the Groin Flap

Patients who have had previous surgery in the groin, including vein stripping, hernia repairs, and lymph node biopsies, may have received injury to the vascular pedicle or alteration of the vascular territory supplied by these vessels. Previous lymphadenitis of the groin may also complicate the dissection of the pedicle.

The amount of skin which can be removed, allowing direct closure, can be evaluated by flexing the hip 45° and pulling the skin together with the fingers. A surprisingly large width of flap may be taken and allow direct closure.

Surgical Technique

1. With the patient supine on the operating table, and a sand bag under the involved buttock, mark the pubic tubercle, inguinal ligament and anterior superior iliac spine (ASIS). The axis of the flap is a line drawn from a point on the femoral artery 2 cm below the inguinal ligament, to and beyond the ASIS (Fig. 2-2 a). However, the flap may be quite successfully taken above or below this line. Angling the axis up towards the ASIS allows the use of either the SEA or SCIA, depending on which proves larger. If a particularly wide flap is required, it is more reliable when extended in a cephalad direction than laterally.

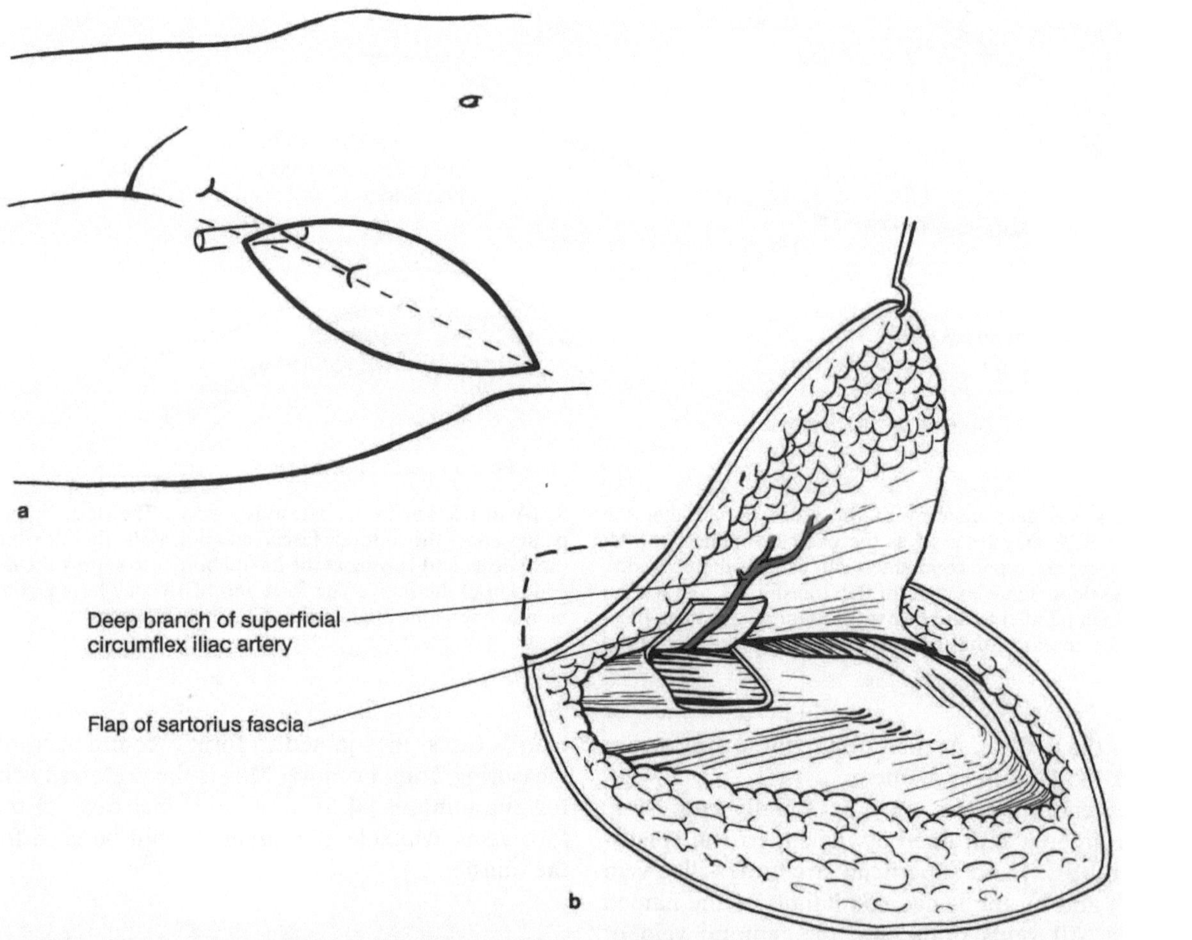

Fig. 2-2. a The surface landmarks for outlining the groin flap are the pubic tubercle, the anterior superior iliac spine (ASIS), the inguinal ligament, and the femoral artery. The flap axis is a line drawn from a point on the femoral artery 2 cm below the inguinal ligament up to and through the ASIS. **b** The flap is elevated from lateral to medial. In order to keep the deep branch of the SCIA in the flap, the dissection must pass under and remove a piece of sartorius fascia

2. Using a pattern taken from the tissue defect, outline the skin flap on this axis with the medial part of the flap over the femoral artery.

3. Incise the superior, lateral and medial skin markings and undermine the flap. If the subcutaneous tissue is thick, a thin layer of subcutaneous fat may be taken in the superior and lateral portion of the flap. However, the full thickness of the subcutaneous fat must be taken from the ASIS to the medial flap margin.

4. Raise the flap from lateral to medial. The lateral margin of the sartorius is partially hidden by the overlying fascia lata. Identify the junction between the sartorius and the tensor fascia lata by palpating the slight groove between them. Go slowly at this point or you will injure the deep branch of the SCIA where it exits from the sartorius fascia to the subcutaneous layer. If the SCIA is not readily visible lateral to the sartorius, it may be identified by transilluminating the flap.

The lateral to medial approach is preferable as it allows identification and tracing of the SCIA or SEA to its origin. This is particularly helpful in those 20% of cases where the SCIA does not enter the femoral artery. The SCIA usually passes superficial to, but may pass through or deep to, the lateral cutaneous nerve of the thigh. Divide and repair this nerve if the artery passes beneath the nerve.

5. Carry the dissection medially, raising a flap of sartorius fascia with the flap, and elevate the deep branch of the SCIA on the deep surface of the sartorius fascia (Fig. 2-2b). Cauterize the small muscular branches to the sartorius before they are inadvertently avulsed.

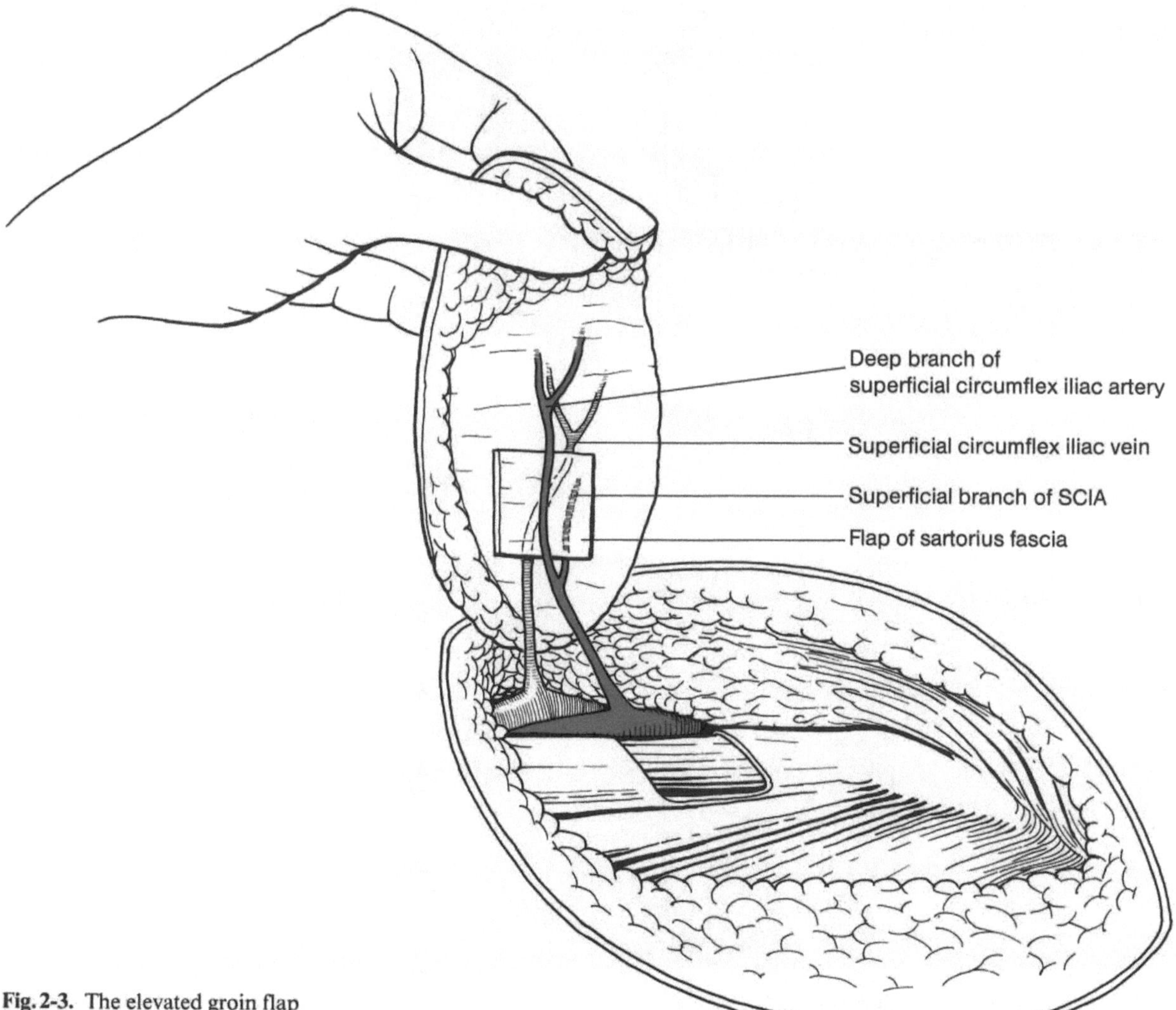

Fig. 2-3. The elevated groin flap with the pedicle still attached

6. At the medial margin of the sartorius, incise its fascia and carry the dissection medially beneath the artery.

If the SEA did not become visible during the superior dissection of the flap, it will become apparent at this point in the dissection, either as an artery joining the SCIA or as a vessel entering the femoral artery superior to the SCIA.

7. Complete the dissection of the medial portion of the flap. Identify the superficial circumflex iliac and superficial epigastric veins and prepare them to their origins.

8. After following both arteries to their origins, select the artery which is larger for the anastomosis. If there is a common trunk, use it unless it is too short to allow a good anastomosis without placing the repair at the Y-junction. Ligate any vessel which will not be used. Select the largest vein and ligate the veins which are not going to be used. Then observe the flap for color, bleeding from the edges, and capillary return. The groin flap normally appears quite pale (Fig. 2-3).

Following removal of the flap, close the donor site in layers over a suction drain with the hip flexed. It is rarely necessary to skin graft this donor site.

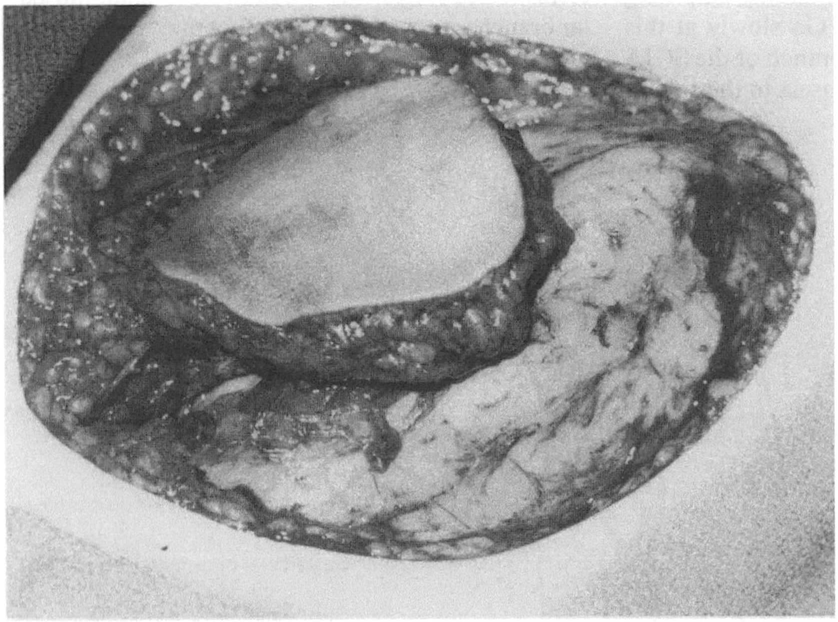

Fig. 2-4. Following dissection of the flap, there is considerable retraction of the skin edges. Nevertheless, direct closure of the donor site is nearly always possible

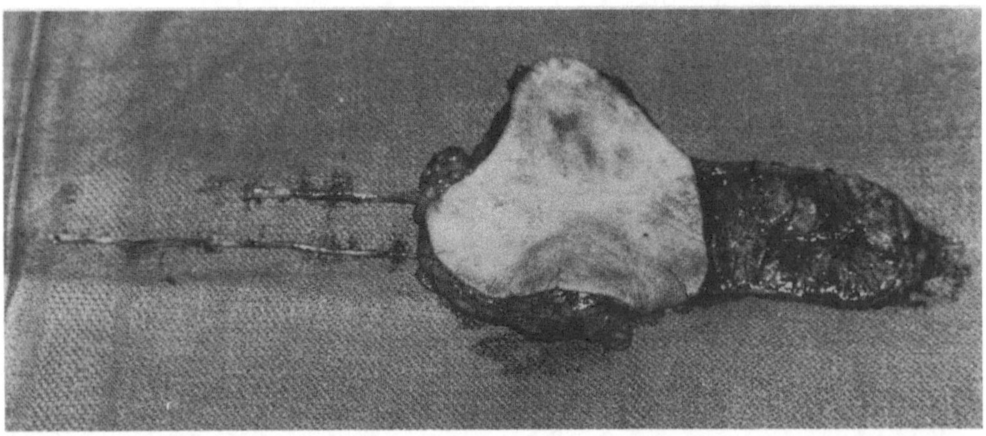

Fig. 2-5. In this groin flap, the short pedicle has been elongated with two vein grafts. The lateral portion of the flap has been de-epithelialized and will be used as a buried flap to provide tissue bulk with a thick layer of subcutaneous fat

References

1. Acland RD (1979) The Free Iliac Flap. Plast Reconstr Surg 64: 30
2. Daniel RK, Taylor GI (1973) Distant transfer of an island flap by microvascular anastomoses. Plast Reconstr Surg 52: 111
3. Harii K, Ohmori K, Torii S, Murakami F, Kasai Y, Sekiguchi J, Ohmori S (1975) Free groin skin flaps. Br J Plast Surg 28: 225
4. Harii K, Ohmori K, Torii S, Sekiguchi J (1978) Microvascular free skin flap transfer. Clin Plast Surg 5 (2): 239
5. Harii K Personal communication
6. McGregor IA, Jackson IT (1972) The Groin Flap. Br J Plast Surg 25: 3
7. Ohmori K, Harii K (1975) Free groin flaps: their vascular basis. Br J Plast Surg 28: 238
8. Smith PJ, Foley B, McGregor IA, Jackson IT (1972) The anatomical basis of the groin flap. Plast Reconstr Surg 49: 41
9. Taylor GI, Daniel RK (1975) The anatomy of several free flap donor sites. Plast Reconstr Surg 56: 243

Chapter 3. Dorsal Foot Flap

The skin on the dorsum of the foot is a reliable donor site for free tissue transfer. As the flap's pedicle is the dorsalis pedis artery, the flap has been called the dorsalis pedis flap. This name is somewhat misleading as the vessels which supply this flap come mostly from the first dorsal metatarsal artery (FDMA). These cutaneous vessels are always adequate for survival of the flap. However, they are small and fragile and must be treated with care. We have used this flap as a free tissue transfer 41 times and many times as a pedicled transfer. In each case, there have been adequate cutaneous branches of the FDMA for perfusion of the flap. We have never discontinued a dorsal foot transfer because of inadequate vascularization of the flap.

This skin flap was one of the first free tissue transfers developed. Following the publications of Gilbert, May, McCraw, Ohmori and Robinson, it enjoyed considerable popularity [1, 5, 6, 7, 8]. However, with the subsequent development of other cutaneous and musculocutaneous flaps, and the recognition of the difficulties associated with the dorsal foot flap, its application is now limited to very specific situations. It is most commonly used as an innervated skin flap and as an osteocutaneous transfer when combined with the second metatarsal. When used on the heel of the foot or on the hand, it provides a thin and very durable innervated tissue cover (Chaps. 18, 21). It can be extended to include the first web space skin or toe pulp to provide an even more versatile innervated reconstruction for the hand. It is particularly valuable when a thin, flexible flap is desired for intra-oral coverage following cancer exterpation (Chap. 14).

There are some disadvantages to this flap. It is a difficult dissection, considerable care must be taken in grafting the recipient site, and the patient must be kept in bed for at least 10 days to obtain a skin graft take. The flap is difficult to dissect because of the awkward location of the plantar communicating branch of the dorsalis pedis artery and the anatomic variations of the first dorsal metatarsal artery. The cutaneous arterial branches of this flap do not come from the dorsalis pedis artery but from the first dorsal metatarsal artery. This artery and the flimsy tissues between it and the skin must be included in the flap. Although skin grafting will take on the dorsum of the foot, the grafts over the extensor retinaculum as well as over the extensor hallucis longus may result in an unstable skin surface which is susceptible to minor repetitive trauma.

As the flap may include the entire dorsum of the foot, flap size is limited by the size of the foot. Our maximum flap size was 9 cm wide and 12 cm in length. However, many feet are not large enough to provide this size of flap. The medial flap margin may extend 2 cm medial to the flexor hallucis longus, and the lateral margin, which has the weakest blood supply, will survive to 1 cm lateral to the fifth extensor tendon. Although branches to the skin from the dorsalis pedis in the area of the extensor retinaculum are not preserved, the skin over this area will survive. Skin grafting the web spaces and the area immediately proximal to these spaces may result in hyperkeratosis in the web and hypertrophic scarring on the distal foot.

Vascular Anatomy of the Foot

One of the most useful areas in the body for the donation of tissues is the foot. It provides skin flaps such as the dorsal foot, web space, and pulp flaps, bone grafts such as the second metatarsal with or without skin, and composite tissue transfers, including joints, toes, and portions of toes. Understanding the arterial vascular pattern of the foot is crucial to the use of the foot as a donor source. Although the standard text book arrangement of the vessels is a starting point for this understanding, the size, branches and common anatomic variations of each of the important arteries in the foot must be appreciated. These arteries are the dorsalis pedis, the first dorsal metatarsal, the first plantar metatarsal, the digital arteries and the communicating arteries (Fig. 3-1, 2) [2, 3].

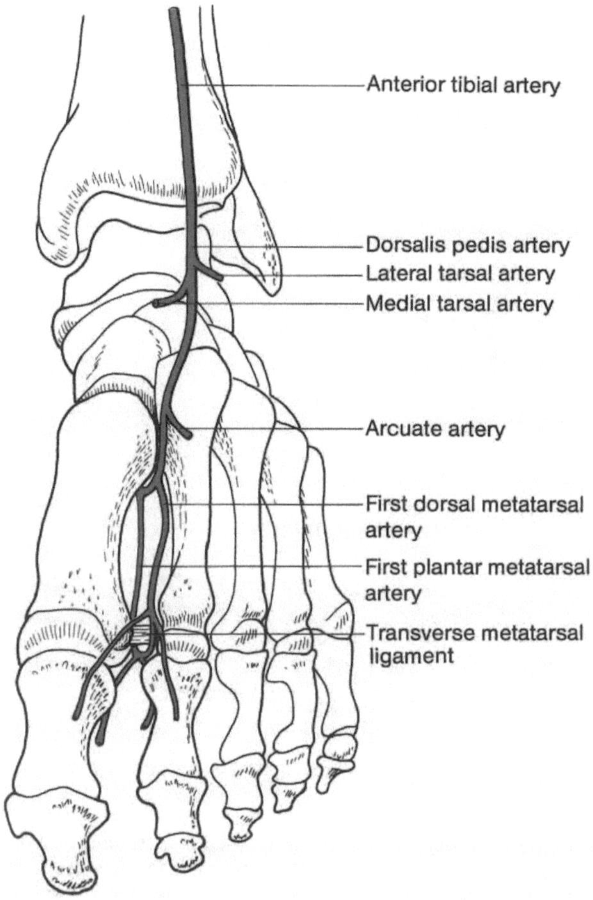

Fig. 3-1. Typical anatomical pattern of the dorsalis pedis artery and its branches. Note the proximal and distal communicating branches which connect the dorsal and plantar systems

The description to follow describes the vascular anatomy, first with respect to the overall arrangement of the arteries and then with attention to the individual vessels and their anomalies. It is applicable to the other foot transfers described in subsequent chapters.

Dorsalis Pedis Artery

Beginning at the ankle joint, the dorsalis pedis is usually a continuation of the anterior tibial artery. It emerges at the ankle from under the extensor retinaculum and extensor hallucis longus and runs lateral to this tendon, in a course directed towards the web space between the first and second metatarsals. It is deeply located, lying on the tarsal ligaments and periosteum as it runs its course over the tallus, navicular, second cuniform, and along the groove between the first cuniform and the base of the second metatarsal. While in this groove, it is crossed obliquely by the extensor hallucis brevis muscle belly. Running with the artery and on its medial side is the deep peroneal nerve.

The medial and lateral malleolar branches arise from the dorsalis pedis artery very near its beginning. One lateral tarsal and one or two medial tarsal branches arise from the middle and distal third of the artery. The arcuate artery may be formed from the lateral tarsal artery or the dorsalis pedis. At the base of the second metatarsal, the laterally directed arcuate artery forms a dorsal arch, giving off the second, third and fourth dorsal metatarsal arteries. The dorsalis pedis ends with a branch to the plantar region called a descending, perforating, or communicating branch which passes through the inter space between the first and second metatarsals. This plantar communicating branch hugs the proximal portion of the inter space and is the major contributing artery to the plantar arch.

In the proximal half of the artery, there are fine branches which pass through the extensor retinaculum on both sides of the extensor hallucis tendon to the overlying skin [4]. However, they are of little practical value, as the interposition of the extensor retinaculum and extensor hallucis longus tendon make the inclusion of these branches in a flap difficult. It is the exception, rather than the rule, to encounter any cutaneous branches from the distal half of the dorsalis pedis artery. The usual diameter of the dorsalis pedis is 2-3 mm. In 3-12% of feet, the dorsalis pedis is absent, and in 3-7%, it is a continuation of the peroneal artery [3].

Venae comitantes are present along the dorsalis pedis artery and are usually large enough for microvascular anastomoses.

First Dorsal Metatarsal Artery (FDMA)

The variations in the location, origin, and course of this artery can create great confusion.

The artery may take its origin from any point on the plantar communicating branch and may lie on or within the first dorsal interosseous muscle. May found it to lie on top of the muscle in 78% of dissections and Gilbert in 66% of dissections. In the other 22-34% of dissections, the origin of the artery was deep within or deep to the interosseous musculature. Its distal course is at the same depth as or shallower than its origin, and it always passes dorsal to the deep transverse metatarsal ligament. This ligament

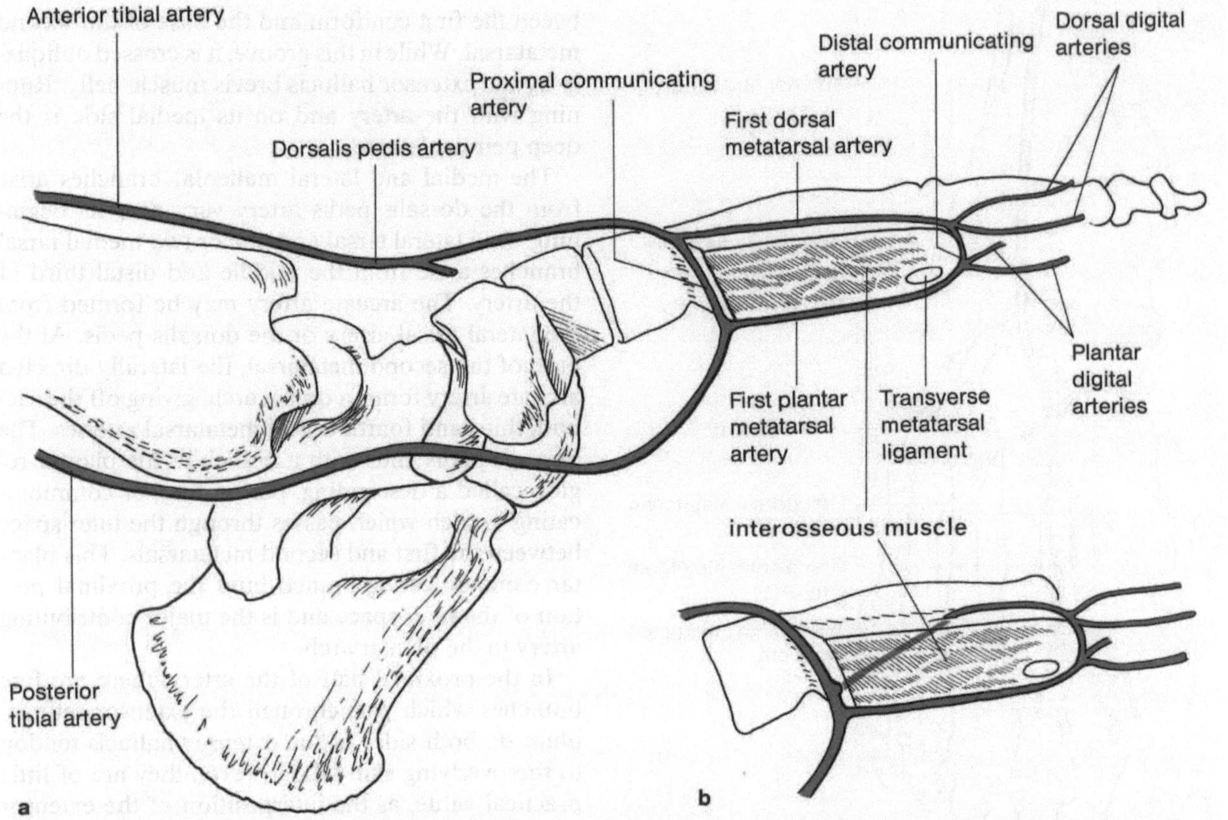

Fig. 3-2. a There are many variations to the 'textbook' arrangement of the vascular anatomy. One of the most important variables to the surgeon who uses the dorsalis pedis-FDMA-digital artery axis is the variable origin and course of the FDMA. **b** The FDMA may have an origin from the communicating branch deep within the interosseous musculature. Following this low origin, the FDMA may rise to the surface of the interosseous muscle as shown here, or pass distally within or deep to the muscle

runs transversely on the plantar aspect, between the head of the first metatarsal and the neck of the second.

There are many branches from this important artery. The small branches to the skin are located at the commencement and termination of the first dorsal metatarsal artery and will support the overlying dorsal foot skin. Some of the muscular branches to the interosseii pass through to supply the metatarsals. Proximal to the deep transverse metatarsal ligament, there is often a small communicating artery to the plantar metatarsal artery. The FDMA continues distally, giving off dorsal digital arteries to the first and second toes, and ends in a distal communicating branch which joins the first plantar metatarsal artery.

There is a marked variation in the location and origin of this distal communicating branch. It may come off the FDMA at or near the bifurcation of the dorsal digital vessels or from one of the digital vessels, and may attach on the plantar surface in a similar varied manner. This connection is critical in the dorsalis pedis FDMA plantar digital vascular axis that is used in toe transfers. There are venae comitantes with the FDMA, but they are usually too small for microvascular repair. Although the vessel is usually 1-1.5 mm in diameter, it is occasionally much smaller.

First Plantar Metatarsal Artery (FPMA)

This artery is usually smaller than the first dorsal metatarsal artery. However, if the FDMA is small, there is a compensatory enlargement of the FPMA.

The FPMA takes origin from the plantar communicating branch of the dorsalis pedis or the plantar arch itself. Occasionally, the FDMA and the FPMA take origin from the same location on the communicating branch, or the FPMA is a branch of the FDMA. Removal of one, with preservation of the other, then becomes impossible. The artery courses distally on the plantar surface of the flexor hallucis brevis and adductor hallucis muscles. This deep location makes surgical accessibility a problem. The first significant branch is an oblique branch from the mid portion of the artery which passes deep to the flexor hallucis longus on its course to the medial side of the first metatarsal. Along with the medial plantar artery, this branch forms the medial digital artery of the great toe. Giving off multiple small muscular branches, the FPMA passes plantar to the transverse metatarsal ligament, receives the distal communicating branch from the FDMA, and produces the plantar digital arteries to the adjacent sides of the great and second toe. Venae comitantes are present but too small for microanastomosis.

Digital Arteries

The dorsal digital arteries are branches of the FDMA and the plantar digital arteries are branches of the FPMA. If there is only one digital artery, although the origin may suggest that it is a dorsal artery, it will usually course in a volar position immediately adjacent to the plantar digital nerve in the usual location of the plantar digital artery. These vessels are 1 mm or less in diameter.

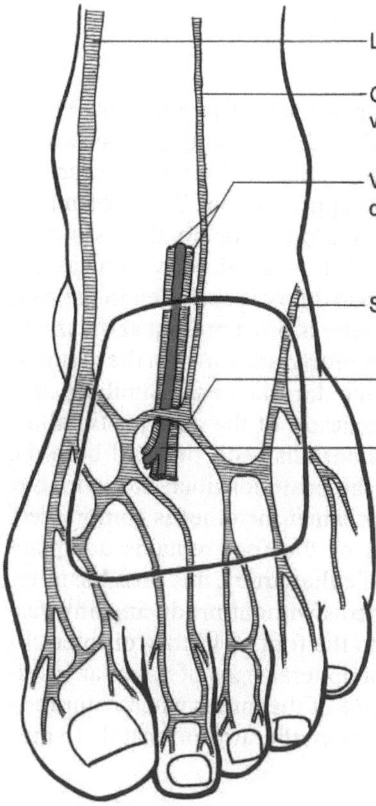

Fig. 3-3. Two venous networks drain the foot; a superficial subcutaneous system and a deep system of venae comitantes. Although either system will drain most transfers, the larger size of the superficial favours its use. Through the cross connections provided by the dorsal venous arch, the distal foot transfers may be drained by any one of three superficial veins: the long or short saphenous or the central foot vein. The distal foot may also be drained through the venae comitantes of the deep system

Venous Supply of the Foot

The venous systems of importance to the surgeon are:

1. the superficial dorsal veins
2. the venae comitantes

Most tissue transfers from the foot can be drained by the superficial dorsal system. Some, but not all, can be drained by the venae comitantes (Fig. 3-3).

The superficial dorsal system begins with small veins on each side of the dorsum of each toe. These veins, located in the dorsal subcutaneous tissues, unite to form dorsal metatarsal veins which form dorsal arches at the level of the proximal metatarsals. The dorsal arches drain medially to the long saphenous vein, which runs anterior to the medial malleolus, and laterally to the short saphenous vein which runs posterior to the lateral malleolus. Proximal to the dorsal arch, there is an irregular dorsal venous network, which frequently gives rise to a central small subcutaneous vein which ascends the ankle and calf midway between the other two veins. On the plantar surface of the foot, the superficial veins are small and form a plantar subcutaneous plexus.

The deep veins of the foot accompany all of the arteries and their branches, draining the deep structures of the foot and forming a complete system of venae comitantes. Both plantar and dorsal superficial systems communicate with the venae comitantes and with each other by subcutaneous and intermetacarpal channels. There are sufficient interconnections between the deep and superficial systems to allow the surgeon to repair the superficial system and provide adequate drainage to the deep structures, including bones, joints and interosseous musculature.

Preoperative Planning

When the dorsalis pedis artery is going to be removed in a transfer, the remaining circulation, through the posterior tibial or the peroneal artery, must be adequate to supply the foot. The presence of both dorsalis pedis and posterior tibial pulses does not ensure that there is forward flow in both vessels.

If the posterior tibial artery is occluded in the calf, the posterior tibial pulse is often present at the medial malleolus through retrograde flow via the communicating branch of the dorsalis pedis. Similarly, it is possible to have occlusion of the anterior tibial artery and still have a dorsalis pedis pulse. If both the dorsalis pedis and the posterior tibial are palpable, and each remains so when the other is compressed, and the circulation of the foot remains adequate with compression of either artery, it is possible to remove the dorsalis pedis without producing any vascular compromise to the foot. A history of intermittent claudication, peripheral signs of vascular insufficiency, or loss of one of the pulses when compressing the other should warn the surgeon that there may be proximal vascular obstruction in the leg. Arteriography and pulse pressure recordings should then be done. Beware of the patient who has had previous polytrauma and may have had a cutdown on the long saphenous vein as this vein will not be suitable for a venous pedicle.

Any one of four veins can be used to drain the flap. These are:

1. the long saphenous vein which is 3-6 mm in diameter and often too large to attach to a recipient vein
2. the central subcutaneous vein which, if present, is 1 to 2 mm in diameter
3. a branch of the lesser saphenous which, although frequently far lateral, is 2-3 mm in diameter
4. the venae comitantes of the dorsalis pedis, which are 1-3 mm in diameter.

Although the venae comitantes of the distal dorsalis pedis are often small when a long pedicle which includes the lower anterior tibial artery is taken, they are at least 2 mm in diameter and ideal for anastomoses. The usual choice is the long saphenous or the venae comitantes. The decision depends upon which vein best fits the location and size of recipient vein.

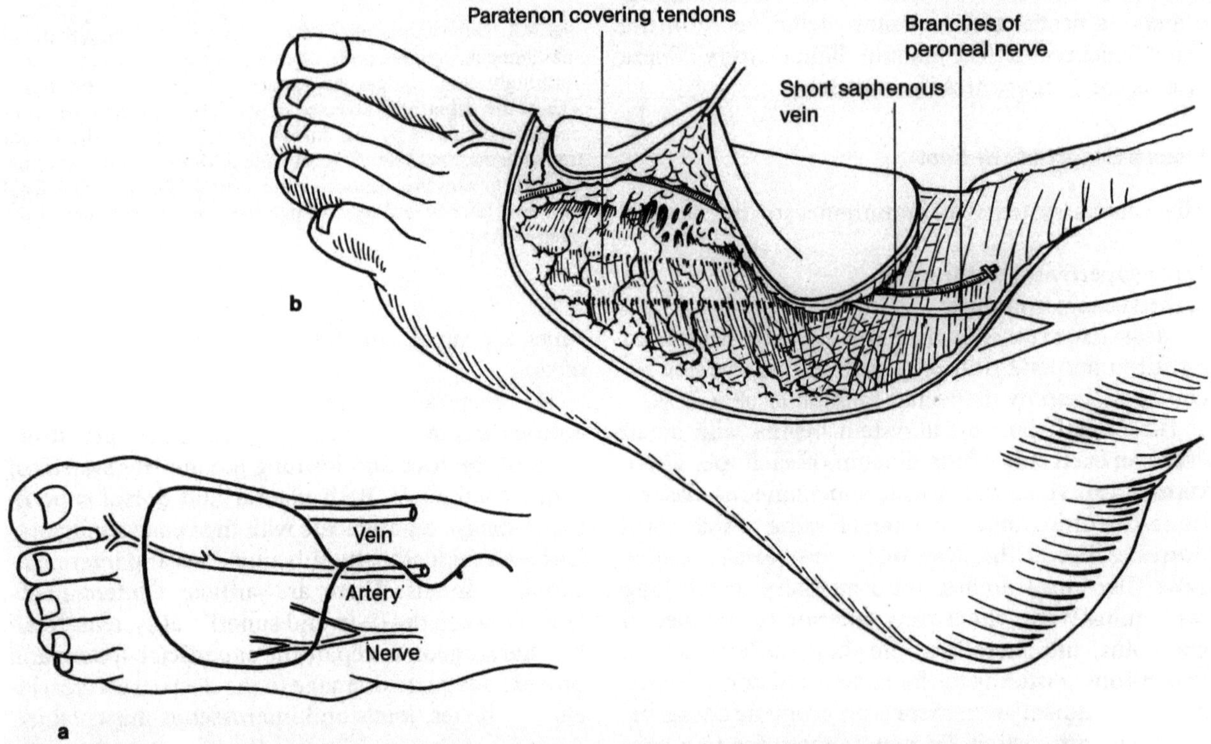

Fig. 3-4. a Outline the dorsalis pedis flap. Expected location of the long saphenous vein, dorsalis pedis artery and the superficial peroneal nerve are marked.
The maximum medial and lateral limits of the flap are outlined. Although the flap may reliably be taken more proximally and distally than shown, skin grafts can be a problem in these areas. **b** Meticulous flap elevation with preservation of the paratenon

Elevating the Dorsal Foot Flap

Surgical Technique

1. Make a pattern of the defect and transfer it to the foot, using the second metatarsal as the longitudinal axis of the flap. Palpate and mark the dorsalis pedis artery and veins (Fig. 3-4 a). Identify the likely location of the superficial peroneal nerves.

2. Incise the skin about the margins of the flap. Watch for and preserve the veins exiting from the skin which might be used for flap drainage. Preserve all veins until the size and location of the recipient vein is known and the most appropriate flap vein can be chosen. Select the superficial vein which is most likely to be used. At the proximal skin incision, identify the superficial branches of the peroneal nerve. Usually there are at least two branches entering the flap along the lateral aspect of the proximal margin. These are preserved if an innervated flap is required.

3. Make the distal skin incision, identifying and dividing the dorsal veins from the toes. Elevate the medial and lateral margins of flap in a plane immediately superficial to the paratenon of the extensor tendons. Elevate the medial flap margin as far as the medial margin of the extensor hallucis longus, and the lateral margin as far as the extensor digitorum longus to the second toe. Keep the paratenon protected from drying out by covering it with damp gauze. Do not use a tourniquet. Its use will accelerate the drying of the paratenon (Fig. 3-4 b).

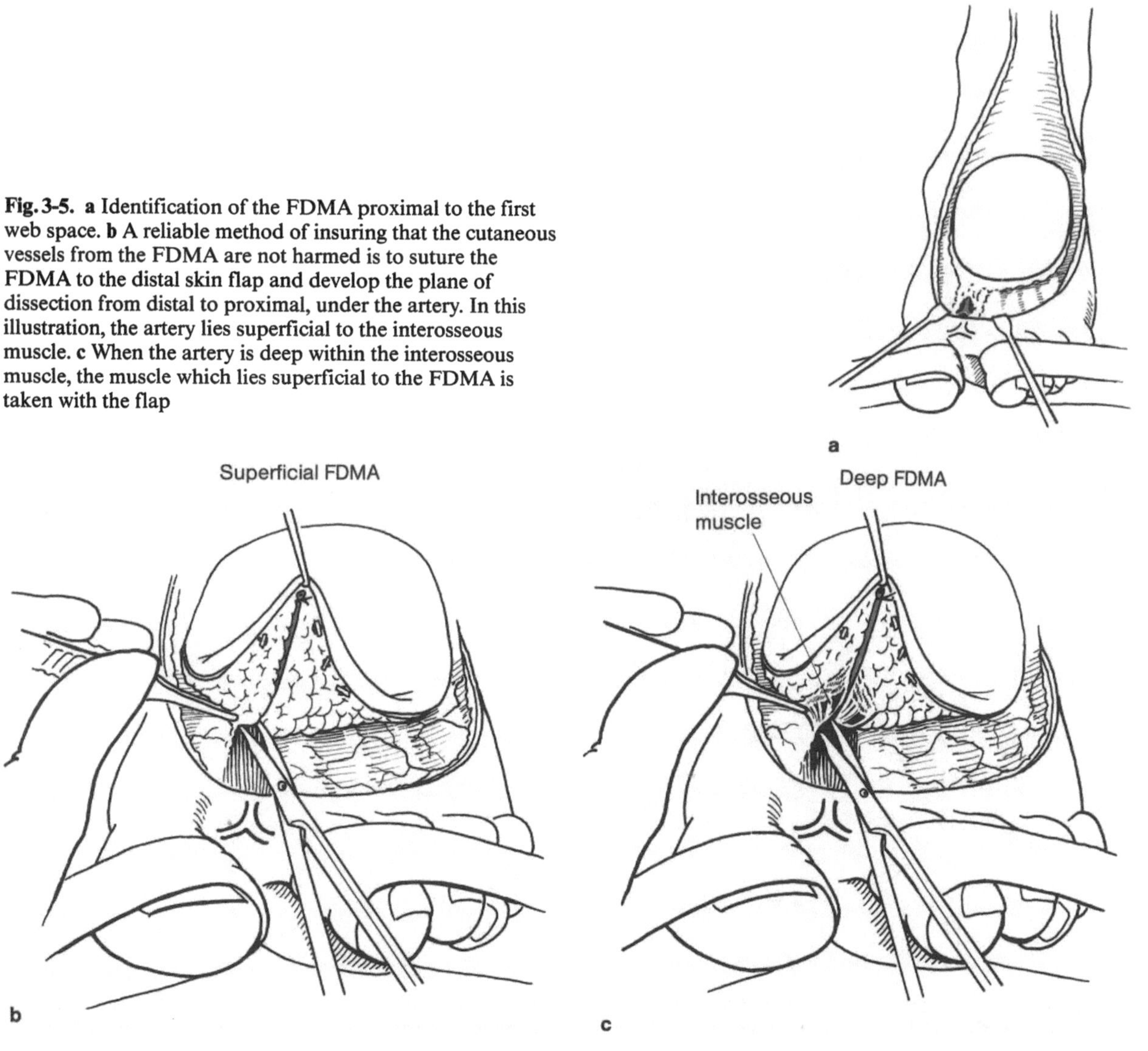

Fig. 3-5. **a** Identification of the FDMA proximal to the first web space. **b** A reliable method of insuring that the cutaneous vessels from the FDMA are not harmed is to suture the FDMA to the distal skin flap and develop the plane of dissection from distal to proximal, under the artery. In this illustration, the artery lies superficial to the interosseous muscle. **c** When the artery is deep within the interosseous muscle, the muscle which lies superficial to the FDMA is taken with the flap

4. The key to the dissection of this flap is keeping the first dorsal metatarsal artery (FDMA) within the flap. When the origin and course of the FDMA lie within the interosseous muscle, it is more difficult to raise the flap. Identify the FDMA in the web space of the first and second toes (Fig. 3-5 a). The thick walled large dorsal toe veins may be mistaken for the distal end of the artery. Do not use the tourniquet. The artery can be identified by its pulsations and spurt. If the artery is not on the surface of the interosseous muscle, dissect into the muscle until it is found. When it is definitely identified, suture ligate the divided artery and suture it to the adjacent edge of the skin flap. This end of the FDMA will pulsate and can be used as a sentinel to assess the integrity of the vascular tree during flap elevation (Fig. 3-5 b).

5. Develop a plane of dissection deep to the FDMA, keeping on the flap all soft tissue located between the first and second extensor tendons and superficial to the artery. The vessels from the FDMA to the skin are in these tissues (Fig. 3-5 b, c). Do the dissection from distal to proximal, spreading the toes to improve visibility. Follow the pedicle proximally under the extensor hallucis brevis and divide this muscle. This muscle does not provide vessels to the flap.

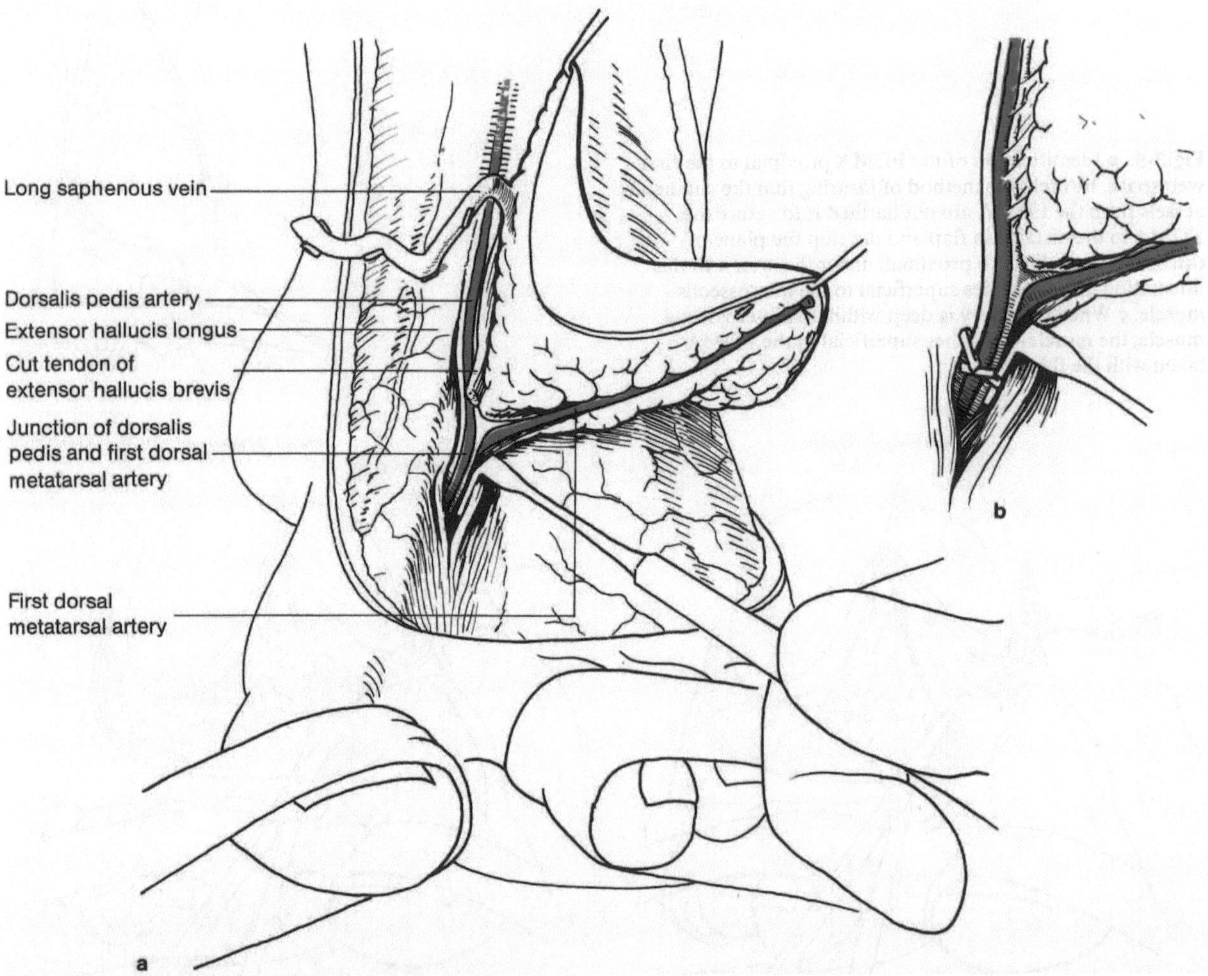

Fig. 3-6. a The FDMA takes origin from the distal portion of the dorsalis pedis, or the plantar communicating branch. **b** Clips are applied to the venae comitantes and the plantar communicating artery distal to the take off of the FDMA

6. The most difficult point of surgical access is the origin of the FDMA, particularly when it has a deep origin from the communicating artery. This is identified best through the distal to proximal dissection of the intermetacarpal space. Clean the junction of the FDMA, dorsalis pedis and its plantar communicating branch until the arterial and venous pattern is clear (Fig. 3-6 a). Then, divide the communicating branch below the take off of the FDMA. Divide both venae comitantes of the plantar communicating branch (Fig. 3-6 b). The flap will then rise out of the metatarsal web space and become free on its proximal pedicle. Metal vessel clips and a tourniquet are useful to make these divisions.

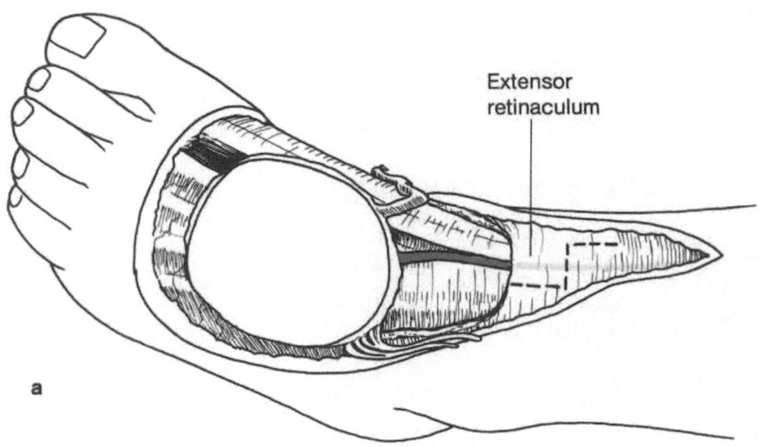

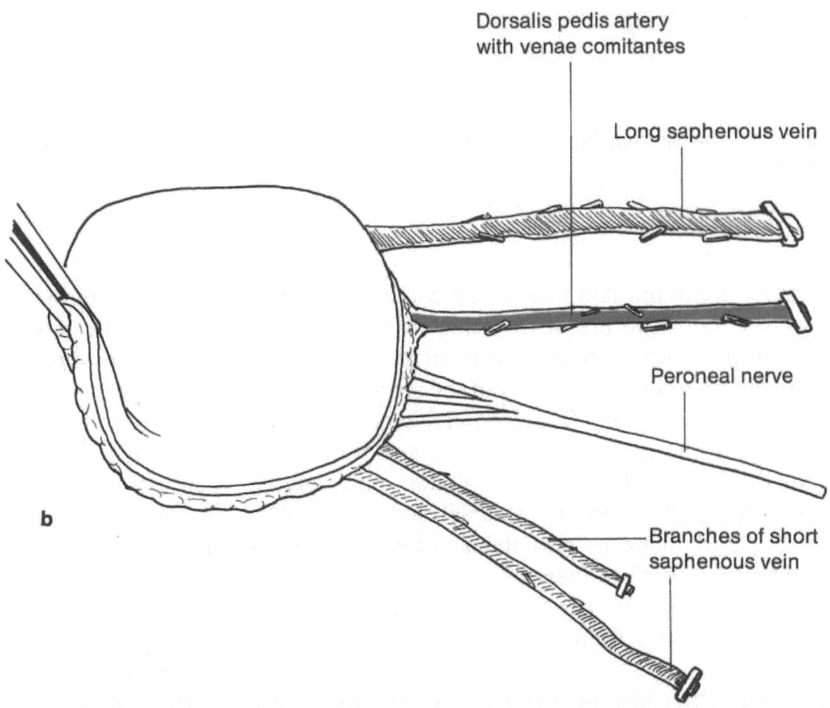

Fig. 3-7. **a** The extensor retinaculum is incised with a step cut to allow preparation of the pedicle. **b** The elevated dorsal foot flap showing three veins which can be used for anatomoses - long saphenous, short saphenous and venae comitantes

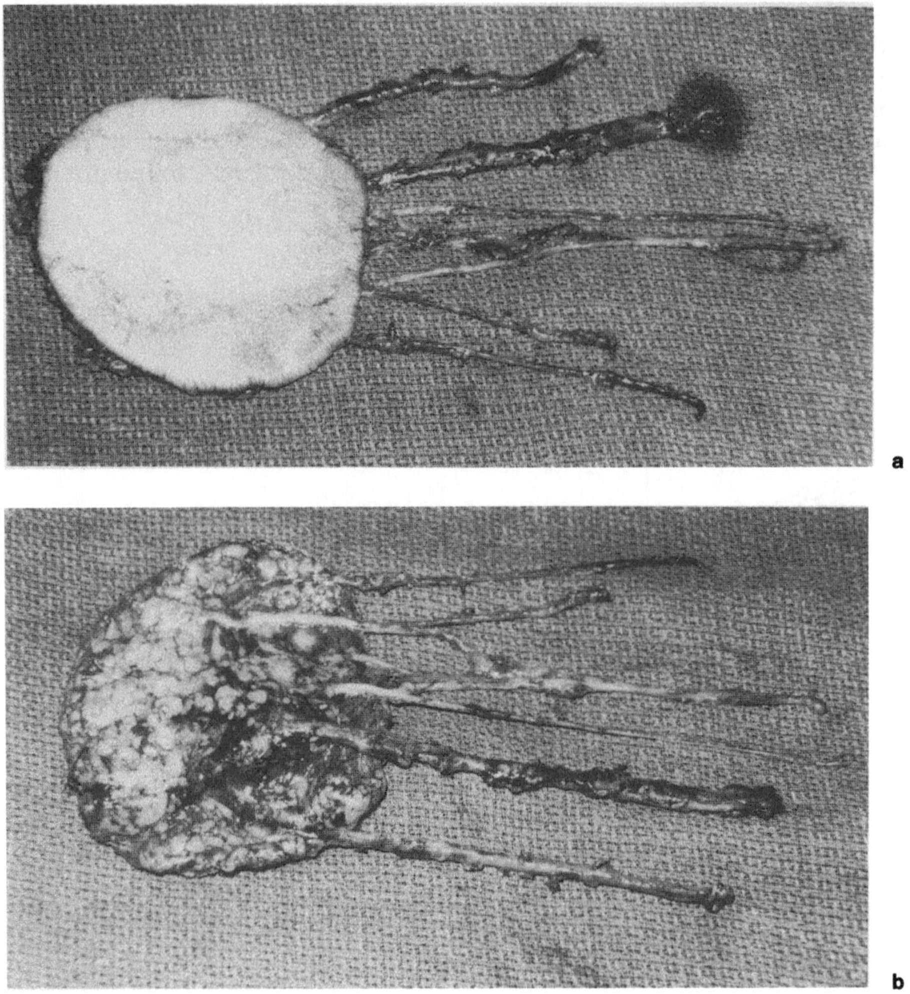

Fig. 3-8. **a** The elevated flap is thin and flexible. The nerves and vessels are the same as in Fig. 3-7 b. **b** There is very little subcutaneous fat

7. Place a curving skin incision proximally from the flap to allow exposure of the selected vein and the dorsalis pedis artery. Make a step cut in the extensor retinaculum to facilitate repair of the retinaculum after removal of the flap (Fig. 3-7 a). Dissect the dorsalis pedis in the proximal tarsal area and follow the pedicle distally. Identify the medial and lateral malleolar, medial and lateral tarsal and the arcuate vessels, and ligate or clip them. There are venae comitantes to each of these branches and all need to be divided carefully. The flap will now be completely detached except for its vascular pedicle (Fig. 3-7 b).

8. Replace the flap on the foot, cover with damp gauze and a dry towel, and allow the circulation to become stabilized. Assess flap color, capillary return, and dermal bleeding after 10–15 minutes. Pulsations will be seen at the distal end of the FDMA where it is sutured to the skin flap. This sentinel of success can also be used to evaluate the pedicle after it has been transferred.

If the skin does not appear to be perfused or the sentinel is not pulsating, either the vessels are in spasm or you have injured the first dorsal metatarsal artery. Lay the flap upside down on the foot, use topical vasodilators and, using magnification, examine the artery. Release any constrictions and repair any damage done to the pedicle.

The key to successful elevation of the FDMA without damage is keeping it within view while dissecting from distal to proximal under the flap.

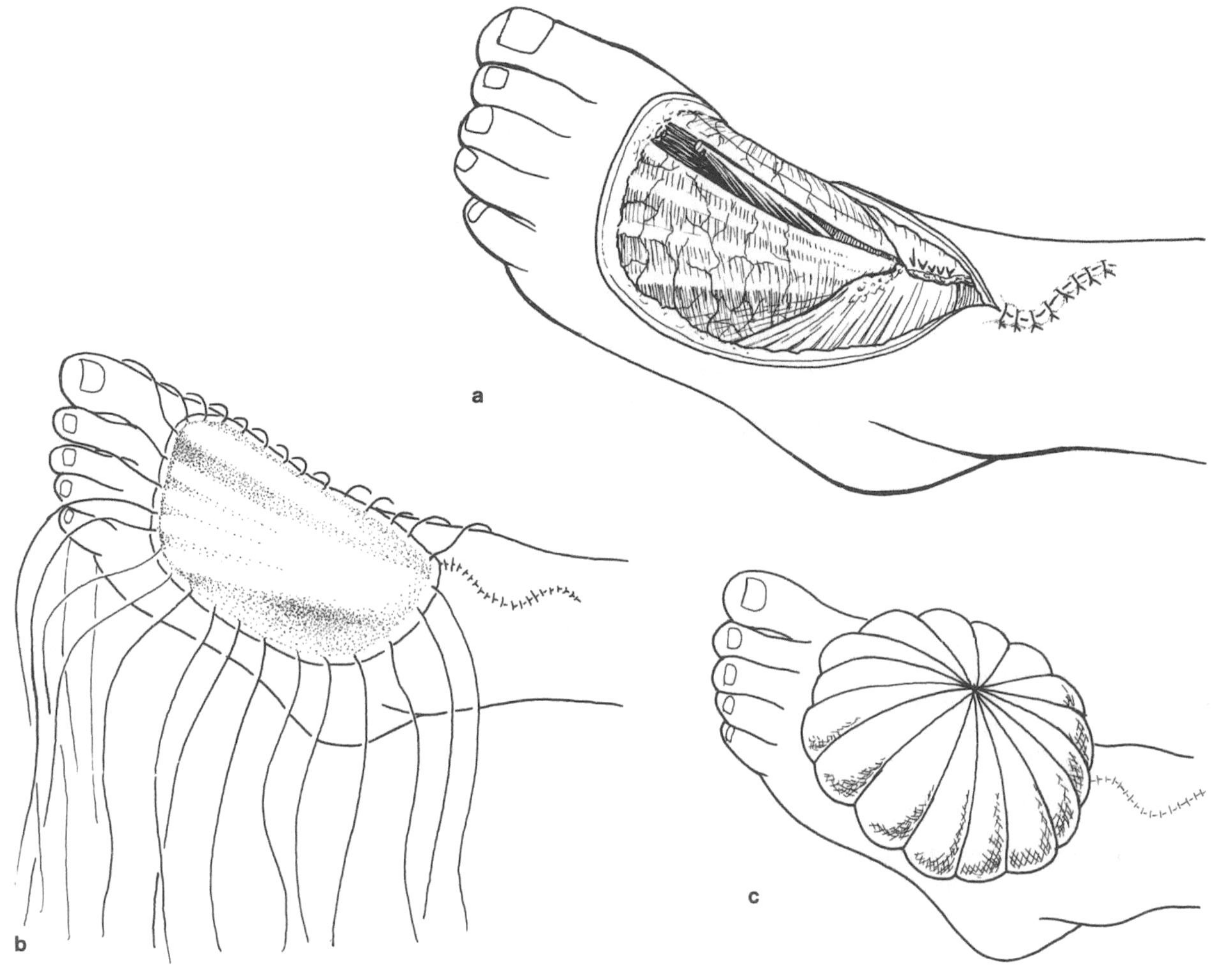

Fig. 3-9. **a** The retinaculum is closed by overlapping the two flaps from the step cut. **b** Application of skin graft and tie over sutures. **c** The bolus tie over must be applied gently

Closing the Dorsal Foot Donor Site

If the donor site is not carefully managed, there will be delayed healing and increased morbidity.

Surgical Technique

1. Obtain complete hemostasis. Repair any rents in the paratenon with fine absorbable sutures. Repair the extensor retinaculum, using the step wise cuts to obtain adequate approximation of the retinaculum over the extensor tendons (Fig. 3-9 a). Problems with skin graft take are often related to damage of the paratenon, either through mechanical trauma or being allowed to dry during surgery.

2. Apply a split thickness skin graft of medium thickness after hemostasis. Gently hold it in place with a molded cotton batten tie over dressing (Fig. 3-9 b, c). As the extensor hallucis longus is quite prominent, an area of pressure concentration may form between the tendon and a tight tie over dressing and the skin graft may not survive.

Splint the ankle, foot and toes to prevent inadvertent movement under the graft. Movements of the extensor tendons post op under a damaged paratenon may contribute to a bad graft take.

3. Elevate the foot and leave the patient in bed with the foot elevated for 10 days. Following 10 days of bed rest, remove the dressing, ambulate the patient gradually with elastic bandage support. After bed rest and dressing removal, use the appearance of the skin graft as an indication for the rapidity of ambulation.

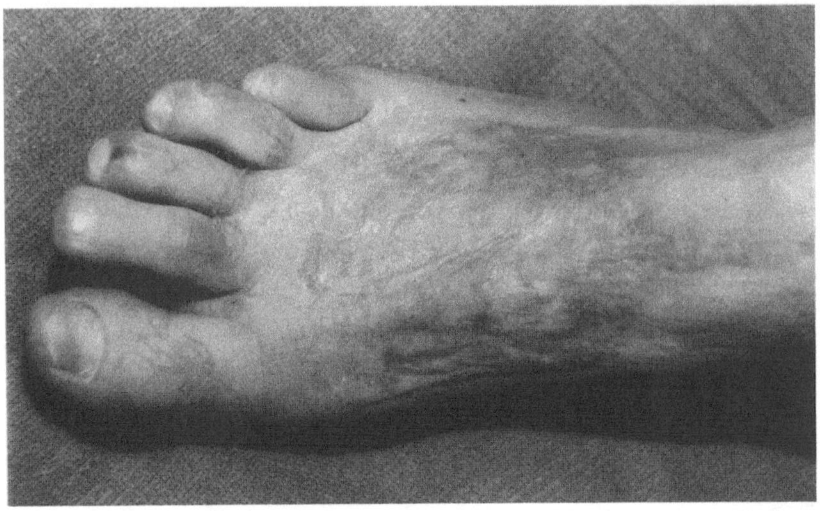

Fig. 3-10. The skin grafted donor site seen one year following surgery

References

1. Gilbert A (1976) Symposium on Microsurgery (ed) Daniller AI, Strauch B. Chapter 25. Composite Tissue Transfer from the Foot: Anatomic Basis and Surgical Technique. C.V. Mosby Co., St. Louis
2. Hollingshead WH (1969) Anatomy for Surgeons: Volume 3 Chapter 9. Harper and Row Pub. New York
3. Huber JF (1941) The arterial network supplying the dorsum of the foot. Anat Record 80: 343
4. Man D, Acland RD (1980) The microarterial anatomy of the dorsalis pedis flap and its clinical applications. Plast Reconstr Surg 65: 419
5. May JW, Chait LA, Cohen BE, O'Brien B McC (1977) Free neurovascular flap from the first web of the foot in hand reconstruction. J Hand Surg 2: 387
6. McGraw JB, Furlow LT Jr (1975) The dorsalis pedis arterialized flap. A clinical study. Plast Reconstr Surg 55: 177
7. Ohmori K, Harii K (1976) Free dorsalis pedis sensory flap to the hand with microneurovascular anastomoses. Plast Reconstr Surg 58: 546
8. Robinson DW (1976) Microsurgical transfer of the dorsalis pedis neurovascular island flap. Br J Plast Surg 29: 209

Chapter 4. Forearm Flap

Introduction

The forearm flap is a particularly useful skin transfer. This is a fasciocutaneous flap which includes the volar forearm skin, the underlying antebrachial fascia and the intermuscular fascia which contains the radial artery and cutaneous branches. Since the flap may include cutaneous nerves, flexor tendons and bone, it is a very versatile flap. When the medial and lateral antebrachial nerves are used, it becomes a well innervated fasciocutaneous flap. With a piece of the underlying radius, it becomes a vascularized osteocutaneous flap. If the palmaris longus and a longitudinal portion of the brachioradialis and flexor carpi radialis are included, it can be used for combined coverage of soft tissue defects and tendon reconstruction [4]. It is likely that with further elucidation of fascial vascular anatomy, many new flaps will be designed. A useful classification and list of currently available fasciocutaneous flaps has been compiled by Cormack and Lamberty.

This tissue transfer, which was developed in the Peoples Republic of China in 1978, at The Ba-Ba Chung Hospital, has quickly become recognized as a very reliable and relatively easy flap to use [10, 14]. Its thin and pliable nature recommended its use to the Chinese surgeons for resurfacing the neck following burn contractures. These same charateristics make it suitable for replacement of intra-oral lining. One half of the forearm diameter and up to 10 cm of the radius may be included for mandibular reconstruction [11].

As an innervated thin flap, it provides good coverage for the sole of the foot or for the palm and digits of the hand. An interesting hemodynamic characteristic of this flap is that the venous drainage may be quite satisfactory in a retrograde direction. Satisfactory retrograde flow has been shown by Mohlbauer and Biemer in the use of the flap as a distally based pedicled flap for hand reconstruction. For transfer to the head and neck or foot, the flap can be elevated while the donor site is being prepared. With the donor site on the arm, the patient can be mobilized quickly and the hospital stay is minimized. The only major limitation to the use of this flap is the cosmetic deformity of the donor site, which many patients and surgeons find unacceptable.

Anatomy of the Forearm Flap

The skin which can be perfused by the cutaneous branches of the radial artery includes the entire volar forearm skin, extending from the subcutaneous border of the ulna around to the radial dorsum of the forearm (Fig. 4-1). Song has had experience with extending the proximal border of this flap to above the elbow. However, most applications will require a flap within the forearm. Over the distal volar fore-

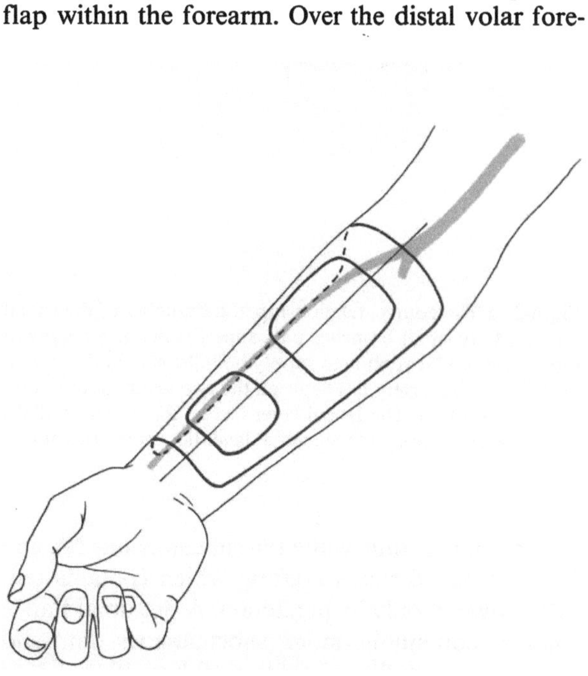

Fig. 4-1. The flap axis is shown by the straight line which is placed slightly medial to the radial artery. The flap may be outlined to include the entire volar forearm skin. However, if a small flap is required, it may be outlined anywhere along the flap axis, as indicated by two of the possibilities illustrated

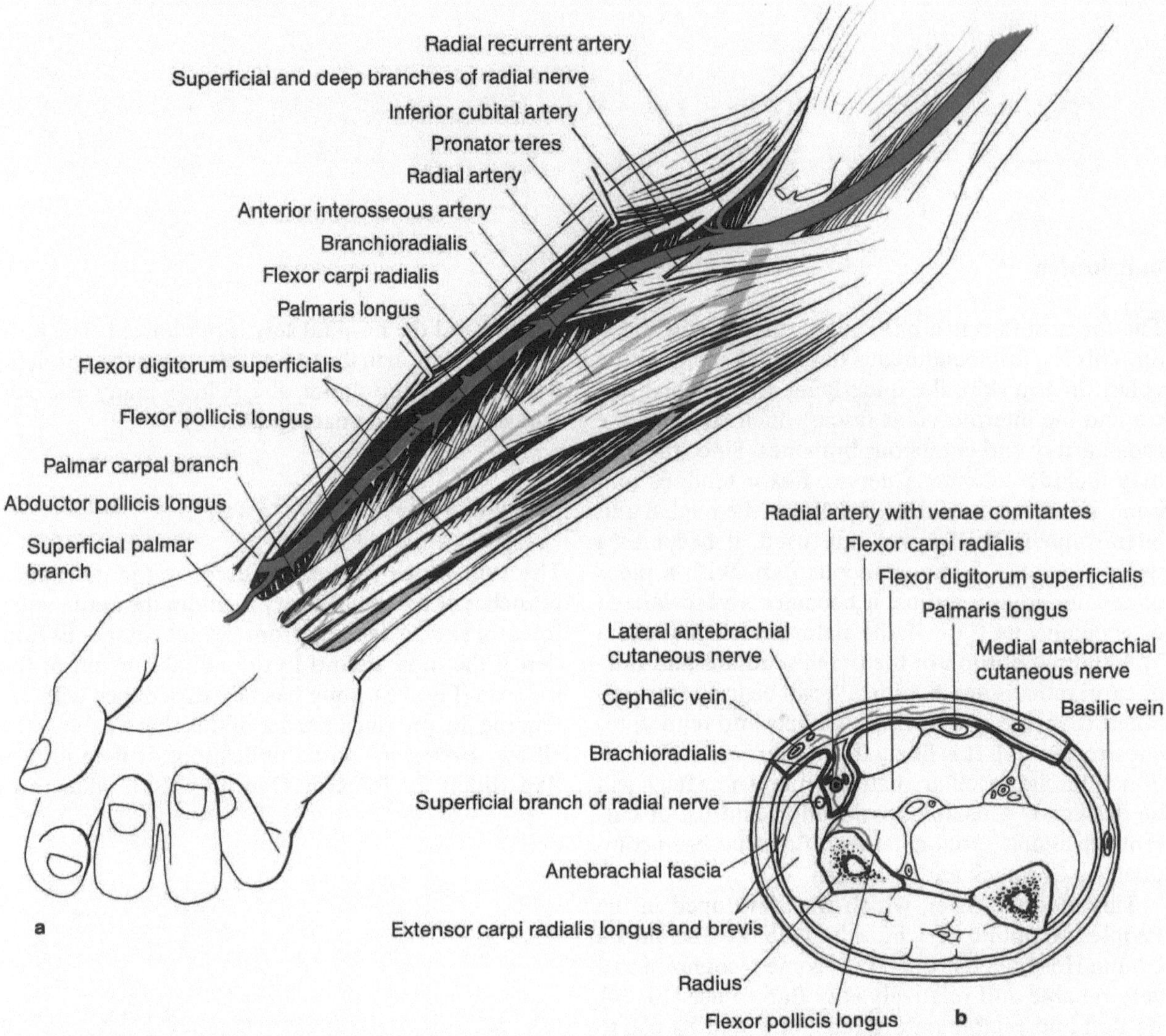

Fig. 4-2. a The course, relationship and branches of the radial artery. Many small branches pass superficially and deeply in the intermuscular septum to supply both the skin and the radius. **b** The radial artery lies between the two layers of the intermuscular septum. The lateral layer lies on the brachioradialis and wrist extensors and the medial layer lies on the flexor carpi radialis and sublimus. The heavy line in the illustration indicates the plane of flap dissection which is deep to the antebrachial fascia and incorporates this fascia and the intermuscular septum in the flap. In this way, the radial artery, with its vessels to the skin, is included in the flap

arm, the flap is thin, with little subcutaneous fat, and leaves a bed for skin grafting which contains tendons covered only by paratenon. A proximal flap is thicker, containing more subcutaneous fat, and leaves muscle bellies as a skin graft bed. If a small or medium sized flap is required, it may be placed on the proximal, middle or distal forearm (Fig. 4-1). The desired thickness of the transfer, the presence of hair on the forearm, the desire of the patient to hide the defect and the need for a long vascular pedicle are the factors which determine the optimum location.

The medial and lateral antebrachial cutaneous nerves enter the proximal margin of the flap in the subcutaneous tissue. They supply sensibility to the volar half of the forearm.

The portion of bone which is available with this transfer is the lateral half of the radius from the insertion of the pronator teres to the flare in the distal radius. This provides a 10 cm length of bone which is primarily cortical and slightly curved, and has a cross section which is one half of a circle. The bone is particularly strong and has been used for hand

and jaw reconstruction. The bone is not designed to carry an intact endosteal supply but to survive on the periosteal contributions of the radial artery.

Vascular Anatomy

Arterial Supply

The entire radial artery from its brachial artery origin to the wrist is available for the transfer. The 2-3 mm diameter of the radial artery ensures a patent vascular anastomosis. For most of its course, the radial artery lies under and adjacent to the brachioradialis. On the artery's medial aspect are the flexor carpi radialis, flexor digitorum sublimus, and on the deep surface, the pronator teres, flexor digitorum sublimus, flexor pollicis longus and pronator quadratus. Lateral to the artery and under the brachioradialis throughout most of its course is the superficial branch of the radial nerve.

After giving off the radial recurrent artery near its origin, and the inferior cubital artery, the radial artery has no named branches until it reaches the wrist where it gives off a superficial palmar branch and a palmar carpal branch. The radial artery then turns laterally to wind around the wrist, deep to the tendons of the abductor pollicis longus and extensor pollicis brevis. Although there are no named branches throughout its course in the forearm, it gives off many cutaneous, muscular and periosteal branches which enable this artery to support skin and bone for a free tissue transfer. The branches which supply the skin are contained in the intermuscular septa between the brachioradialis and the flexor carpi radialis, and rise to the surface to lie on the antebrachial fascia over these muscles. The largest of these branches is the inferior cubital artery. It takes origin 4 cm below the intercondylar line and supplies the proximal forearm fascia and overlying skin. Sometimes it arises from the radial recurrent artery rather than the radial. This artery is not usually included in the flap unless a proximally located flap is required [5]. The branches to the bone pass deep to the radial artery in a condensation of fascia. They supply the bone by direct branches and by musculo periosteal branches which pass through the flexor pollicis longus musculature.

In 750 upper extremity dissections, McCormick found both radial and ulnar arteries present 100% of the time. The only anomaly of the radial artery was a high take off from the brachial artery above the elbow which occured 14% of the time. However, arteries with this high origin had a normal course within the forearm. The ulnar artery provides the dominant supply to the hand through the superficial palmar arch and will usually supply the entire hand. However, in view of the many variations of palmar anatomy, the ulnar artery cannot be assumed to supply all of the hand. In over 10% of Coleman and Anson's dissections, there were no branches of the superficial palmar arch to the thumb and index. In 50% of dissections, the deep arch which originates from the radial artery did not connect to the ulnar artery. If both of these variations are present in a hand, the thumb and index will likely depend upon the radial artery for their perfusion [12, 13]. If a forearm flap is used in patients with these variations, the radial artery may need to be reconstituted with a vein graft to ensure the circulation to the radial side of the hand.

Venous Drainage

Adequate venous drainage for this transfer is provided by either the subcutaneous or the deep venous systems. There are 3 subcutaneous veins which may be used to drain the transfer. The basilic vein originates on the ulnar dorsal side of the hand and runs proximally on the ulnar border of the forearm. It is usually too far medial to be included in the flap. The cephalic vein takes origin on the radial dorsal side of the hand, and curves around the wrist to run on the radial volar surface of the forearm. This vein lies in the usual territory of the flap and has a diameter averaging 3.5 mm. The median forearm vein runs up the anterior surface of the forearm and is frequently small and less reliable for transfer. Near the elbow, the median cubital vein forms an oblique connection between the basilic and cephalic veins and a connection with the deep venae comitantes of the forearm.

On either side of the radial artery are paired venae comitantes which provide a good venous outflow through the deep system. Either the cephalic vein or a vena comitans is the preferred vein for microvascular transfer.

Alternate Vascular Pedicles for the Forearm Flap

Both the inferior cubital artery and the ulnar artery have been used to transfer fasciocutaneous forearm flaps [5]. The large size of the ulnar artery favours its use as a vascular pedicle.

There is one dominant cutaneous branch of the ulnar artery to the overlying fascia and skin which is located at the junction of the middle and proximal third of the forearm. Lovie described a flap based upon this fasciocutaneous system with reliable clinical experience. Using the proximal ulnar forearm rather than the radial forearm has the advantage that the donor site is more easily hidden by the patient, and the flap is less hairy and thinner than the radial arm donor site. The disadvantage is that there are few cutaneous branches, often only one and occasionally none. In view of the possibility that there are no cutaneous vessels, Morrison recommends that the flap should be raised from the ulnar aspect. If a cutaneous branch is not seen, the flap should continue to be raised from ulnar to radial in order to include the fascial septum to the radial artery and convert it to a proximal radial artery flap.

Elevating the Forearm Flap

Using Allen's test, assess the ability of the ulnar artery to supply the hand. Examine the cutaneous forearm veins with a proximal venous tourniquet in place to identify their pattern and ensure that there has been no venous injury through previous trauma or venipuncture. If bone is to be taken, a plain x-ray is required to evaluate the shape and size of the radius.

Surgical Technique

1. Mark the course of the radial artery and the superficial veins. The flap axis is slightly medial to the course of the radial artery. Using a pattern taken from the recipient site, transfer the size and shape of the defect and the location of the recipient structures, including nerves and vessels. Position this pattern in a suitable location along the flap axis (Fig. 4-3 a).

2. Incise the flap down to the underlying fascia. Identify and prepare the subcutaneous veins and nerves which will be used in the transfer.

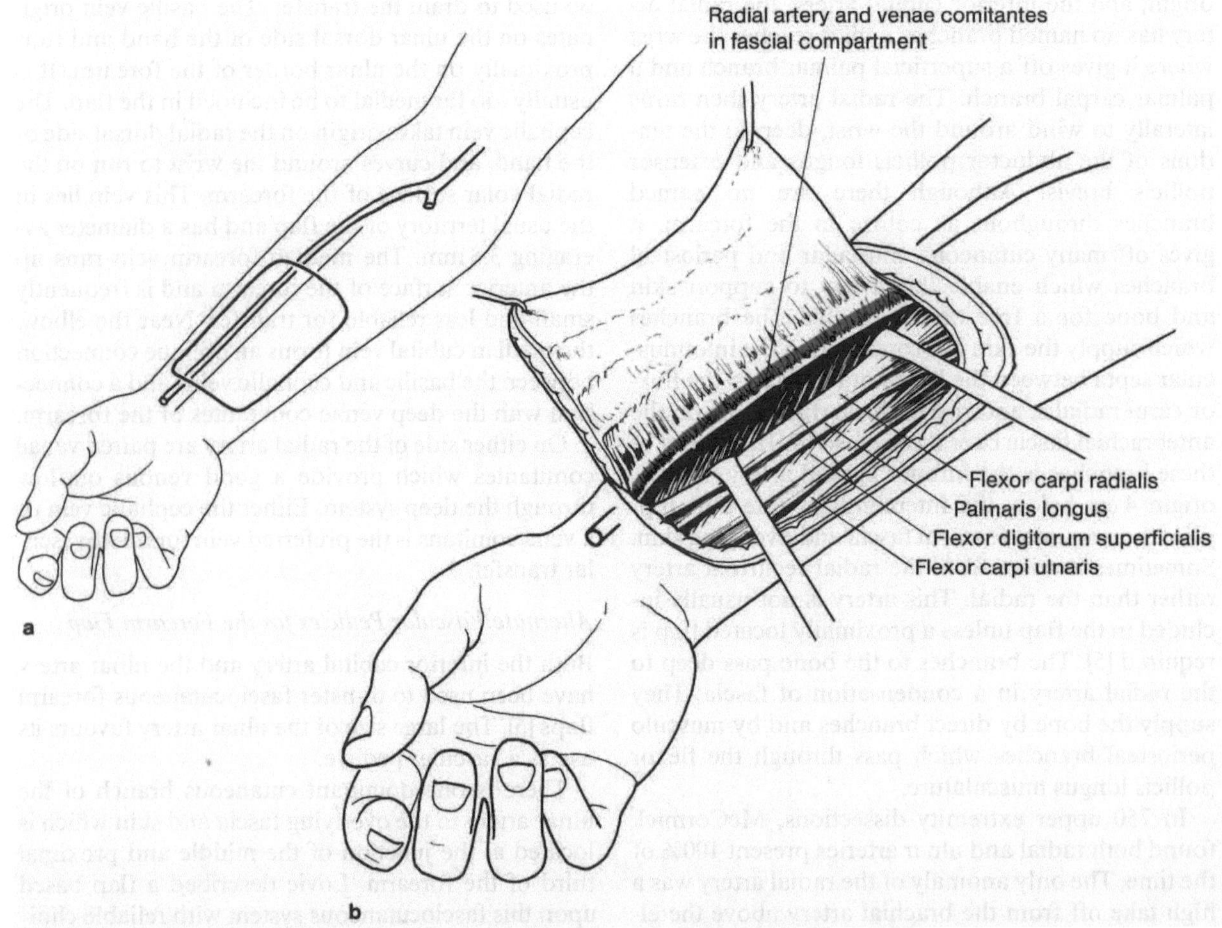

Fig. 4-3. a A medium sized, distally located skin flap. **b** The flap is raised sub-fascially to the lateral border of the flexor carpi radialis. The dissection then turns deeply to include the intermuscular septum in the flap

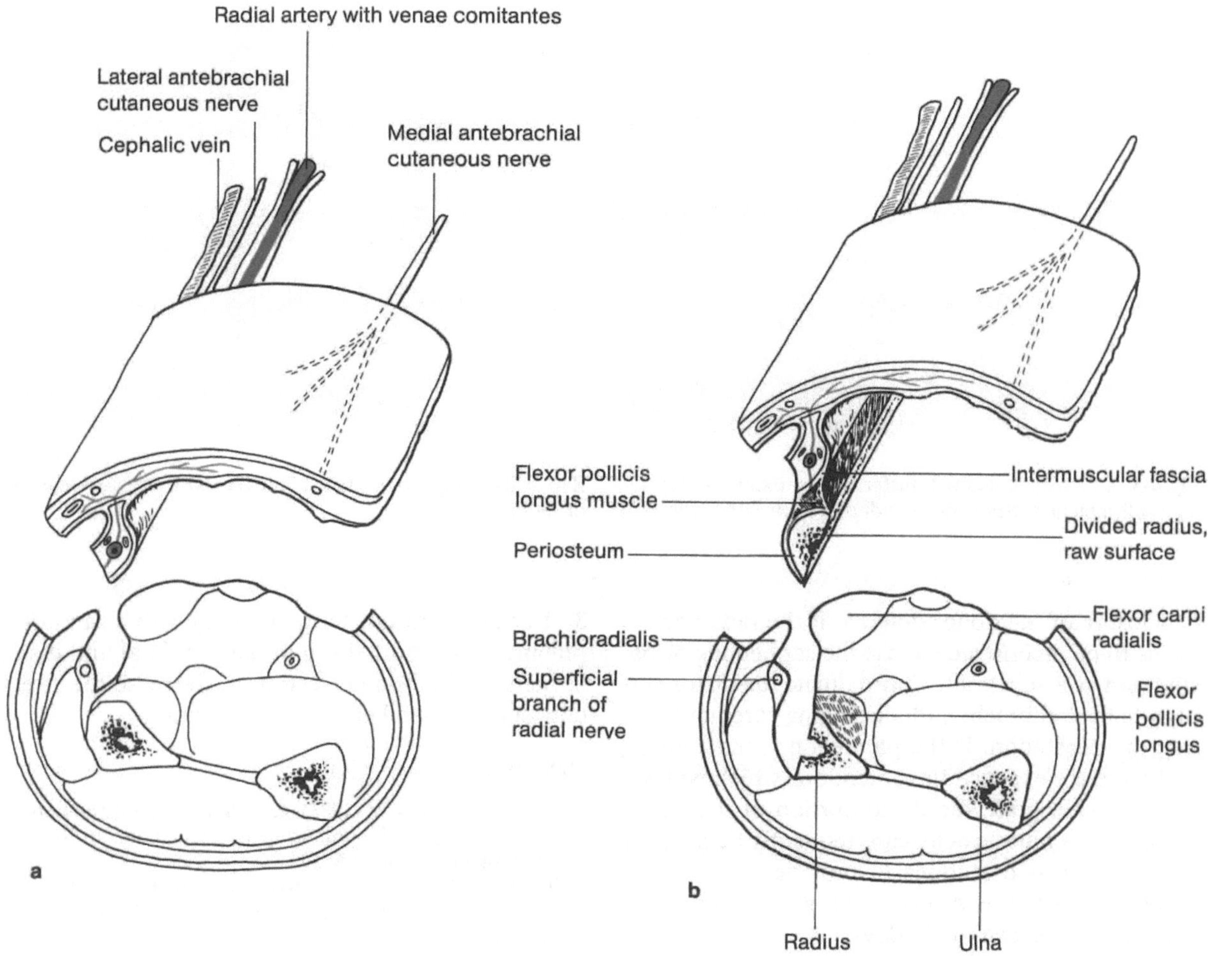

Fig. 4-4. a The radial artery and its branches to the skin lie in the intermuscular septum. Either the cephalic vein or a vena comitans is commonly used to drain the flap. Both the lateral and medial antebrachial nerves are available for flap innervation. **b** By carrying the dissection deeply on both sides of the radial artery, and keeping intact the deep branches of the radial artery to the flexor pollicis longus and the radius, the surgeon may include the lateral half of the radius as an osteocutaneous transfer

3. Carry the skin incision through the underlying antebrachial fascia and lift the flap subfascially. Dissect from the medial and lateral sides of the flap towards the fascial septum, leaving a bed of muscle proximally and tendons with intact paratenon distally.

4. When approaching the 'space' between the flexor carpi radialis and the brachioradialis, retract these two muscles and carry the dissection deeply, hugging the muscle bellies (Fig. 4-3 b). Keep the dissection between the muscle and the intermuscular fascia. This procedure creates a longitudinal curtain of fascia hanging between the two muscles and connecting the skin to the radial artery. Observe the artery in the depth of the fascial curtain and the superficial branch of the radial nerve lying laterally under the brachioradialis.

5. Spread the flexor carpi radialis and brachioradialis apart with retractors and divide the radial artery and venae comitantes distally. Develop a plane of dissection under the radial artery, working from distal to proximal, along its entire length. The flap will now be free except for the proximal pedicle (Fig. 4-4 a). The separation of the radial artery from its bed requires the cautery of multiple small vessels which pass from the artery to the surrounding muscles, especially the flexor pollicis longus, flexor digitorum superficialis, and the area of insertion of the pronator teres. Release the tourniquet and evaluate the circulation to the flap.

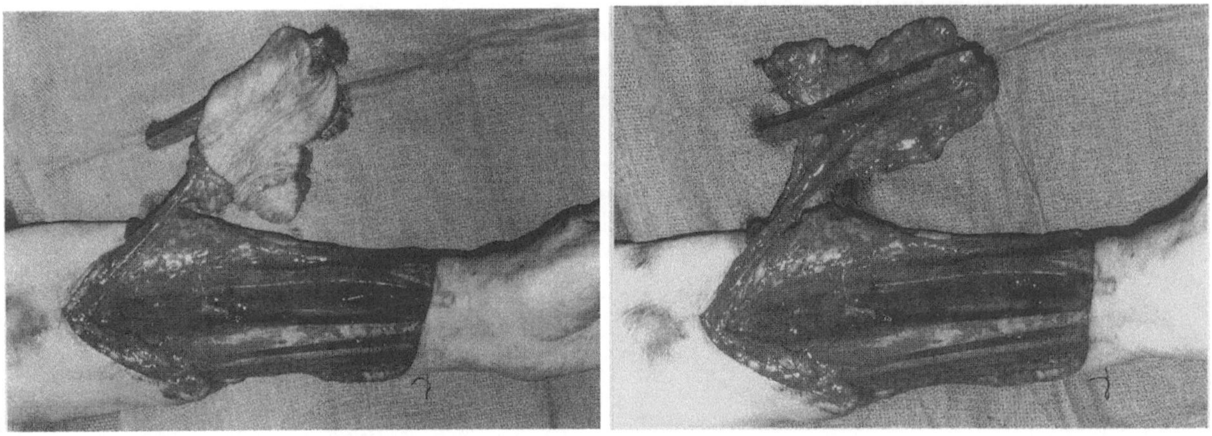

a b

Fig. 4-5. a Osteocutaneous transfer with proximal radial artery still attached. Segment of radius is seen under the skin flap. **b** Showing deep surface of the flap with attached segment of radius

6. Closure of the donor defect - If the radial artery needs to be reconstructed, use the saphenous or basilic vein as a vein graft. Approximate the flexor carpi radialis and brachioradialis, taking care not to injure the paratenon. If the paratenon is inadequate, and there are exposed flexor tendons which will not accept a skin graft, the distal portion of the flexor carpi ulnaris muscle belly can frequently be brought over the exposed tendons to provide an adequate bed for a graft take. Apply a skin graft and a splint and elevate the arm for 10 days.

Taking an Osteocutaneous Flap

Surgical Technique

1. Good exposure is required to identify the position of the shaft of the radius to allow an accurate longitudinal split. The maximum length of bone which may be removed extends from the distal flare of the radius to the pronator teres insertion. Expose the lateral and postero-lateral surfaces of the radius by elevating the brachioradialis and extensor carpi radialis brevis and longus.

2. Carry the dissection on the medial side of the intermuscular fascia through the musculature over the radius, dividing the pronator teres, flexor digitorum sublimus and flexor pollicis longus directly on top of the midline of the bone. In this way, muscular and musculo-periosteal vessels to the lateral half of the radius will remain connected to the radial artery (Fig. 4-4b).

3. Divide the radius longitudinally with a saw, after placing a drill hole through the proximal and distal corners of the bone resection to decrease the stress concentration and chance of a fracture.

References

1. Biemer E, Stock W (1983) Total thumb reconstruction: A one stage reconstruction using an osteocutaneous forearm flap. Br J Plast Surg 36: 52
2. Coleman SS, Anson BJ (1961) Arterial patterns in the hand based upon a study of 650 specimens. Surg Gynecol Obstet 113: 409
3. Cormack GC, Lamberty BGH (1984) A classification of fascio-cutaneous flaps according to their patterns of vascularization. Br J Plast Surg 37: 80
4. Foucher G, van Genechten F, Merle N, Michon J (1984) A compound radial artery forearm flap in hand surgery: an original modification of the Chinese forearm flap. Br J Plast Surg 37: 139
5. Lamberty BGH, Cormack GC (1982) The forearm angiotomes. Br J Plast Surg 35: 420
6. Lovie MJ, Duncan GM, Glasson DW (1984) The ulnar artery forearm free flap. Br J Plast Surg 37: 486
7. McCormack LJ, Cauldwell EW, Anson BJ (1953) Brachial and ante brachial arterial patterns: a study of 750 extremities. Surg Gynecol Obstet 96: 43
8. Morrison Personal communication
9. Muhlbauer W, Herndl E, Stock W (1982) The forearm flap. Plast Reconstr Surg 70: 336
10. Song R, Gao Y (1982) The forearm flap. Clin Plast Surg 9: 21
11. Soutar DS, Scheker LR, Tanner NSB, McGregor IA (1983) The radial forearm flap: a versatile method for intra oral reconstruction. Br J Plast Surg 36: 1
12. Weathersby HT (1954) The volar arterial arches. Anat Record 118: 365
13. Weathersby HT (1955) The artery of the index finger. Anat Record 122: 57
14. Yang Guofan et al (1981) Forearm free skin flap transplantation. Nat Med J China 61: 139

Chapter 5. Scapular Flap

The scapular flap has become a favorite cutaneous transfer for many reasons. The circumflex scapular artery (C.S.A.) provides a constant pedicle which is relatively long, large and easy to prepare. The skin is thick and hairless with less subcutaneous fat than the groin. The donor site can be closed directly and the donor defect is relatively good. However, a tight donor site closure will result in a spread scar and its high location on the back is not acceptable to many women.

This flap was developed by dos Santos and clinically applied by Gilbert. Many authors, including Barwick, Urbaniak, Hamilton and Godina, have found the flap to be a useful addition to the armamentarium of free skin transfers.

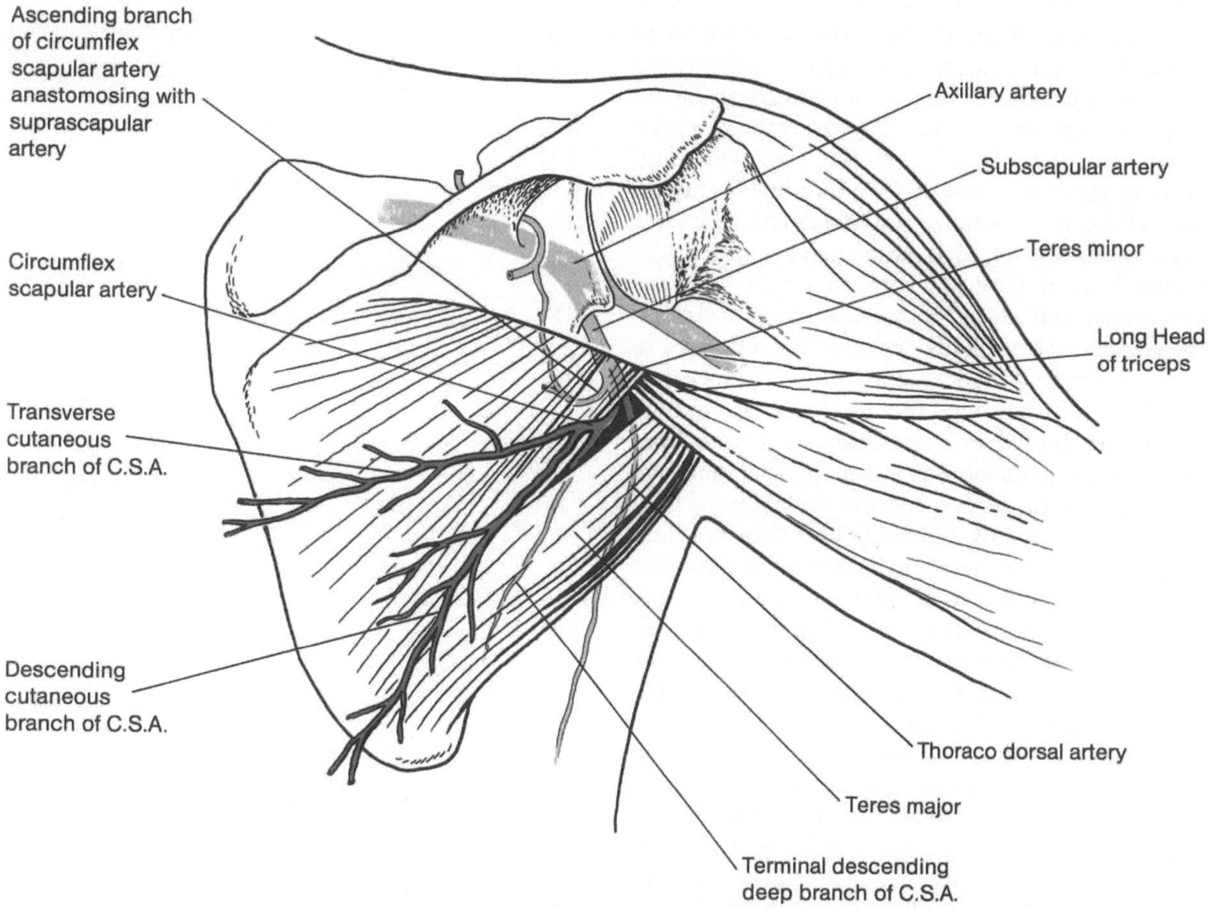

Fig. 5-1. The pedicle for the scapular and parascapular flaps is the circumflex scapular artery (C.S.A.). A branch of the subscapularis artery, the C.S.A., enters the back through the triangular space and gives off one deep and two cutaneous branches. The scapular flap is based on the transverse cutaneous branch of the C.S.A. and the parascapular flap is based on the descending cutaneous branch of the C.S.A.

In view of its ease of use, it is often preferred over the groin flap, when a skin only flap is required. The thick skin and thin layer of fat recommend its use for coverage of the sole of the foot. In addition, Bosse has reported that this flap can be taken with the lateral border of the scapula as a reliable osteocutaneous flap.

Vascular Anatomy of the Scapular and Parascapular Flap

The subscapular artery, which is 3-4 mm in diameter, takes origin from the third part of the axillary artery, passes inferiorly, and terminates in two arteries, both of which are important for free tissue transfers (Fig. 5-1). The thoracodorsal artery is used to carry the latissimus dorsi transfer. The circumflex scapular artery (C. S. A.) carries the scapular flap. The C. S. A. winds posteriorly around the subscapularis, and passes through the muscular triangle created by the teres minor and major and the long head of the triceps. During its course, it gives off muscular branches to the subscapularis, infra-spinatus, and teres musculature. There are two terminal branches: a deep descending branch, running deep to the teres major, along and supplying the lateral border of the scapula, and a cutaneous branch which hugs the teres minor as it passes to the subcutaneous tissues. The cutaneous branch divides into two: a transverse and a descending branch, either of which may supply a flap. Godina found that the transverse branch was not present in 3 of 28 dissections, but noted that the descending branch was always present, and recommended using the descending branch for the flap. However, dos Santos, Urbaniak and Gilbert found the transverse branch to be constant in over 100 dissections, and dos Santos noted it to be 1.5-2.5 mm in diameter. The initial concept of the scapular flap was to orient it transversely and base it on the transverse cutaneous branch of the C. S. A. When the descending cutaneous branch was identified as a constant branch, it allowed an obliquely oriented flap to be designed inferior to the scapular flap. This obliquely oriented flap is called the parascapular flap (Fig. 5-2).

The C. S. A. is 2.5-3.5 mm in diameter and provides a pedicle which is 4-8 cm in length. This artery is accompanied by two venae comitantes which provide adequate drainage for both flaps. Often, the venae comitantes join to form one vein in the triangular space. However, the presence of many venous branches in the depth of the triangular space may present difficulty in developing an unbranched end of vein for anastomosis.

The maximum area of skin which is reliably perfused by these branches is unknown. Hamilton reported a successful 24 cm long scapular flap which crossed the mid line of the back. However, flap tip necrosis sometimes occurs when the transverse flap is taken as far as the mid line. For an oblique parascapular flap, Shaw has reported a maximum possible length of 30 cm.

Elevating the Scapular and Parascapular Flap

Surgical Technique

The flap may be taken with the patient prone, or lying on the contralateral side with the arm draped free so that it can be abducted to facilitate the dissection of the pedicle.

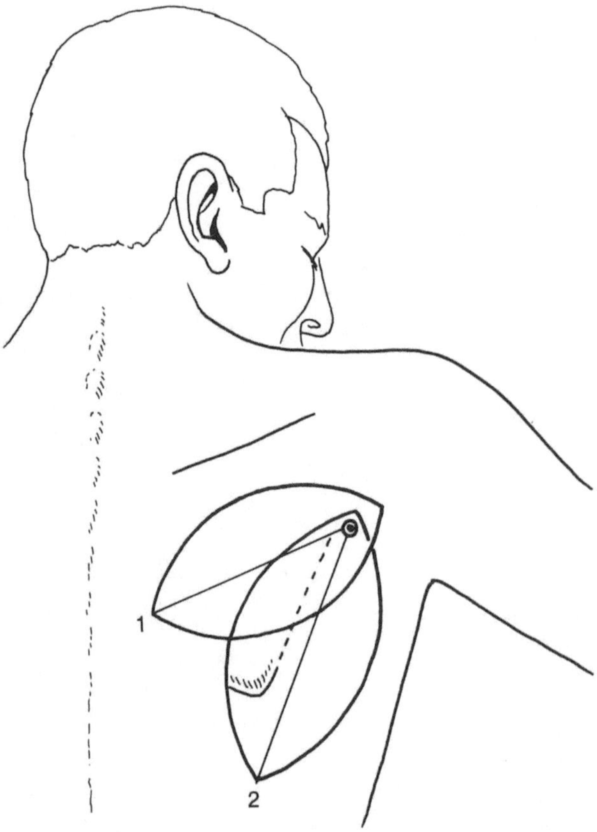

Fig. 5-2. The flap landmarks are the spine, angle, lateral border of the scapula and a palpable depression between the teres minor and major. This depression marks the mid point of the lateral margin of the scapula (dot). The scapular flap axis and its vessel lie parallel to the spine of the scapula and equidistant from the spine and the angle [1]. The parascapular flap axis and its vessel lie along the lateral margin of the scapula [2]

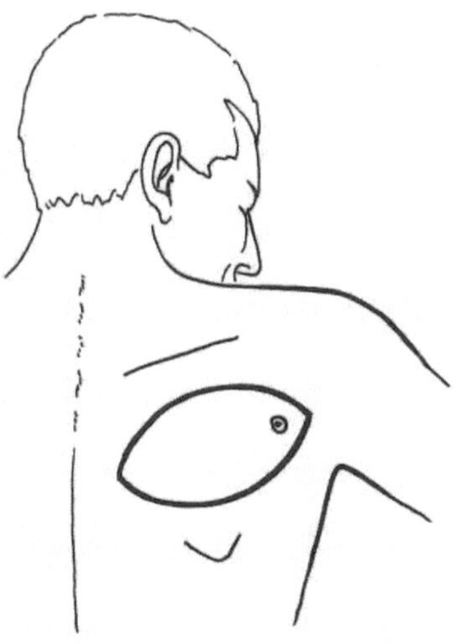

a

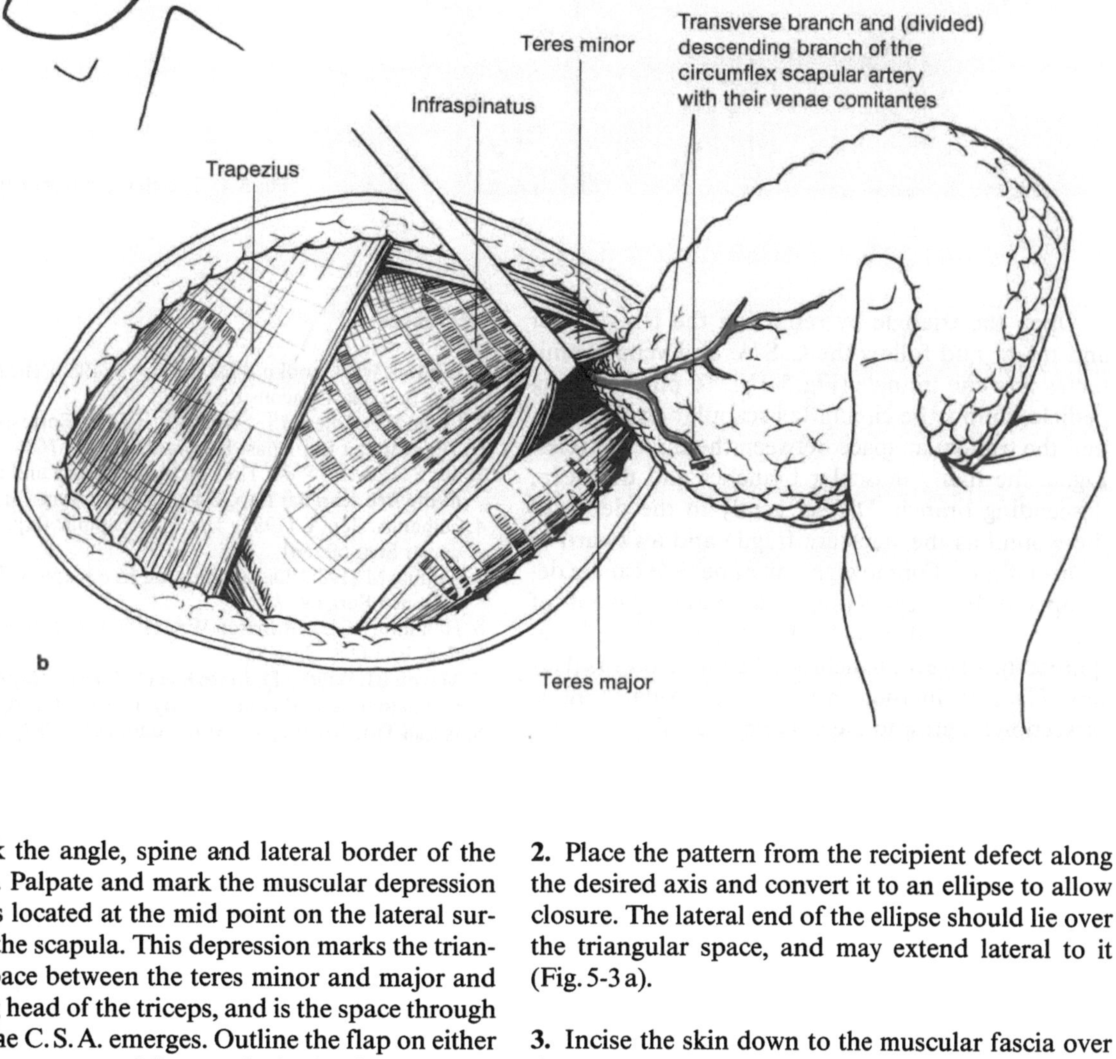

b

Fig. 5-3. a Outline of scapular flap. **b** The flap is elevated from medial to lateral, superficial to the muscular fascia, revealing the cutaneous branches of the C.S.A. The transverse cutaneous branch is the main supply and the descending branch has been ligated. Retraction of the teres minor demonstrates the pedicle

1. Mark the angle, spine and lateral border of the scapula. Palpate and mark the muscular depression which is located at the mid point on the lateral surface of the scapula. This depression marks the triangular space between the teres minor and major and the long head of the triceps, and is the space through which the C.S.A. emerges. Outline the flap on either a transverse or an oblique axis, both of which pass through this point. The transverse axis lies parallel to the spine of the scapula and equidistant to the spine and the angle. The oblique axis lies along the lateral edge of the scapula (Fig. 5-2). The choice of axis is determined by the thickness of the subcutaneous tissue, the skin laxity which facilitates closure, and the desire to hide the scar.

2. Place the pattern from the recipient defect along the desired axis and convert it to an ellipse to allow closure. The lateral end of the ellipse should lie over the triangular space, and may extend lateral to it (Fig. 5-3 a).

3. Incise the skin down to the muscular fascia over the medial two thirds of the flap. Elevate the flap from medial to lateral, just superficial to this fascia. As the dissection approaches the triangular space, the cutaneous branches of the C.S.A. will become apparent on the deep surface of the flap.

4. When the artery is visible, and its position clear, complete the medial skin incision.

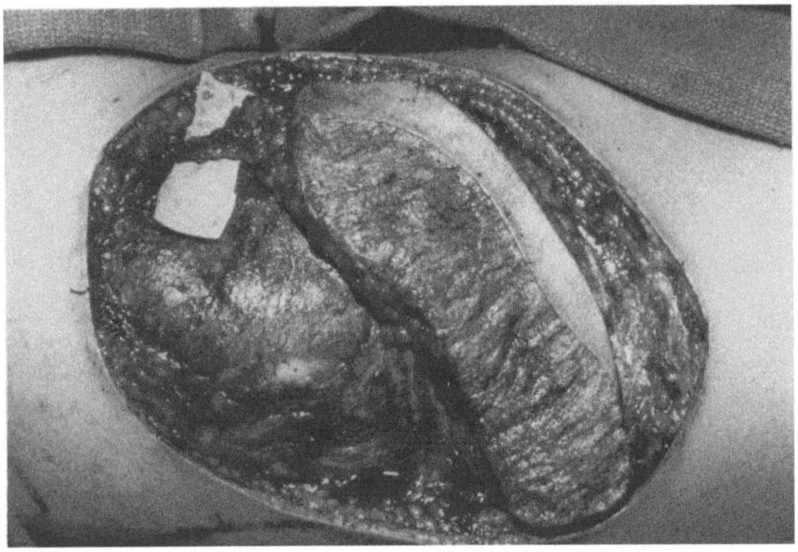

Fig. 5-4. The elevated parascapular flap

5. Open the triangle by retracting the teres minor and major and follow the C.S.A. and venae comitantes into the triangle (Fig. 5-3b). To obtain a long pedicle, follow the circumflex scapular artery down into the triangular space between the three muscles. Ligate the many muscular branches and the deep, descending branch. Dissect gently in the depth of the wound as the veins are fragile and awkward to control if torn. Four to eight cm of pedicle can be developed if the artery is prepared up to the takeoff of the thoracodorsal branch. If a longer pedicle is required, the dissection includes the thoraco-dorsal artery. Place an incision in the lateral axilla to allow dissection anterior to the latissimus dorsi.

6. Assess the viability of all areas of the flap prior to dividing the pedicle.

7. Close the defect by undermining and advancing the skin edges.

References

1. Barwick WJ, Goodkind DJ, Serafin B (1982) The free scapular flap. Plast Reconstr Surg 69: 779
2. Colen SR, Colen HS, Shaw WW (1982) Correspondence: The scapular flap. Plast Reconstr Surg 70: 768
3. dos Santos LF (1984) The vascular anatomy and dissection of the free scapular flap. Plast Reconstr Surg 73: 59
4. Gilbert A, Teot L (1982) The free scapular flap. Plast Reconstr Surg 69: 601
5. Godina M (1982) Discussion: the free scapular flap. Plast Reconstr Surg 69: 786
6. Hamilton SGL, Morrison WA (1982) The free scapular flap. Br J Plast Surg 35: 2
7. Mayou BJ, Whitby D, Jones BM (1982) The scapular flap - an anatomical and clinical study. Br J Plast Surg 35: 8
8. Nassif TM, Vidal L, Povet JL, Baudet J (1982) The parascapular flap: a new cutaneous microsurgical free flap. Plast Reconstr Surg 69: 591
9. Teot L, Bosse JP, Moufarrege R, Papillon J, Beauregard G (1981) The scapular crest pedicled bone graft. Int J Microsurgery 3: 257
10. Urbaniak JR, Koman LA, Goldner RD, Armstrong NB, Nunley JA (1982) The vascularized cutaneous scapular flap. Plast Reconstr Surg 69: 772
11. Urbaniak JR (1984) Discussion: The vascular anatomy and dissection of the free scapular flap. Plast Reconstr Surg 73: 604

Muscle Transfers

In the late 19th century, Iginio Tansini used skin flaps from the posterior lateral chest to cover mastectomy defects. The distal portion of these flaps always failed. After taking his clinical problem to the anatomy dissection table, he recognized that the skin over the posterior lateral chest wall received its blood supply from branches passing through the latissimus dorsi muscle to the overlying skin [4, 9]. This was the first clinical recognition of the concept of muscular perforators' supplying circulation to the overlying skin. Using this concept, he developed the latissimus dorsi musculocutaneous flap for skin coverage following radical mastectomy. In spite of the discovery of this revolutionary procedure, the musculocutaneous concept did not become understood and accepted until Orticochea described the gracilis musculocutaneous flap. A few years later, the latissimus dorsi was again 'discovered' and its tremendous versatility and usefulness appreciated [6]. With the identification of the robust thoraco-dorsal pedicle, it was just a short step from pedicled flap to free tissue transfer.

In a few short years, most of the muscles of the body have been assessed for their usefulness as pedicled and free tissue transfers [5]. The availability of muscle and myocutaneous flaps has greatly increased the range of flaps available for free tissue transfer. With their large, long and predictable pedicles, and robust blood supply, they have become the most common transfer used in reconstructive microsurgery.

Mathes and Nahai observed five different patterns of vascular anatomy in skeletal muscles [3]. This classification assists the surgeon in determining the suitability of a muscle for transfer. The basic requirement for microvascular transfer is that the portion of muscle transferred be perfused by a pedicle with an adequate size for anastomosis. When transferring an entire muscle, a single pedicle muscle or one with a dominant pedicle must be used. A vena comitans is always used for venous return.

With a myocutaneous flap, branches of the muscle's arterial pedicle perforate the muscle to supply the overlying skin flap. As these perforators are always accompanied by venae comitantes, venous return from the skin flap is not a problem. Since the skin is perfused by a fascial and subdermal plexus from the perforators, the cutaneous flap may extend beyond the muscle margins.

When the bulk of a myocutaneous flap is undesirable, or the donor site cannot be closed directly, a muscle only transfer should be used. The muscle is a good bed for a split thickness skin graft which provides a durable and fairly acceptable appearance. Muscles have also been used as free tissue transfers to supply a functional contracting tissue for reconstruction of the extremities and for facial paralysis reconstruction.

The selection of a muscle for free tissue transfer depends upon the size and shape of the defect, the recipient vessel size and location, the functional expendability of the muscle, the ease of muscle elevation and the need for an attached cutaneous segment. I have selected three muscles for inclusion in the book: the gracilis, latissimus dorsi and rectus abdominis. These three will reconstruct 99% of soft tissue defects and manage most functional muscle problems. The entire muscle or just a small segment of each may be used. Each muscle can be taken with an attached reliable cutaneous segment. When the entire muscle is employed, the latissimus dorsi will cover huge defects, the rectus abdominis medium to large long defects, and the gracilis small to medium defects. There are other muscles available for transfer, both for cover and function. These include the pectoralis minor and major, the serratus anterior, tensor fascia lata, gluteus maximus, rectus femoris, and the gastrocnemius [1, 7].

References

1. Hill HL, Nahai F, Vasconez L (1978) The tensor fascia lata myocutaneous free flap. Plast Reconstr Surg 61: 517
2. Manktelow RT, McKee NH, Vettese T (1980) An anatomical study of the pectoralis major muscle as related to functioning free muscle transplantation. Plast Reconstr Surg 65: 610

3. Mathes SJ, Nahai F (1981) Classification of the vascular anatomy of muscles: experimental and clinical correlation. Plast Reconstr Surg 67: 177
4. Maxwell GP (1980) Iginio Tanzini and the origin of latissimus dorsi musculocutaneous flap. Plast Reconstr Surg 65: 686
5. McCraw JB, Dibbell DG (1977) Experimental definition of independent myocutaneous vascular territories. Plast Reconstr Surg 60: 212
6. Olivari N (1976) The latissimus flap. Br J Plast Surg 29: 126
7. Orticochea M (1972) The musculo-cutaneous flap method: an immediate and heroic substitute for the method of delay. Br J Plast Surg 25: 106
8. Takayanagi S, Tsukie T (1982) Free serratus anterior muscle and myocutaneous flaps. Ann Plast Surg 8: 277
9. Tanzini I (1906) Sopra il mio nuovo processo di amputazione della mammaella. Reforma Medica 12: 757

Chapter 6. Gracilis

The gracilis muscle is a long strap-like muscle which lies on the medial thigh (Fig. 6-4). The neophyte microvascular surgeon will enjoy using this muscle. It is relatively easy to elevate, and has a reliable neurovascular pedicle.

The muscle can be used to solve soft tissue coverage problems and to provide functioning muscle transfers. Small tissue defects can be filled readily by using a small piece of the muscle centered on the vascular pedicle, and larger defects can be handled by transplanting the entire muscle (Fig. 6-1). Functional muscle deficits can be accurately reconstructed by transplanting all or a portion of the muscle (see Chap. 17, 19).

Although originally described as a pedicled musculocutaneous flap by Orticochea and McCraw, and then as a free musculocutaneous transfer by Harii, the muscle is often raised as a free tissue transfer without the skin paddle [1, 2, 3]. The thick fat of the medial thigh is frequently too bulky for soft tissue coverage and has few perforators. Injection studies by Young, in our institution, identified a constant perforator exiting from the muscle at the level of the dominant vascular pedicle. As more distal perforators are only occasionally present, perfusion of a skin flap over the middle or distal portion of the muscle is unreliable. In many coverage situations, it is preferable to transfer the muscle without the skin paddle and apply a split thickness skin graft directly to the muscle.

The muscle is particularly useful for transfer as a functioning muscle. It has a single, easily repairable

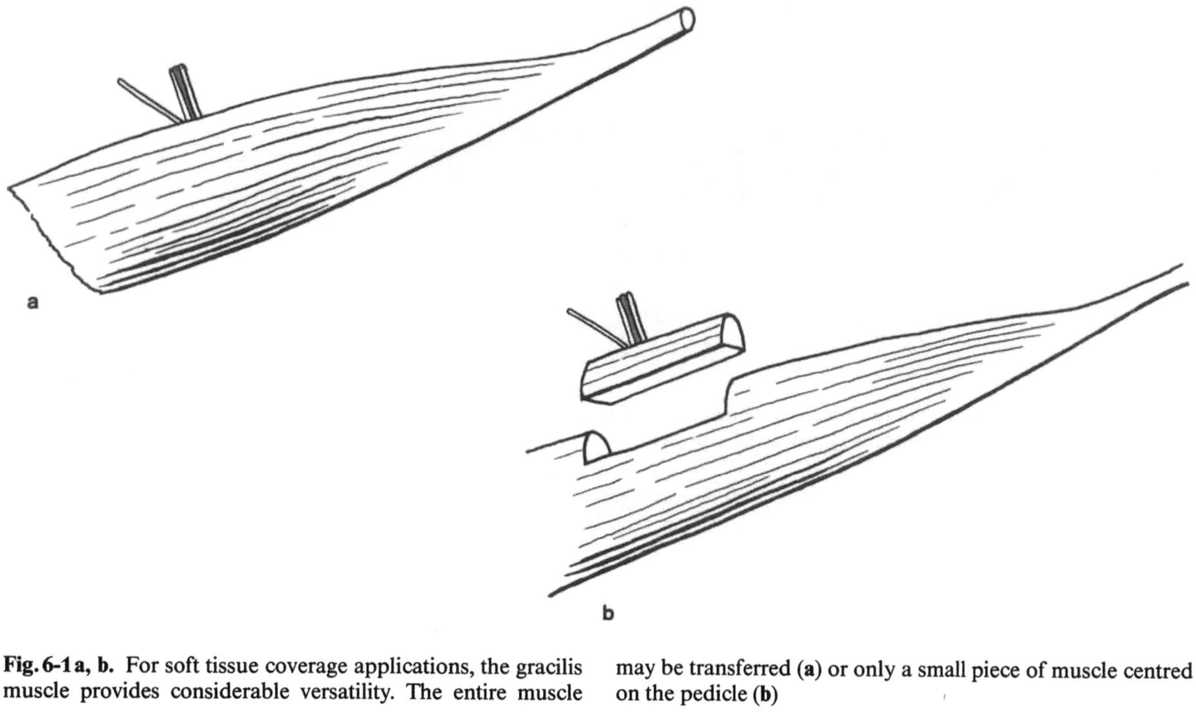

Fig. 6-1 a, b. For soft tissue coverage applications, the gracilis muscle provides considerable versatility. The entire muscle may be transferred (**a**) or only a small piece of muscle centred on the pedicle (**b**)

motor nerve. The long length of the muscle and the individual muscle fibres allows replacement of many skeletal muscle defects and provides a good range of muscle excursion. The long tendon of insertion and short fibrous origin facilitate its use in many anatomic locations (Fig. 6-2). Transfer of only a portion of the muscle is useful in facial paralysis (Fig. 6-3). Fortunately, this muscle can be removed without any noticeable functional loss and the incision on the upper aspect of the medial thigh produces an easily hidden scar.

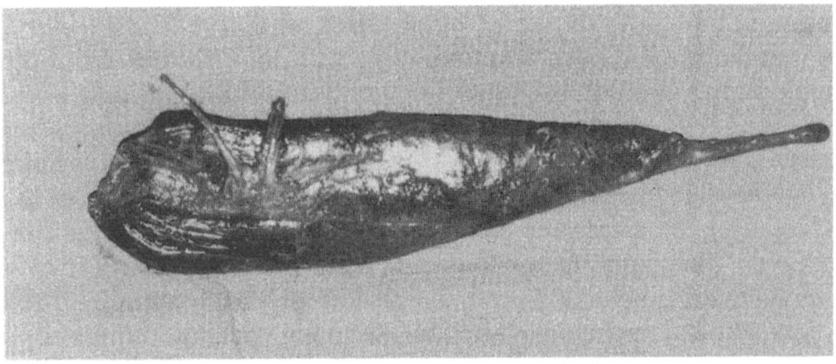

Fig. 6-2. Deep surface of gracilis muscle. Occasionally the neurovascular pedicle enters the central portion of the deep surface as shown here, rather than the anterior portion of the deep surface

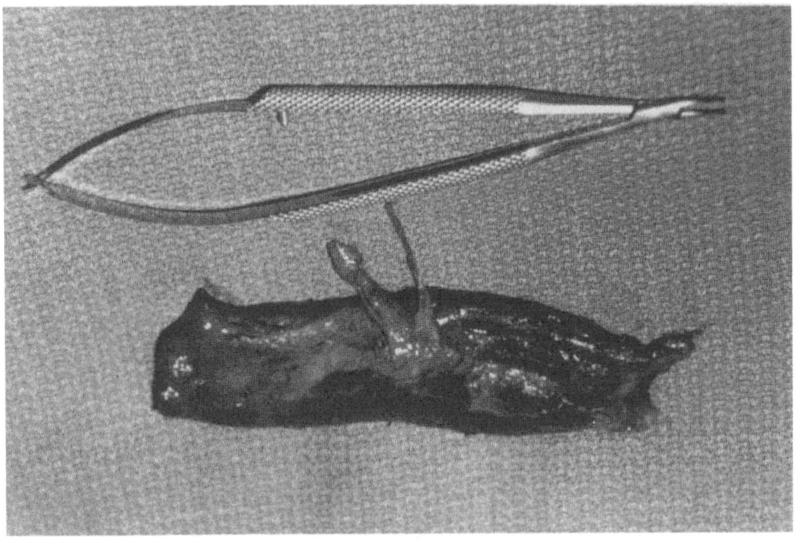

Fig. 6-3. A 2 × 10 cm segment of the gracilis has been removed from the rest of the muscle and placed beside a microsurgical needle driver. This segment contains the neurovascular pedicle

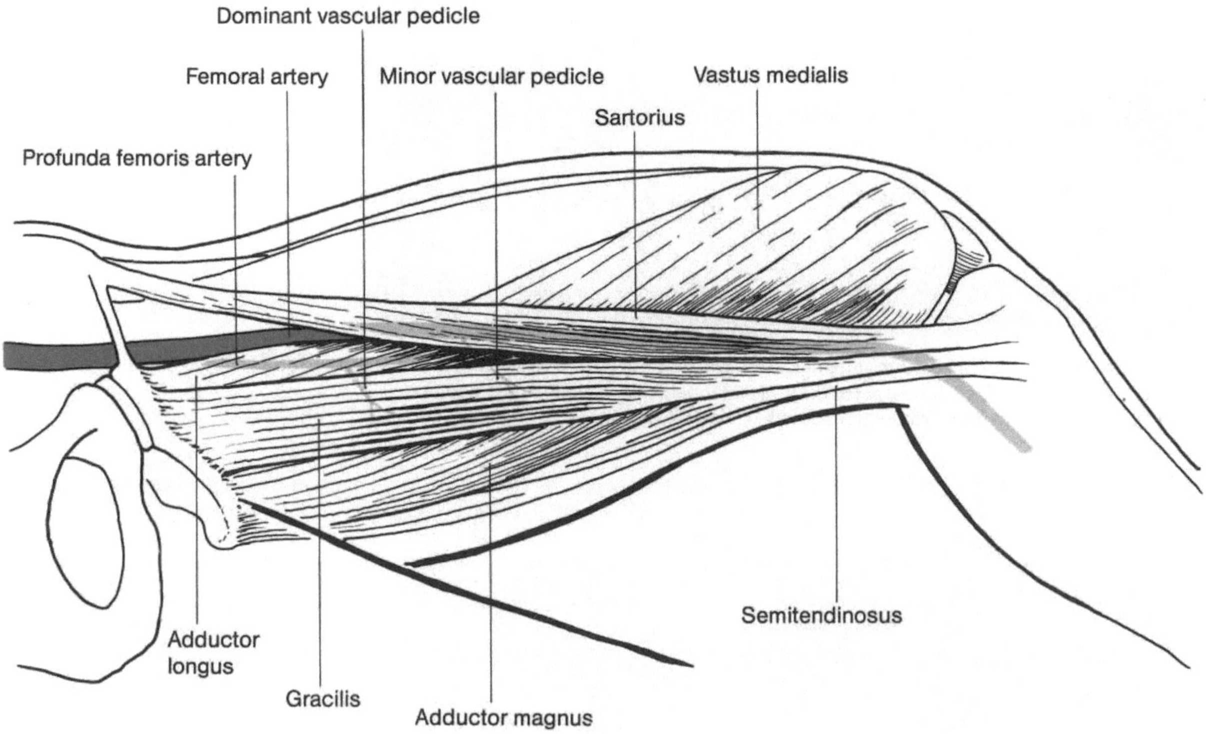

Fig. 6-4. Anatomical relationships of the gracilis muscle and the locations of the proximal vascular pedicles

Anatomy of the Gracilis Muscle

The gracilis muscle lies immediately under the deep fascia of the medial thigh (Fig. 6-4). Its origin is a short thin aponeurosis from the body of the pubis and the inferior ramus. It is inserted through a long oval tendon into the shaft of the tibia, on the medial lip of the tibial tuberosity. Its tendon of insertion may be palpated with some difficulty just anterior to the semitendinosis and semimembranosus. The muscle belly lies posterior to the adductor longus and sartorius and superficial to the adductor magnus.

The dominant vascular pedicle is usually located 9 cm (6-12 cm) from the origin and enters the muscle on the anterior aspect of the deep surface. Although the external arterial diameter ranges from 1-2 mm, if the pedicle is taken above its adductor longus muscle branches, it is usually at least 1.5 mm. There is always a pair of venae comitantes on each side of the artery, one of which is larger than the artery and occasionally as large as 4 mm. The artery usually takes origin from the profunda femoris or medial femoral circumflex artery. However, this junction is barely visible in the usual surgical dissection. Rarely, the dominant vascular pedicle is a double pedicle with two arteries and two venae comitantes running side by side. One to four secondary minor pedicles, branches of the femoral artery, are present. A distal minor pedicle may be the only blood supply to the most distal few centimeters of muscle. The intramuscular arterial anatomy, as studied by Young, commonly consists of a series of longitudinal vessels linked together at each pedicle (Fig. 6-5).

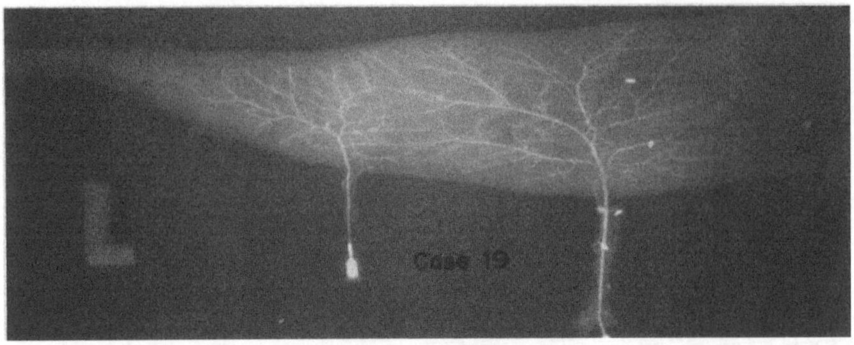

Fig. 6-5. Radiograph of a barium sulphate arterial injection study of the dominant *(right)* and a secondary vascular pedicle. Note the branching pattern from each pedicle of vessels and the connections between the longitudinal vessels from each pedicle (S. Young)

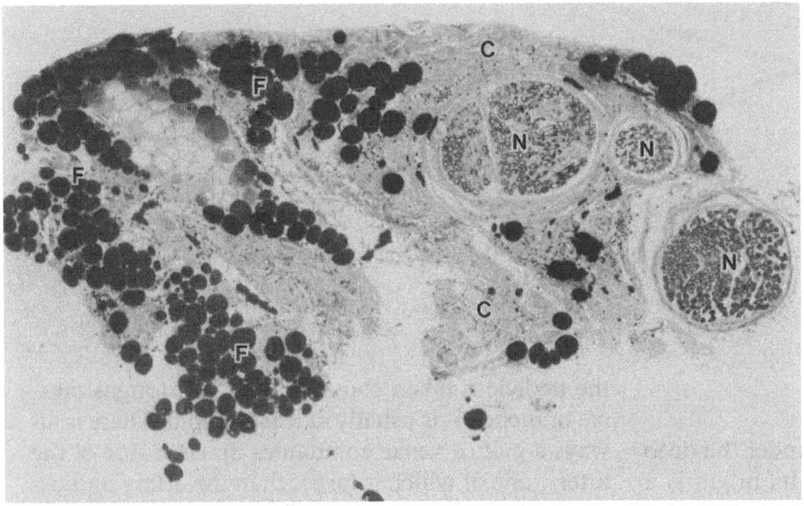

Fig. 6-6. Cross section of gracilis motor nerve. One micron epon embedded, toluidine blue stain. Reproduced 50 ×. Note the large amount of fatty tissue (F) and connective tissue (C) in this 3 fascicle nerve

The single motor nerve lies between the adductor longus and magnus muscles. It is a branch of the obturator and enters the muscle obliquely just proximally to the dominant pedicle. Two to seven fascicles are present. The usual number is 3. In operative procedures, the fascicles of the motor nerve have been separated from each other, individually stimulated, and the portion of muscle which contracted observed. In this way, the muscle can usually be divided into two longitudinal, separately functioning neuromuscular territories. The most common pattern of functional muscle division is the control of the anterior 25-50% of the muscle by a single fascicle. The posterior 50-75% of the muscle is under the control of the remaining fascicles. There is usually slight overlap in neural control of the two territories. Occasionally three separate territories are present. The motor nerve contains a large amount of fat and loose connective tissue. For reasonable alignment of fascicles, a nerve repair should use fascicular suturing (Fig. 6-6).

The pattern of the muscle fibres has been studied by Fish in our institution (Fig. 6-7). In the proximal three fifths of the muscle belly, the fibres are parallel in a strap muscle configuration. In the distal two fifths, the muscle fibres insert sequentially into the tendon which lies along the posterior border of the muscle. The muscle fibres in the posterior part of the muscle belly are shortest and insert into the most proximal tendon, and the long anterior muscle fibres insert into the most distal tendon. The muscle belly is 5-6 cm wide and 32 cm long with a mean muscle fibre length of 24 cm.

When only the muscle insertion has been detached to allow freedom of excursion, our experience with intra-operative gracilis motor nerve stimulation is that a shortening of at least 12-15 cm is produced in an adult gracilis muscle when the motor nerve is stimulated. Based upon our clinical experience, it is likely that the muscle, after transplantation, is capable of producing at least a 10 cm range of excursion with good power.

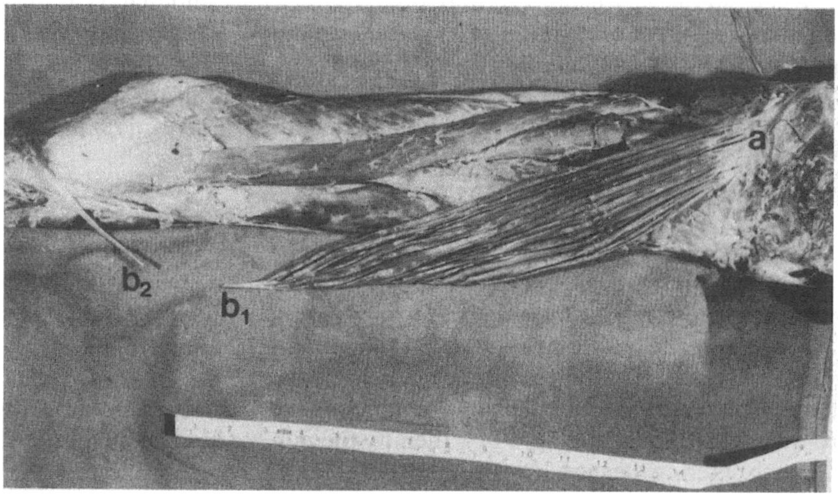

Fig. 6-7. Cadaver dissection of medial aspect of right thigh. Gracilis muscle origin (**a**) and divided tendon (*b1, b2*). The muscle fibres have been dissected into groups of fibres to better visualize the position and length of individual muscle fibres. The short posterior fibres insert most proximally into the gracilis tendon and the long anterior fibres most distally (Fish, J. and McAvoy, G)

Elevating the Gracilis Muscle Transfer

1. With the patient lying supine, prep the leg from above the groin to below the knee and drape it free. Position the leg with the hip in moderate abduction and external rotation and the knee slightly flexed. Stand on the side of the operating table opposite to the donor leg.

2. The surface landmarks are the insertion of the adductor longus tendon into the adductor tubercle and the tibial tubercle. Draw a line between these two structures, marking the upper border of the gracilis muscle (Fig. 6-8 a).

3. When not taking a cutaneous flap, place the incision 2 cm below the anterior muscle margin over the proximal half of the muscle. Carry the incision through the superficial fascia to the fascia lata. Place your finger on the adductor longus tendon to identify the juncture of the gracilis and adductor and incise the fascia lata along this juncture.

4. Elevate the skin and fascia over the entire muscle. Identify and develop the posterior muscle border and separate the gracilis from the adductor magnus.

Dissect a plane between the adductor longus and gracilis. Retract the adductor longus and identify the dominant neurovascular pedicle found 6–12 cm from the pubic tubercle (Fig. 6-8 c). Identify the motor nerve entering the muscle on its deep surface, just proximally to the neurovascular pedicle. It lies on the adductor magnus and is loosely attached to it.

5. Dissect the desired length of the muscle belly and identify minor pedicles. Usually, the first minor pedicle is found at least 10–15 cm distally to the dominant pedicle.

6. Complete the dissection of the pedicle. A headlight and loop magnification are helpful. Preserve the cutaneous branch to the medial thigh and the motor branch to the adductor longus, both of which lie on the posterior surface of this muscle. Place two right angle retractors under the adductor longus, one on each side of the dominant pedicle and lift the adductor longus (Fig. 6-8 c). Divide the multiple side branches which enter the adductor longus (Fig. 6-9 a, b). With good elevation of the adductor longus, an additional 3 cm of pedicle can be obtained to provide a total pedicle length of 6–7 cm.

Separate the deep surface of the pedicle from the adductor magnus. Look for the branch which occasionally goes to this muscle from the deep surface of the pedicle.

7. Divide the muscle distally and then proximally, dividing minor pedicles as necessary. If the full muscle with tendon is required, retrieve the tendon through a transverse incision over the proximal ham strings (Fig. 6-8 b).

8. After proximal division of the muscle, leave it in situ without tension on the pedicle to observe the adequacy of muscle perfusion.

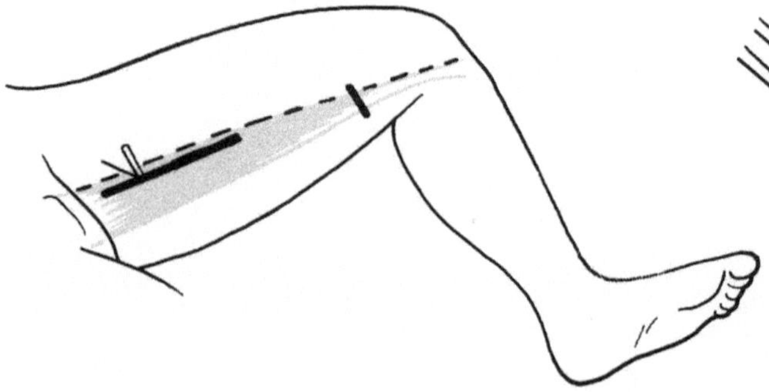

Fig. 6-8. a With the hip flexed, abducted and externally rotated, and the knee flexed, a line drawn between the easily palpable adductor longus tendon and the tibial tubercle, marks the anterior border of the gracilis muscle. The entire muscle and tendon may be removed through the incisions illustrated by solid lines

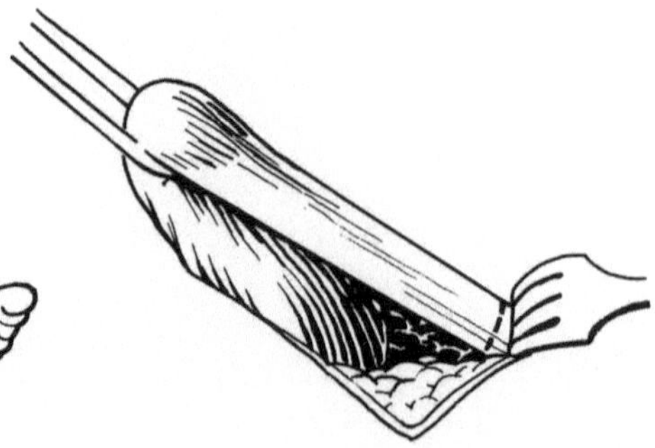

Fig. 6-8. b The tendon of the gracilis muscle is retrieved through a transverse incision just proximal to the knee. This tendon lies immediately anterior to the easily palpable tendons of the semimembranosis and semitendonosis muscle

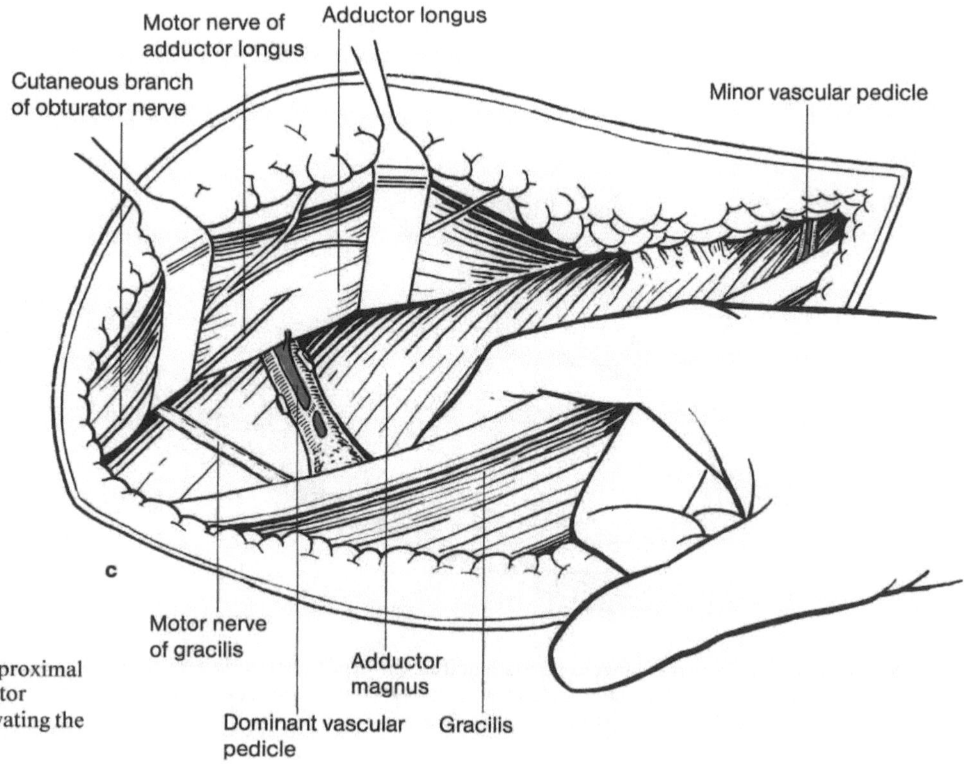

Fig 6-8. c The dominant proximal vascular pedicle and motor nerve are exposed by elevating the adductor longus muscle

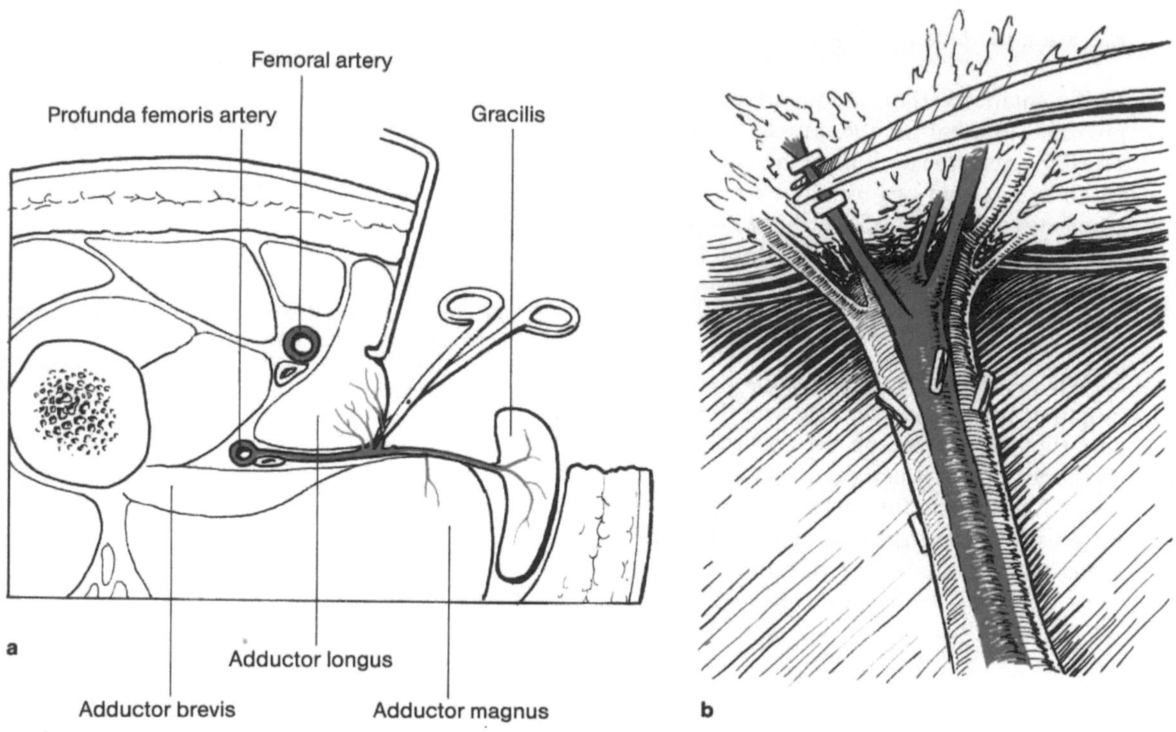

Fig. 6-9. a Branches of the vascular pedicle must be divided in order to obtain the full length of pedicle. A group of branches always enter the deep surface of the adductor longus. There is an inconstant branch on the deep surface of the pedicle which supplies the adductor magnus. **b** The branches entering the deep surface of the adductor longus must be carefully identified and divided. There is a minimum of one arterial and two venous branches present. If these branches are divided, the pedicle can be isolated up to its origin, providing a 6–7 cm pedicle length

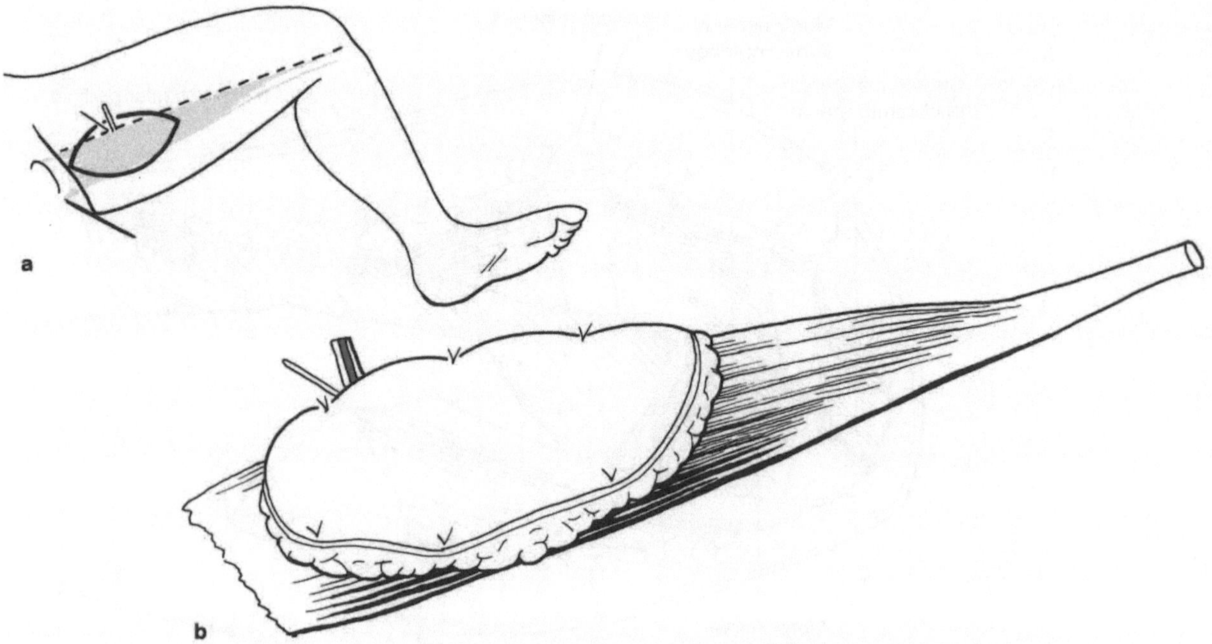

a

b

Fig. 6-10 a, b. When a myocutaneous flap is required, the skin flap is outlined directly over the muscle at its proximal end. There is a constant cutaneous perforator at the level of the dominant vascular pedicle

Elevating the Gracilis Myocutaneous Transfer

1. If a cutaneous flap is required, outline it over the proximal one half of the muscle belly (Fig. 6-10 a). The flap axis is the midline of the muscle. A skin flap width of 8–10 cm can usually be removed and still allow direct closure of the thigh. When measured from the pubis, a skin flap length of 15 cm will survive. Although survival distal to this point will sometimes occur, it is uncertain.

2. When developing a cutaneous flap, it is important to centre the flap directly over the muscle to ensure that the perforators are included. First, incise the intended distal margin of the flap and carry the dissection down to the gracilis. When the location of the muscle is confirmed, the flap can be redrawn to a more anterior or posterior position if necessary.

As the connections between the muscle and the subcutaneous fat are tenuous, sutures should be placed between the superficial fascia or dermis and the muscle to prevent shearing of the skin flap on the muscle (Fig. 6-10 b). These may be removed following the transfer and prior to inserting the skin flap.

References

1. Harii K, Ohmori K, Sekiguchi J (1976) The free musculocutaneous flap. Plast Reconstr Surg 57: 294
2. McCraw JB, Dibbell DG (1977) Experimental definition of independent myocutaneous vascular territories. Plast Reconstr Surg 60: 212
3. Orticochea M (1972) The musculocutaneous flap method: an immediate and heroic substitute for the method of delay. Br J Plast Surg 25: 106

Chapter 7. Latissimus Dorsi

The latissimus dorsi muscle is a dependable and versatile muscle for free tissue transfer. It is easily elevated, has a large surface area, and the thoraco dorsal artery provides a large, long and reliable pedicle. First described as a pedicled musculocutaneous flap by Tansini in 1906, it did not enjoy popularity as such until the publications of Olivari, Muhlbauer, McCraw and others. After Baudet described the use of the latissimus dorsi as a free tissue transfer, this muscle became one of the most popular flaps for free tissue transfer.

The muscle has excellent characteristics for coverage. It is thin and flat and may easily be molded to cover any shape or fill any defect. Of all the muscles available, it provides the largest possible soft tissue coverage. Although the entire muscle may be transferred, the postero-inferior margin may not survive as its primary blood supply is left behind. Frequently, only a portion of the muscle is required. If the anterior half of the muscle is used and the motor nerve is left in place, the remaining portion of muscle will continue to function. A large skin flap may be taken as there are many reliable perforators. Nevertheless, when the chest wall is skin grafted, it is cosmetically very unsatisfactory. Therefore, when used as a myocutaneous transfer, the skin flap is usually limited to a maximum width of 10 cm which allows direct closure of the donor site. When the latissimus dorsi is used to cover large skin defects, it is usually taken as a muscle only transfer with a skin graft applied directly to the muscle.

Although its most common application is coverage using the muscle alone, it has great reconstructive versatility. Since the dominant artery to the serratus anterior is a branch of the thoraco dorsal, preservation of this branch allows both the serratus anterior and the latissimus dorsi muscles to be taken on the common thoraco dorsal pedicle. If kept attached to the serratus anterior, a vascularized rib may be taken with this transfer.

Removal of the muscle is associated with minimal weakness which is rarely of functional significance. Nevertheless, persons who are active in skiing, tennis and throwing sports may notice a decrease in strength. If the serratus anterior is removed, winging of the scapula can be expected. Buncke's experience is that if the upper half of the serratus is preserved and only the lower half removed, winging of the scapula will not result.

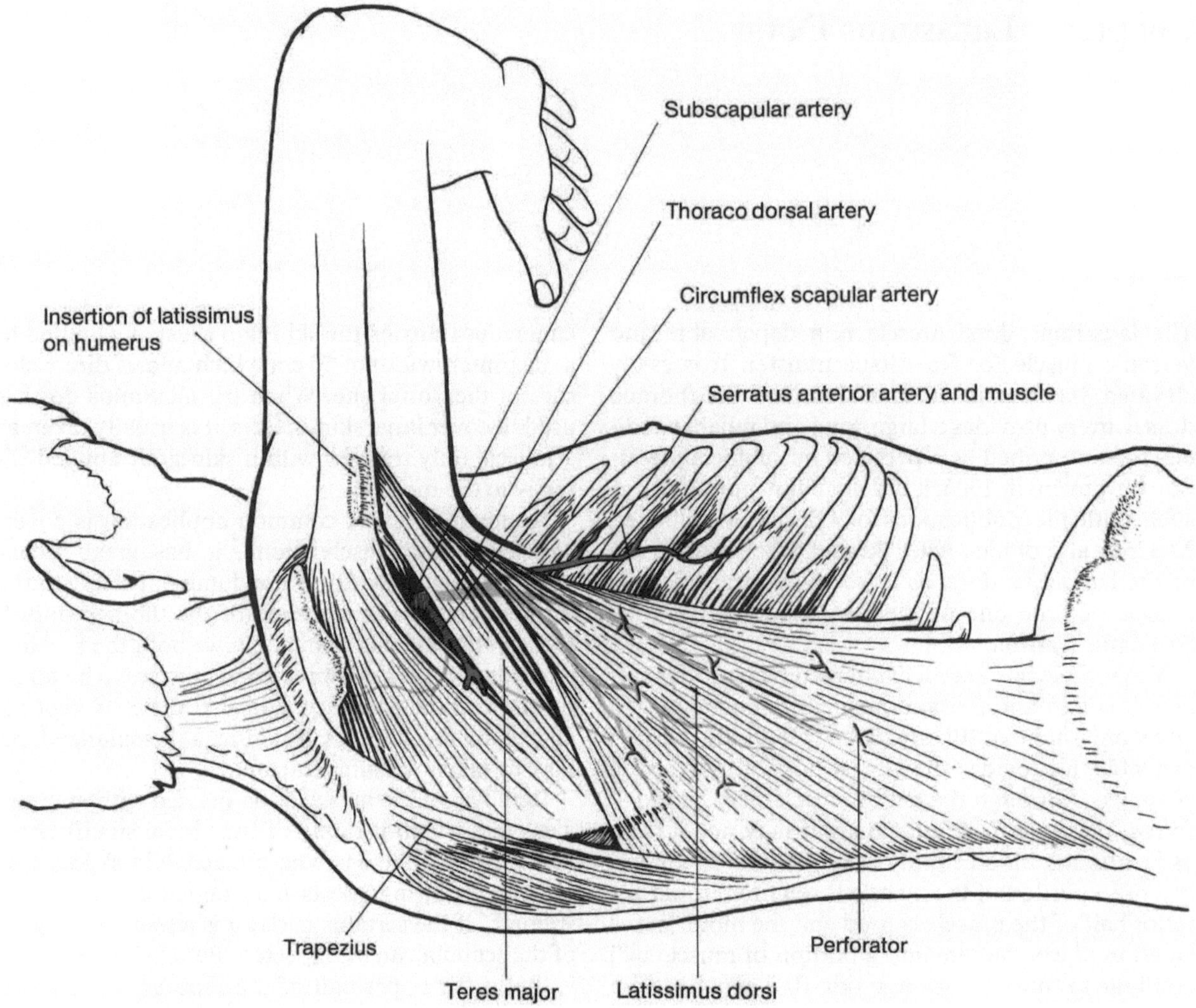

Fig. 7-1. The anatomical relationship of the latissimus dorsi and its vascular pedicle

Anatomy of the Latissimus Dorsi Transfer

This fan-shaped flat muscle takes origin through the thoraco lumbar fascia from the lower six thoracic and the lumbar vertebrae and from the posterior and lateral portion of the iliac crest and the anterior aspect of the lower three ribs (Fig. 7-1). With the teres major, it forms the posterior axillary fold, wrapping around this muscle and twisting 180° to insert into the medial lip of the bicipital groove on the humerus. The superior border of the muscle overlaps and attaches to the inferior angle of the scapula. The upper medial border of the muscle is covered by the inferior portion of the trapezius. The remainder of the muscle is subcutaneous. This is a strap muscle with long fibres extending the full length of the muscle.

The dominant vessel supplying the latissimus dorsi is the thoraco dorsal artery, a terminal branch of the subscapular. Shortly after its take off, the subscapular divides into two branches, the circumflex scapular artery and the thoraco dorsal artery. The circumflex scapular artery, the larger of the two, passes posteriorly around the lateral border of the scapula. The thoraco dorsal artery leads directly to the latissimus dorsi and follows a course along and under the anterior margin of the muscle, entering the muscle 2 cm posterior to the muscle border. Along the way, it supplies branches to the serratus anterior muscle and the chest wall. The serratus branch can supply the muscle if the thoraco dorsal artery is interrupted. This situation has occurred in many patients who have had radical mastectomy with loss of the thoraco dorsal artery in the axillary node dissec-

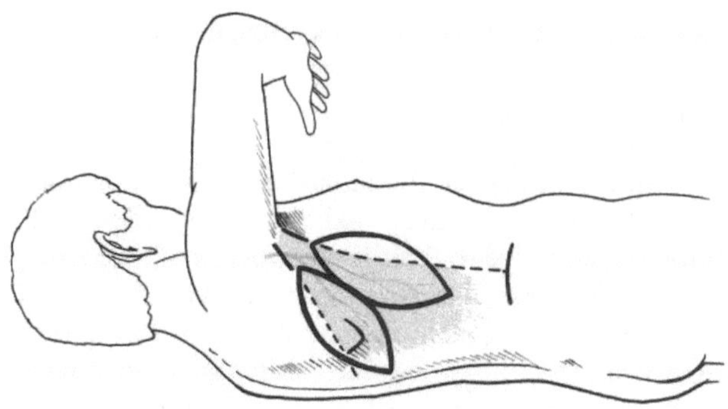

Fig. 7-2. The anterior margin of the muscle lies under a line drawn between the anterior aspect of the posterior axillary fold and the mid lateral point on the iliac crest. The superior margin of the muscle lies under a line between the posterior aspect of the posterior axillary fold and a point 4 cm above the inferior angle of the scapula

Cutaneous perforators are clustered over the two intramuscular branches of the thoracodorsal artery. These branches parallel the anterior and the superior border. If a small to medium cutaneous flap is required, it may be placed over either intramuscular vessel for maximum incorporation of perforators

tion. Fisher has reported that the muscle can be transferred based entirely on the serratus pedicle, and I have had this experience in one case. When the flap is based on the serratus pedicle, the direction of the arterial and venous flow is reversed.

The thoraco dorsal artery is 1.5-4.0 cm in diameter and is the primary supply of the lateral and superior two thirds of the muscle [1]. The primary supply of the medial and distal muscle is the perforating branches of the segmental intercostal arteries. The surgeon should be prepared for peculiarities in the origin of the thoraco dorsal artery. Either a separate origin from the axillary or an origin from a common trunk with other branches of the axillary artery may occur. There are two venae comitantes with the thoraco dorsal artery which join to form a single large thoraco dorsal vein (3-5 mm) prior to entering the subscapular vein. The subscapular artery and vein usually run together, although, on occasion, the artery may separate from the vein and take origin higher in the axilla than the vein.

The neurovascular hilum is 8-9 cm from the axillary artery and enters the deep surface of the muscle 1.5-3.0 cm from the anterior border. The muscle is innervated by the thoraco dorsal nerve, a branch of the posterior cord. The nerve passes behind the axillary artery and quickly joins the vascular pedicle and enters the muscle with the artery. The vessels and nerve usually bifurcate and then run together on the deep surface of the muscle. One branch runs parallel behind the anterior border of the muscle and the second parallel and below the superior border of the muscle. Tobin found a bifurcating neurovascular pedicle in 94.5% of 110 cadaver dissections and Bartlett found this bifurcation in 86% of 50 cadaver dissections. This bifurcation provides the anatomic basis for separating the latissimus muscle into two separately functioning neuromuscular units. Each of these two units can be transferred in the same reconstruction, or only one unit can be transferred, leaving the remaining muscle to provide its normal function.

Skin flaps may be outlined anywhere on the muscle and will survive well. However, the greatest concentration of perforators lies over the two intra muscular branches of the thoraco dorsal artery which run parallel to the anterior and superior margins of the muscle (Fig. 7-2). An additional concentration of perforating vessels lies parallel to the spine along the medial margin of the muscle. These branches of the posterior intercostal arteries supply cutaneous flaps which are based upon the medial segments of latissimus muscle. The particularly generous supply of perforators along the anterior muscle margin allows a large skin flap to be raised on a narrow strip of anterior muscle margin. This strip may be as narrow as 3-4 cm as long as it includes the anterior branch of the thoraco dorsal artery. It will support a skin flap which extends at least 4-6 cm on either side of the muscle.

Elevating the Latissimus Dorsi Muscle Transfer

Surgical Technique

1. With the patient in the lateral decubitus position (Fig. 7-3 a), prep the chest, axilla and shoulder, and drape the arm free to facilitate exposure of the pedicle. Care must be taken that there is neither excessive nor prolonged abduction of the shoulder during the dissection. It is also possible, although more awkward, to raise the flap with the patient turned onto his/her back, abdomen or any position in between.

2. Draw a line from the posterior axillary fold to the midline of the iliac crest. This marks the anterior margin of the muscle which lies further anteriorly than is usually appreciated. With the arm abducted, the neurovascular hilus is 10 cm from the axillary artery along this line. Draw the superior muscle margin as an oblique curving line from the humeral insertion to a point 4 cm above the inferior angle of the scapula.

3. If a cutaneous flap is required, it may be designed over any portion of the muscle (Fig. 7-2). However, the anterior margin is usually preferable. Using a pattern taken from the recipient tissue defect, which includes the location of the recipient vessels, outline a skin flap over the anterior portion of the muscle (Fig. 7-3 b). Pinch a large fold of skin at the flap site and determine the amount of skin which can be removed and still allow direct closure.

4. For pedicle dissection, a right handed surgeon will be better positioned facing the patient's back when removing the right latissimus.

Incise the skin flap in its proximal position and identify the anterior margin of the flap (Fig. 7-3 c). If you have misjudged the position of the anterior margin of the muscle, it can now be re-drawn and the skin flap outline repositioned as necessary. Incise the entire skin flap down to the latissimus musculature and lateral chest wall. If the flap is small or loosely attached to the muscle, tack it to the muscle with some sutures around the periphery to prevent shearing strains to the perforators.

5. Develop a plane between the lateral chest wall and the muscle, using sharp and blunt dissection. If this is begun 12 cm distal to the humeral origin, your plane of dissection will be distal to the vascular pedicle and hilum and proximal to the muscle's fusion with the serratus anterior. Do not look for the pedicle now. It will be easier to find and prepare at a later stage when the muscle is detached distally. Divide the muscle's attachment to the serratus anterior and the lower three ribs (Fig. 7-4).

6. Allowing for some muscle retraction, mark the maximum length of muscle required and divide the latissimus inferiorly and medially. Cauterize the large posterior perforators of the intercostal vessels before they retract.

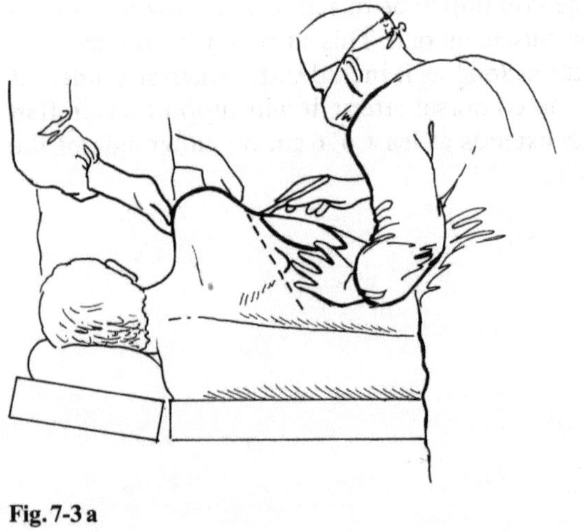

Fig. 7-3 a

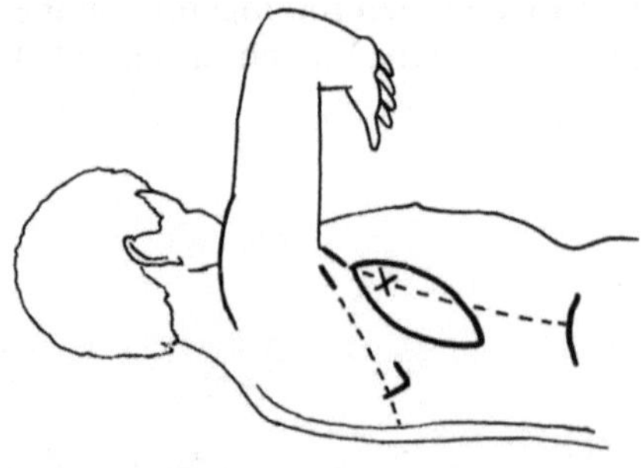

Fig. 7-3 b

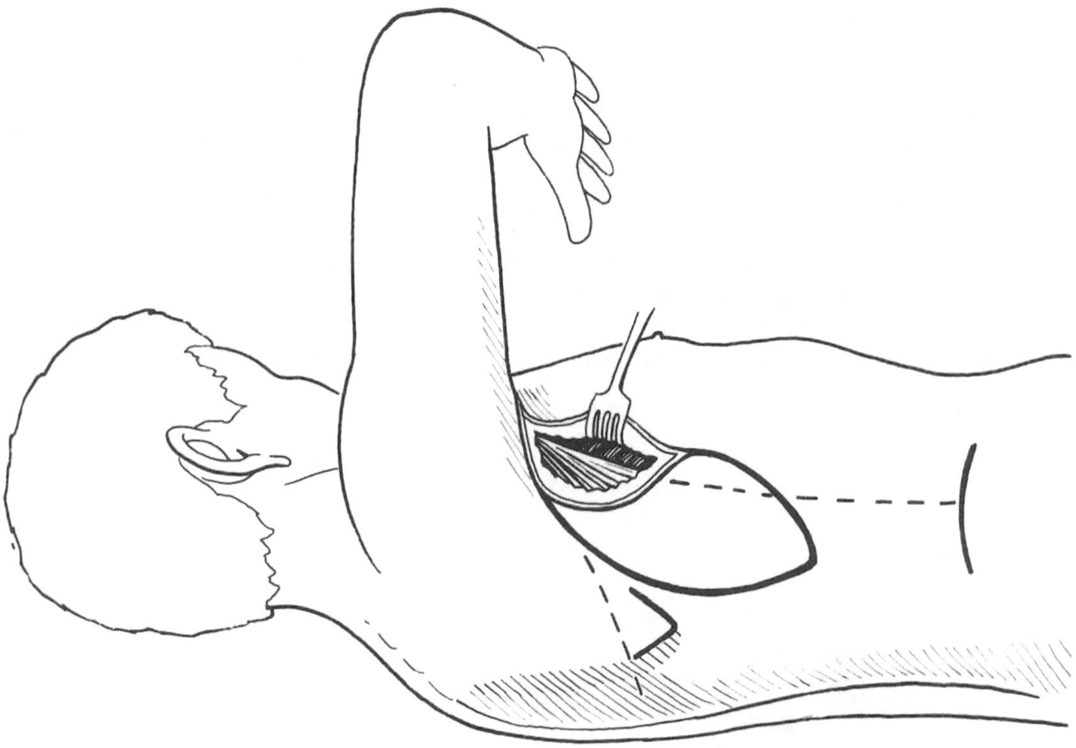

c

Fig. 7-3. **a** Convenient access to the muscle and its pedicle is provided by the lateral decubitus position with the arm draped free. **b** The cutaneous flap is marked parallel to and overlapping the anterior margin of the muscle. The pedicle enters at 'x'. The perspective for this and subsequent drawings is that of the surgeon who is looking down on the patient, as shown in Figure 3a. **c** An incision over the proximal part of the skin flap allows confirmation of the exact location of the muscle's anterior margin

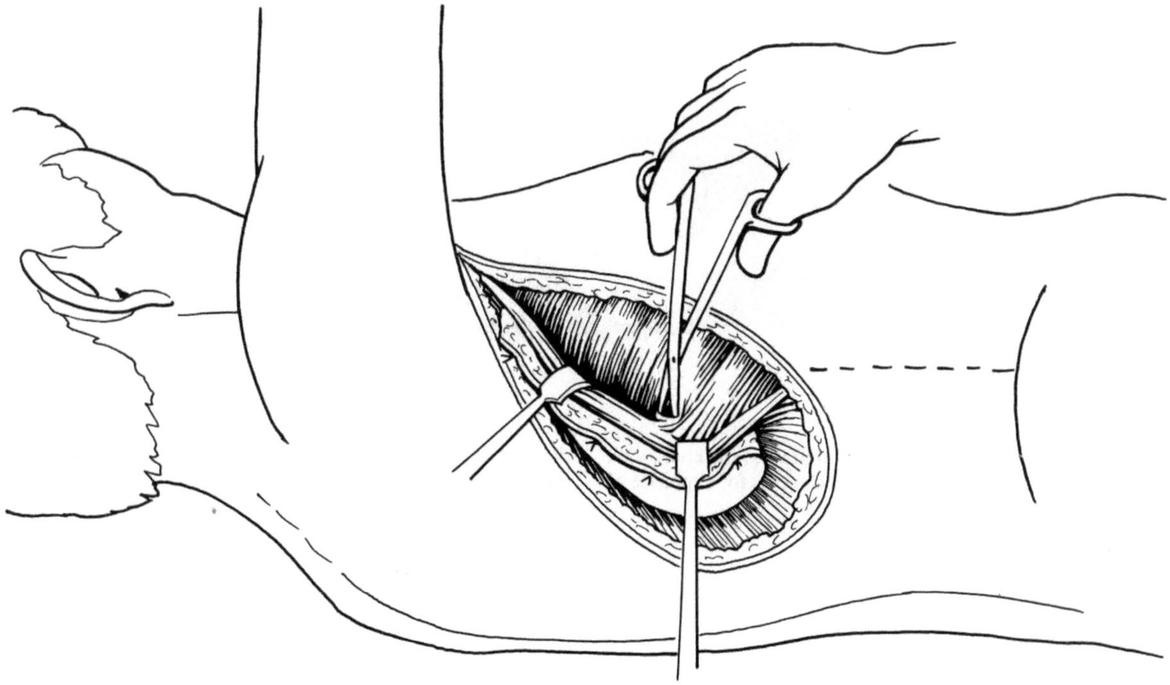

Fig. 7-4. Division of the attachments of the latissimus dorsi to the serratus anterior at the lower portion of the anterior muscle margin

7. Lift the flap towards the head to expose the pedicle (Fig. 7-5 a). Palpate the neurovascular pedicle where it enters the muscle, surrounded by fatty connective tissue. Follow the pedicle, dissecting proximally towards the axillary artery and vein. Leave the fatty tissue around the pedicle for support. The long thoracic nerve to serratus anterior is not usually exposed. However, be aware of its location just anterior to the thoraco dorsal pedicle on the chest wall. Identify and divide the arterial and venous branches to the serratus anterior and chest wall.

The size and distance of the recipient vessels from the defect determine the length of pedicle required and the necessity of including the large subscapular artery and vein in the pedicle.

8. Unless the tendon of insertion and the bulky muscle entering the tendon are required in the transfer, divide the muscle just above the neurovascular hilum.

After complete separation of the muscle except for the vascular pedicle, leave the muscle in situ without tension and observe the adequacy of perfusion of the entire muscle and cutaneous flap.

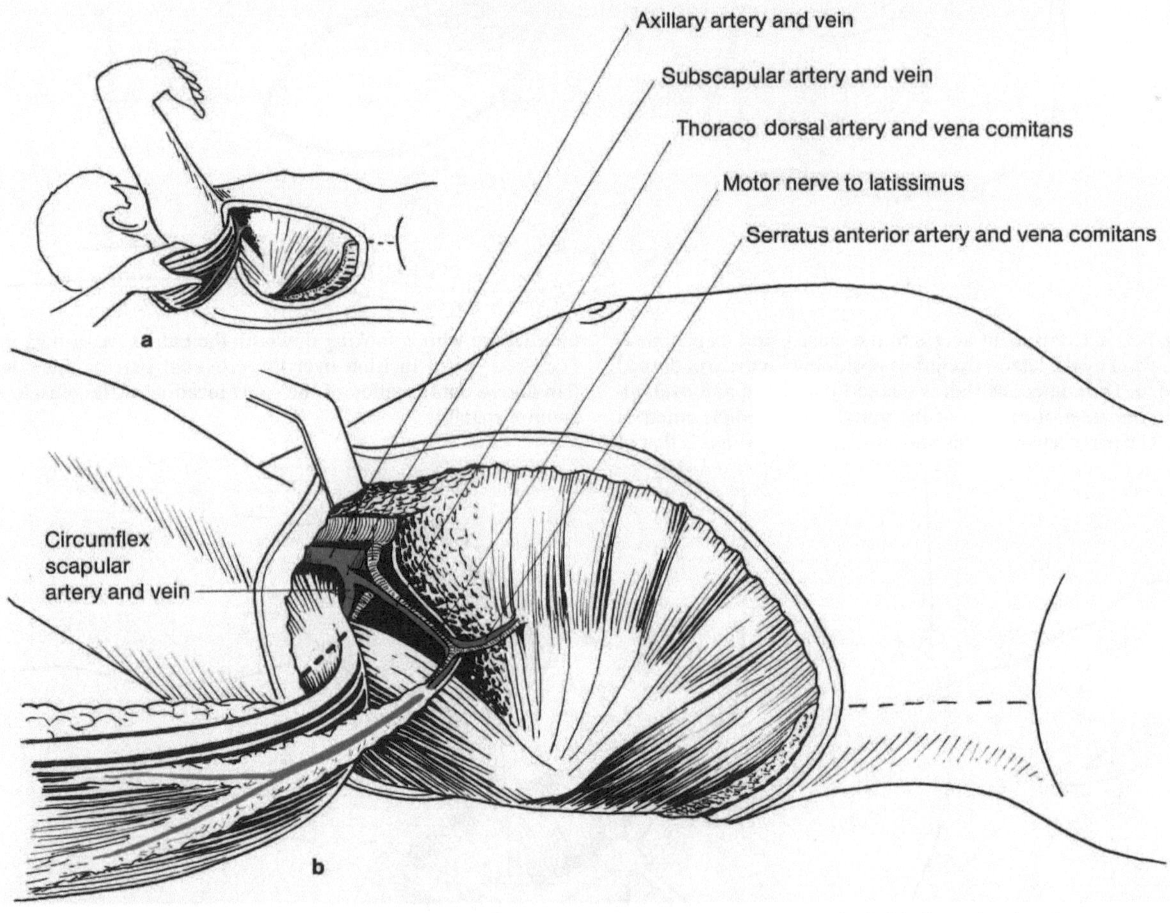

Fig. 7-5 a, b. After the muscle is separated from the chest wall, it can be lifted cranially to provide good access for exposure of the pedicle. The muscle is divided proximal to the neurovascular hilus (dotted line)

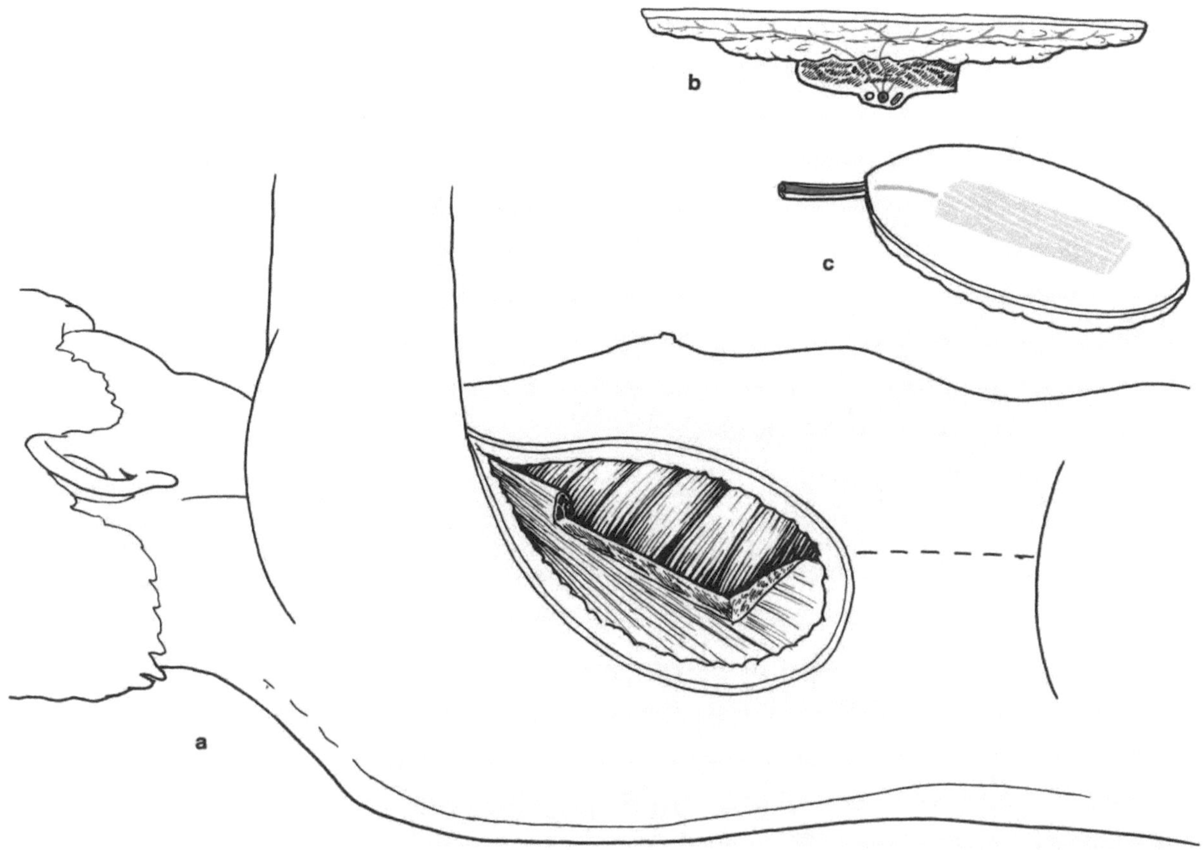

Fig. 7-6 a-c. The concentration of myocutaneous perforators along the anterior margin of the muscle allows a large cutaneous flap to be based on a small strip of anterior margin of the muscle. To further minimize the bulk, the skin flap is raised with only the superficial layer of subcutaneous fat at the margins (**b**)

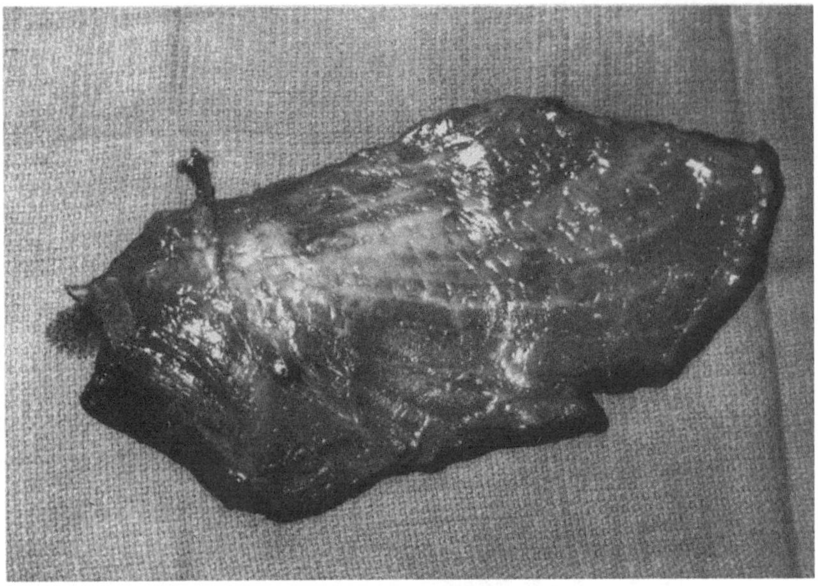

Fig. 7-7. Deep surface of the latissimus dorsi muscle after elevation and separation from the patient. Pedicle is seen in upper left

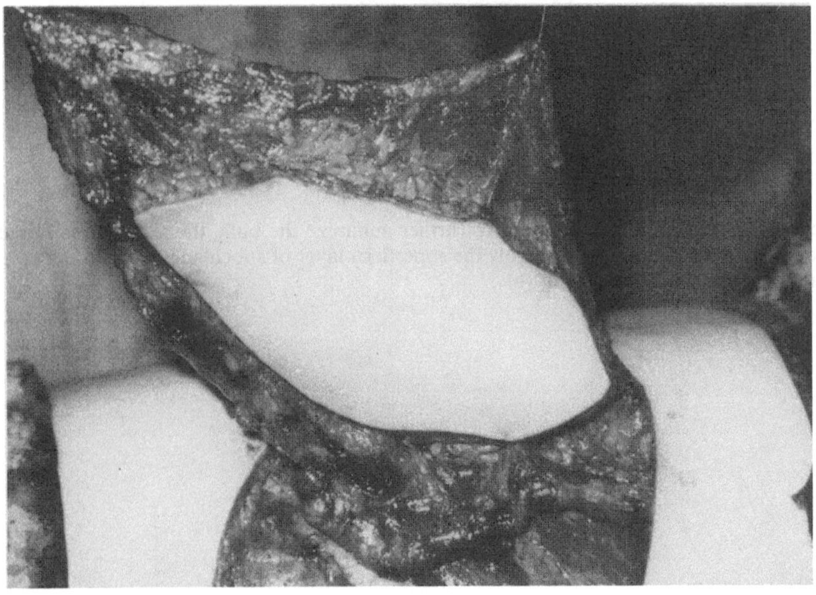

Fig. 7-8. Myocutaneous latissimus dorsi with cutaneous paddle sutured to muscle surface. Muscle's origin and pedicle are still attached in the axilla

References

1. Bartlett SP, May JW, Yaremchuk JM (1981) The latissimus dorsi muscle: a fresh cadaverous study of the primary neurovascular pedicle. Plast Reconstr Surg 67: 631
2. Baudet J, Guimberteau J, Nascimento E (1976) Successful clinical transfer of two free thoraco dorsal axillary flaps. Plast Reconstr Surg 58: 680-688
3. Fisher J, Bostwick J, Powell RW (1983) Latissimus dorsi blood supply after thoraco dorsal vessel division: the serratus collateral. Plast Reconstr Surg 72: 502
4. Mahoney J Personal communication
5. McCraw JB, Penix JO, Baker JW (1978) Repair of major defects of the chest wall and spine with the latissimus dorsi myocutaneous flap. Plast Reconstr Surg 60: 341
6. Muhlbauer W, Olbrisch R (1977) The latissimus dorsi myocutaneous flap for breast reconstruction. Chir Plast. 4: 27
7. Olivari N (1976) The latissimus flap. Br J Plast Surg 29: 126
8. Tanzini I (1906) Sepra il mio nuovo processo di amputazione della mammaella. Reforma Medica 12: 757
9. Tobin GR, Shusterman M, Peterson GH, Nichols G, Bland KI (1981) The intramuscular neurovascular anatomy of the latissimus dorsi muscle: the basis for splitting the flap. Plast Reconstr Surg 67: 637

Chapter 8. Rectus Abdominis

In reconstructive flap surgery, there is considerable interest in the epigastric artery axis. This axis, supplied above by the superior epigastric artery and below by the deep inferior epigastric artery (DIEA), supplies the rectus abdominis muscle and a huge area of abdominal skin. Its value for pedicled flaps based on the superior vessel was particularly appreciated by Brown, Mathes and McCraw. Its most common application on the superior vessel is for breast reconstruction as a myocutaneous flap. Usually the skin flap is taken from the lower abdomen, in the abdominoplasty region [4, 5, 7, 9]. The ability of the superior epigastric artery to carry all of the ipsilateral lower abdominal skin and at least half of the contralateral skin has amazed reconstructive surgeons. However, increasing experience has shown that, when using the superior epigastric artery, the higher the skin flap is based on the rectus musculature the more reliable is its perfusion. Since the DIEA is twice the diameter of the superior epigastric artery and is the dominant blood supply to the rectus abdominis muscle, the DIEA is the preferred pedicle for free tissue transfer [3, 8].

The application of this muscle and its cutaneous territories as a free tissue transfer is just beginning to be appreciated. The muscle is useful for coverage alone or can be taken with a variety of attached skin paddles. The size of the muscle places its coverage ability between that of the gracilis and the latissimus dorsi. It is particularly useful for long narrow defects.

The only recognized complication of removing this muscle is abdominal herniation if the anterior rectus sheath is removed and not adequately repaired below the arcuate line. The long term effect of removing the rectus abdominis muscle is unknown. It is possible that some patients may eventually develop attenuation of the sheath and bulging of the abdominal wall. However, removal of this muscle has not created a functional problem for even the very physically active person.

Anatomy of the Rectus Abdominis Transfer

The rectus abdominis muscle is a long, strap like muscle divided transversely by three tendinous intersections, fibrous bands which are adherent to the anterior rectus sheath. The muscle arises from the symphysis pubis and crest of the pubis and inserts into the cartilages of the 5th, 6th and 7th ribs (Fig. 8-1). With contraction, it compresses and supports the abdominal viscera and flexes the spine. The muscle is enclosed in a strong fascial sheath which is formed in its central portion by the aponeurosis of the internal oblique, which divides into two lamellii. One of these passes behind the rectus, blending with the aponeurosis of the transversus, and the other passes in front of the rectus, blending with the aponeurosis of the external oblique. These fascial layers, the anterior and posterior rectus sheaths, fuse together along the midline to form the linea alba. The anterior rectus sheath is present over the entire length of the muscle. However, the posterior rectus sheath ends with the formation of the arcuate line at the level of the anterior superior iliac spines. Inferior to this line, the aponeuroses of the transversus abdominis and internal oblique lie anterior to the rectus abdominis muscle. Below the arcuate line, this muscle lies in direct contact with the transversalis fascia and parietal peritoneum. The innervation of the rectus is through segmental branches of the 7th to 12th intercostal nerves, which enter the lateral margin of the rectus sheath. The muscle is 7-10 cm in width and up to 30 cm in length. It is thin and flat, providing good soft tissue coverage for long defects such as large anterior tibial defects. Short segments of the muscle may be taken for smaller defects.

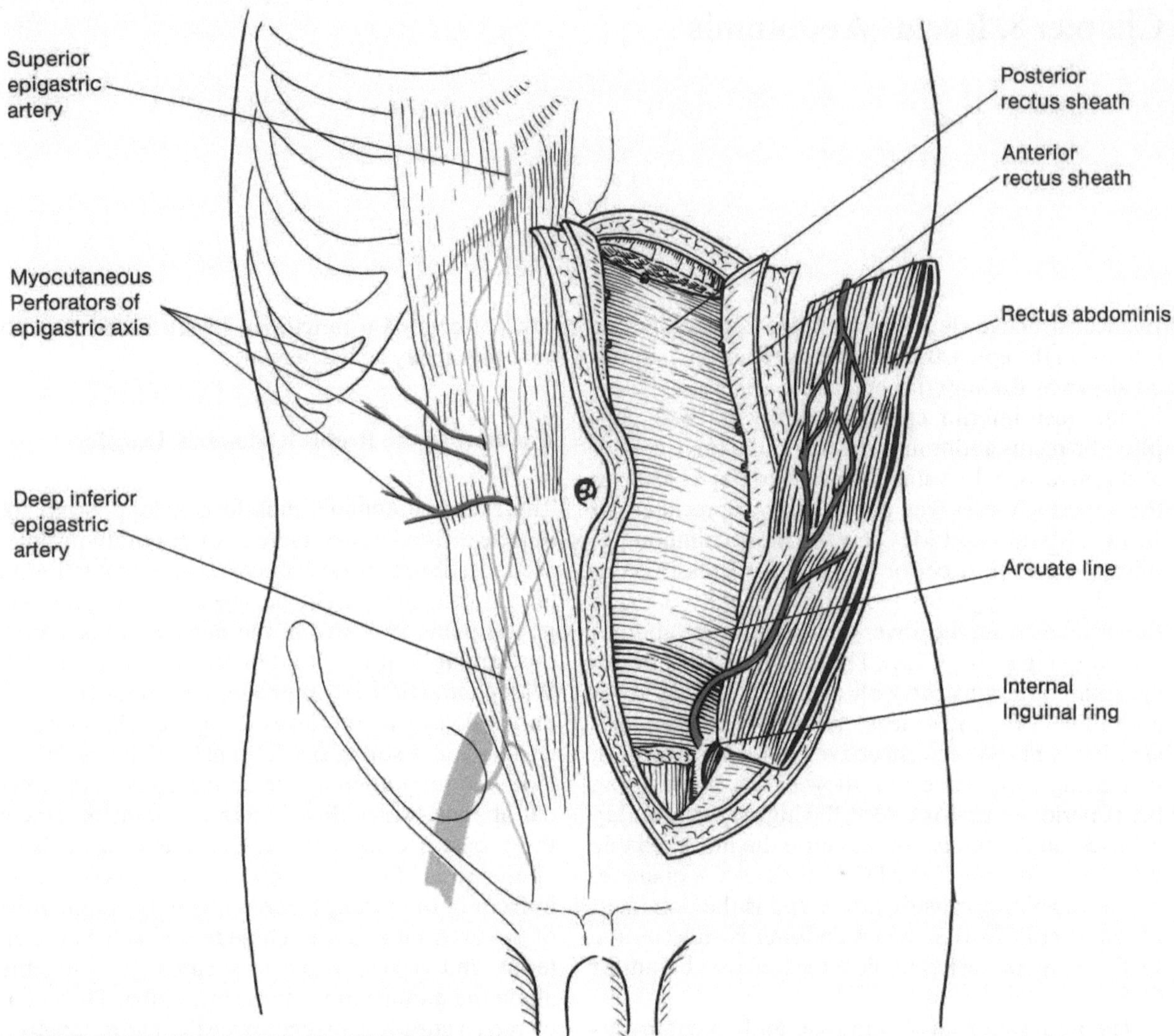

Fig. 8-1. The anatomy of the rectus abdominis muscle

Vascular Anatomy

The vascular anatomy has been thoroughly studied by Boyd. The average diameter of the deep inferior epigastric artery is 3.4 mm at its origin, twice the size of the superior epigastric artery. The DIEA originates from the medial aspect of the external iliac artery, opposite and proximal to the origin of the deep circumflex iliac artery, and ascends obliquely towards the rectus abdominis. It lies in an extra peritoneal position, deep to the transversalis fascia, along the medial margin of the deep inguinal ring. On occasion, the DIEA will arise from the femoral artery just below the inguinal ligament or as a common trunk with a distally located obturator artery. Ascending under the rectus abdominis musculature, it enters the rectus sheath at the arcuate line and lies on the deep surface or within the rectus abdominis muscle. It ascends to a point halfway between the umbilicus and the xyphi sternum to terminate in an arborization with the superior epigastric vessels (Fig. 8-1). Two branches are given off prior to entering the rectus abdominis musculature. These are the pubic branch and a muscular branch to the lower rectus. Frequently, the artery divides into 2-3 branches as it passes cephalad on the posterior aspect of the rectus muscle. The venous drainage of this flap occurs through the DIEA venae comitantes which drain into the external iliac vein. This system is constant and of an adequate size for anastomoses. If there are two veins, the average diameter is 2.5 mm, and if only one, the average diameter at the iliac vein is 4.4 mm.

The dominant blood supply of the anterior ab-

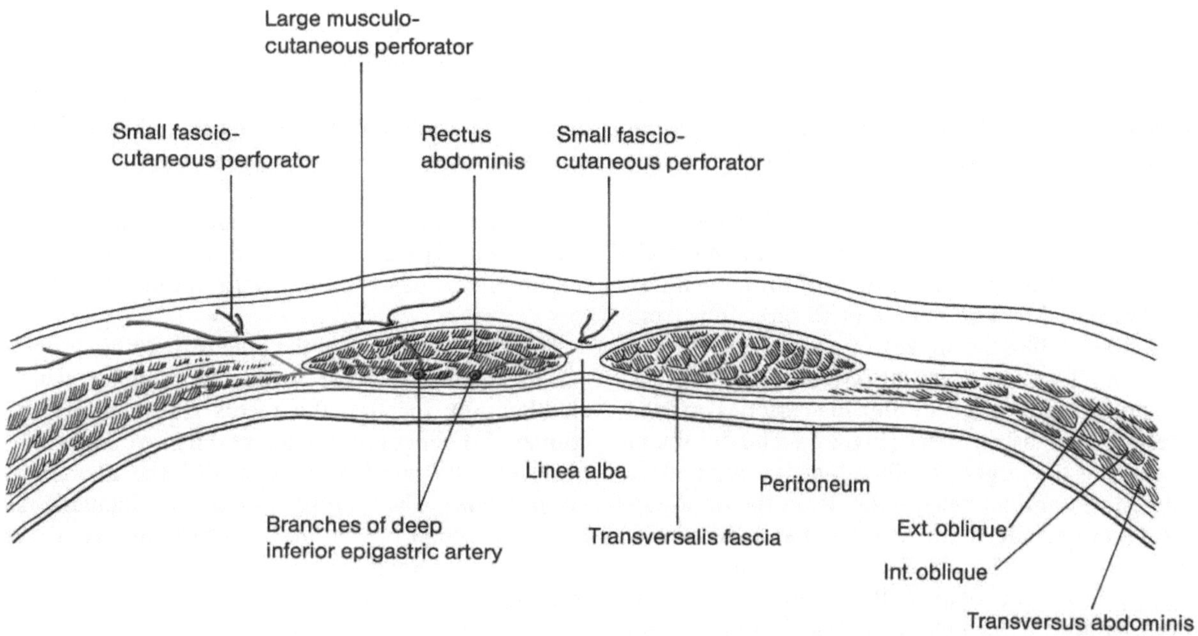

Fig. 8-2. Cross section of middle portion of the anterior abdominal wall showing the location of two subdivisions of the DIEA and their branches. The small fasciocutaneous perforators in the linea alba and linea semilunaris are not important in the construction of skin flaps. However, the large centrally placed para-umbilical musculocutaneous perforators provide a rich vascular supply to the overlying and adjacent skin

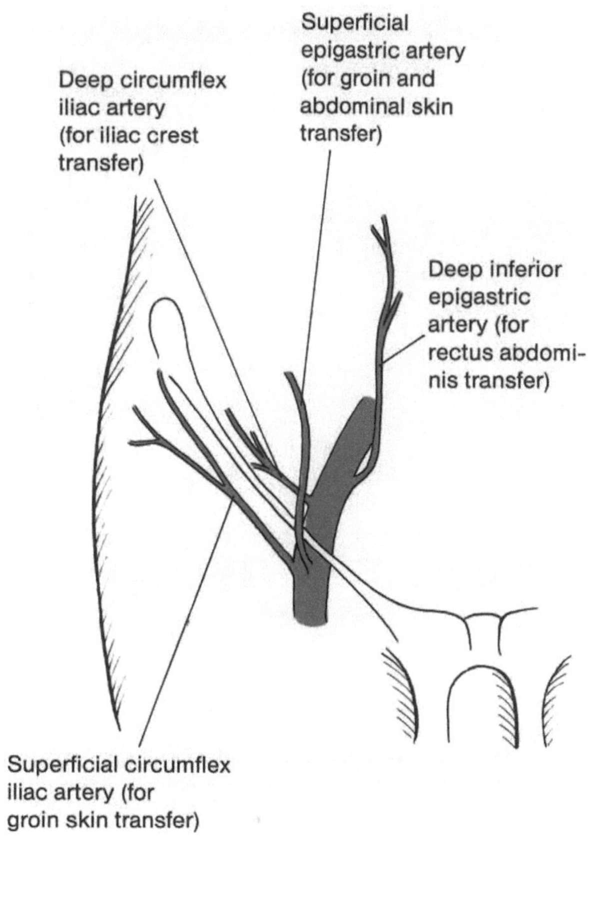

Fig. 8-3. The relationships of the four groin arteries which are used in free tissue transfers

dominal skin flows through musculocutaneous perforators of the epigastric artery axis (Fig. 8-2). The cadaver injection studies of Boyd, Taylor and Corlett have identified a para-umbilical concentration of musculocutaneous perforators (Fig. 8-4). This concentration explains the improved skin perfusion when the flap is placed in a para-umbilical location. After passing through the rectus sheath, these vessels lie on and within the deep surface of the subcutaneous abdominal fat and radiate in all directions from the umbilicus like the spokes of a wheel. They connect with all adjacent arterial systems, including the deep and superficial circumflex iliac arteries and the superficial epigastric artery (Fig. 8-5). The dominant direction of the large musculocutaneous perforators is superiorly and laterally at 45° from the para-umbilical area, parallel to the segmental abdominal vessels and nerves. The presence and course of these large perforators prompted Pennington and Taylor to design an oblique cutaneous flap from the para-umbilical area. The axis of the cutaneous paddle ascends from the umbilicus at a 45° angle to the midline and is based on a piece of the underlying abdominal musculature. However, their ink stain injection studies suggest that the entire anterior abdominal skin could be raised on the perforating branches of the rectus abdominis muscle and a cutaneous flap could be designed to radiate in any direction from the umbilicus based on the para-umbilical perforators.

The other branches of the epigastric artery are relatively small. There are segmental branches which exit laterally through the rectus sheath along the course of the incoming segmental nerves. They connect with the terminal branches of the intercostal arteries and also supply small fasciocutaneous branches which pierce the linea semilunaris. There are also fasciocutaneous branches which exit through the linea alba.

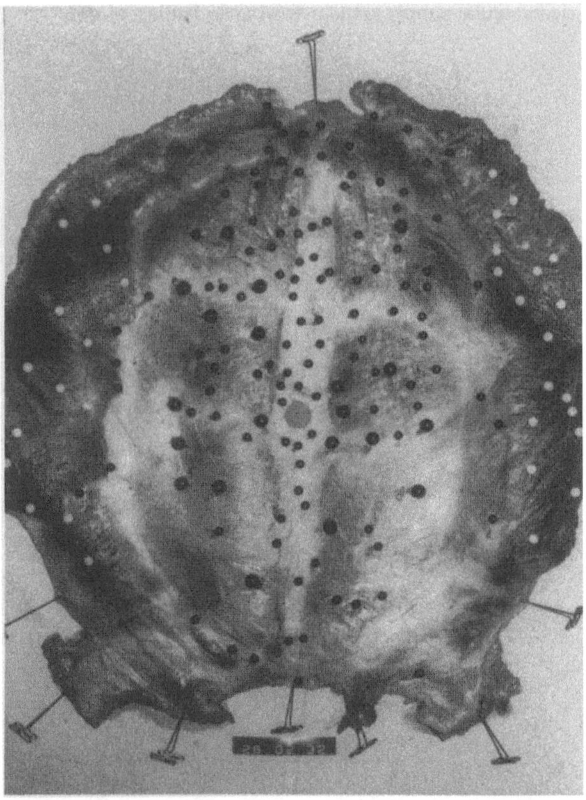

Fig. 8-4. Entire anterior abdominal wall with fat removed. Perforators larger than 0.5 mm are marked with a large light or dark circle. Smaller perforators are marked with small circles. Note the para-umbilical concentration of large perforators in the third of the rectus abdominis musculature (from Boyd JB, Taylor GI, Corlett R)

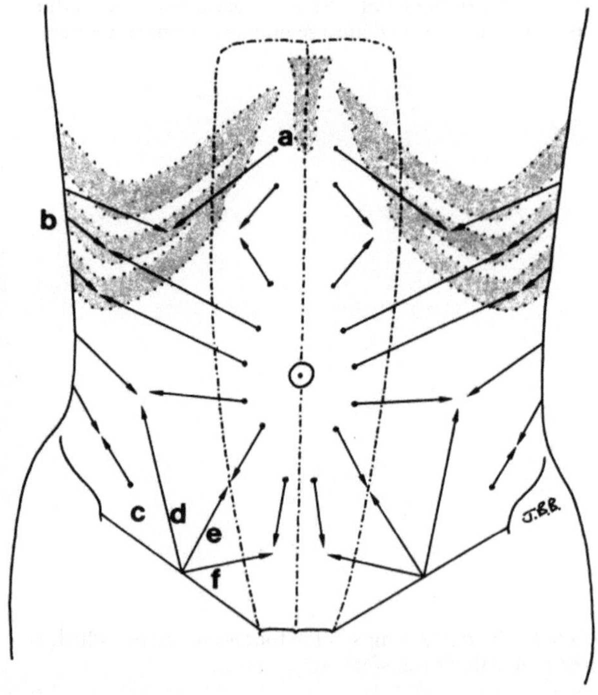

Fig. 8-5. Arrows radiating from the umbilicus indicate the direction of arterial flow within the abdominal skin and subcutaneous tissue from the large musculocutaneous perforators as revealed by cadavre injection studies. The para-umbilical perforators communicate with *a* the superior epigastric artery; *b* cutaneous branches of the lateral intercostal arteries; *c* perforators of the deep circumflex iliac artery; *d* superficial circumflex iliac artery; *e* superficial inferior epigastric artery; *f* the external pudental artery. (from Boyd JB, Taylor GI, Corlett R)

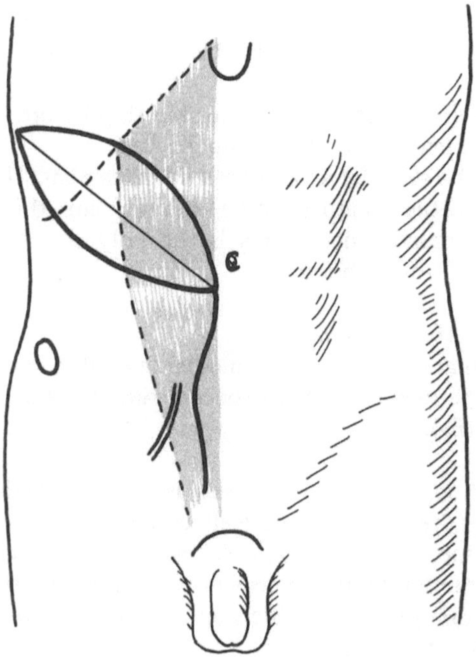

a

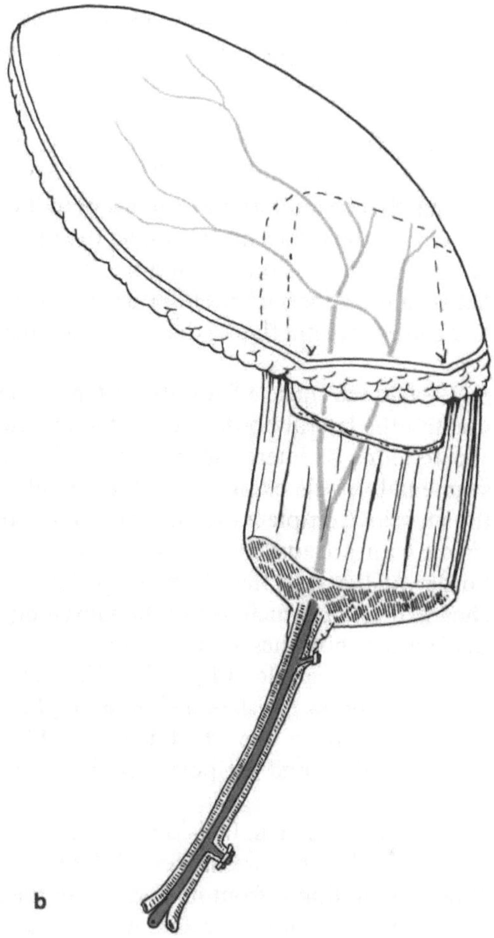

b

Fig. 8-6. a Preoperative markings for the para-umbilical rectus abdominis myocutaneous transfer. To incorporate the large obliquely placed para-umbilical perforators, the flap is outlined on an axis which lies at 45° to the midline and passes 3 cm below the umbilicus. **b** Rectus abdominis myocutaneous transfer. The minimum amount of muscle and fascia which must be taken to ensure reliable skin flap transfer is the portion of rectus abdominis musculature and anterior rectus sheath which lies deep to the skin flap

Elevation of the Rectus Abdominis Transfer

If there has been previous surgery in the groin, particularly a hernia repair, an angiogram may be necessary to ensure that the DIEA is patent. Abdominal scars which traverse the intended flap will prevent its use.

Surgical Technique

A. Myocutaneous Transfer

1. Note the location of the xyphi sternum, pubis, ASIS and costal margin. Mark the expected location of the rectus abdominis muscle and the site of entrance of the DIEA into the sheath (Fig. 8-6 a). The artery enters halfway between the umbilicus and the pubis on the lateral margin of the muscle. The lateral border can usually be palpated where it lies halfway between the midline and the anterior superior iliac spine. Be wary of the patient with a diastasis of the rectus, which will displace the muscle further laterally than normal.

2. To obtain a long pedicle and a maximum vascular supply from the perforators, outline the cutaneous flap on an axis which passes upwards and laterally at 45° from the umbilicus. According to Taylor, it can be taken as far as the mid axillary line to place at least one third of the flap over the lower chest wall. Using a pattern from the defect, place the flap along this line, beginning at the umbilicus. The maximum width of the flap is determined by the laxity of the skin, as the donor site is closed directly. Be sure that a generous portion of the medial aspect of the flap overlies the rectus in the region of the para-umbilical perforators.

3. Incise the flap to the fascia and elevate the skin flap from lateral to medial. Preserve the areolar layer on the under surface of the subcutaneous fat up to the linea semilunaris which marks the lateral border of the rectus muscle. Be cautious at this point. If the lateral rectus border is missed, you will pass on to the sheath and into the perforators.

4. Incise the rectus sheath transversely, parallel to the upper margin of the skin flap, and carry the rectus sheath incision inferiorly adjacent to the linea alba. Divide the rectus muscle along the upper border of the sheath incision, ligating the interconnections between the superior and inferior epigastric vessels, and suture the skin flap to the fascia and muscles.

5. Elevate the muscle from its posterior sheath and identify the lateral border. Incise the anterior rectus sheath along its lateral border and divide the many segmental vessels exiting from the lateral border of the muscle. Complete the anterior rectus sheath excision with a transverse incision along the inferior border of the skin flap. A piece of anterior rectus sheath, through which passes the musculocutaneous perforators, now lies between the muscle and the isolated skin paddle (Fig. 8-6b). This lower transverse incision in the sheath should be placed above the arcuate line, a line which is not visible until the muscle is lifted and the posterior sheath visualized.

6. Use a para median incision over and through the rectus sheath to expose the rest of the rectus muscle. When separating it from its bed, ligate the multiple medial and lateral perforators which pass from the muscle to the sheath. Lift the muscle from its sheath and note the DIEA on the deep surface passing laterally to exit from the sheath just below the arcuate line. To obtain the maximum pedicle length, carry the pedicle dissection extraperitoneally to the external iliac artery.

7. Divide the rectus muscle below the point at which the DIEA exits from the sheath. To decrease the bulk of the transfer, remove all the rectus muscle up to the point at which the DIEA begins to arborize.

8. Observe the perfusion of the skin flap before ligating the pedicle and removing the flap.

Close the skin defect by direct advancement. The anterior rectus sheath must be carefully closed below the arcuate line as this is the only structure which will prevent herniation.

B. Rectus Muscle Alone

1. Flap marking - Mark the medial and lateral borders of the rectus and the expected site of entrance of the DIEA.

2. Use a longitudinal median skin incision down the middle of the rectus sheath. Reflect the sheath laterally and medially off the muscle, using sharp dissectors for the tendinous intersections. A Pfannenstiel or abdominoplasty type incision can be used for a more easily hidden scar.

3. When the desired length of muscle has been exposed, divide the upper end. Separate it from its sheath beginning at the upper end. Identify and divide segmental branches exiting from the muscle. Note the DIEA in the lower portion of the posterior surface of the muscle.

4. Below the arcuate line, separate the muscle carefully from the transversalis fascia. Do not enter the peritoneum.

5. Divide the muscle transversely at its origin. The inferior epigastric artery can easily be followed in its extraperitoneal position to the external iliac artery. Observe the perfusion of the muscle before ligating the artery and vena comitans (Fig. 8-1 a).

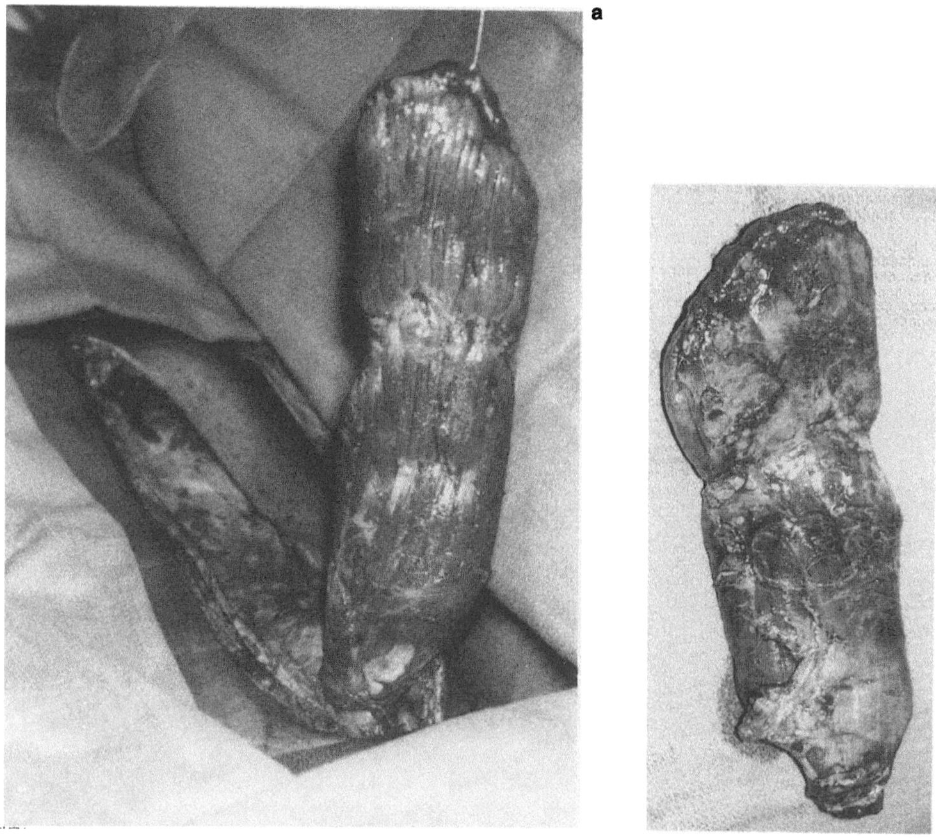

Fig. 8-7. **a** Rectus abdominis muscle, attached by its pedicle and elevated above its bed. **b** Deep surface of rectus abdominis muscle. Vascular pedicle is seen in upper left

References

1. Boyd JB, Taylor GI, Corlett R (1984) The vascular territories of the superior epigastric and the deep inferior epigastric systems. Plast Reconstr Surg 73: 1
2. Brown RG, Vasconez LO, Jurkiewicz MJ (1975) Transverse abdominal flaps and the deep epigastric arcade. Plast Reconstr Surg 55: 416
3. Bunkis J, Walton RL, Mathes SJ (1983) The rectus abdominis free flap for lower extremity reconstruction. Ann Plast Surg 11: 373
4. Drever, JM (1981) Total breast reconstruction. Ann Plast Surg 7: 54
5. Hartrampf CR, Scheflin M, Black KW (1982) Breast reconstruction with a transverse abdominal island flap. Plast Reconstr Surg 69: 216
6. Mathes SJ, Bostwick J III. (1977) A rectus abdominis myocutaneous flap to reconstruct abdominal wall defect. Br J Plast Surg 30: 282
7. McCraw JB, Dibbell DJ, Carraway JH (1977) Clinical definition of independent myocutaneous vascular territories. Plast Reconstr Surg 60: 341
8. Pennington DG, Lai MF, Pelly AD (1980) The rectus abdominis myocutaneous free flap. Br J Plast Surg 33: 277
9. Robbins TH (1979) Rectus abdominis myocutaneous flap for breast reconstruction. Aust NZ J Surg 49: 527
10. Taylor GI, Corlett R, Boyd JB (1983) The extended deep inferior epigastric flap: a clinical technique. Plast Reconstr Surg 72: 751

Bone Transfers

A vascularized bone graft is a transfer of a bone or portion of a bone in which the circulation is maintained by microvascular anastomoses. As the endosteal and periosteal circulation is maintained, the bone remains alive after its transfer and responds to biological stresses like a normal bone. The mechanism of healing at the ends of the graft is similar to the healing which occurs at an osteotomy, with primary bone union occurring between the graft and recipient bone rather than the graft undergoing creeping substitution as occurs in non-vascularized bone grafts. The response of the graft to physical stress is similar to that of normal bones. In the extremity, weight bearing will result in bone hypertrophy.

Vascularized bone grafts are used when conventional grafting techniques are unlikely to succeed. Standard bone grafts are likely to be unsuccessful when the bone defect is extensive and when the bone graft bed is scarred, contaminated or radiated. The type of case which will benefit from a vascularized bone graft includes congenital conditions such as tibial pseudarthrosis, and large, long bone and mandibular defects following trauma and tumor resections.

The donor sites which I have chosen for inclusion in this book are the fibula, metatarsal and iliac crest. We have had experience with 97 vascularized bone grafts. Of these, 1 was a radius, 19 fibulae, 28 metatarsals and 49 iliac crests. There are, however, other donor sites which are useful, including the rib, lateral margin of the scapula, a portion of the humerus, and portions of the toe phalanges.

Chapter 9. Fibula

The fibula is the longest bone which may be transferred by microsurgical techniques. It provides a relatively straight piece of well-vascularized bone which readily fits into long bone defects. The pedicle, being large and reliable, is suitable for microvascular anastomoses. Although a skin flap can be taken with the bone transfer, it must be very narrow to allow direct closure of the defect. Skin grafting a wide defect produces a cosmetically undesirable result. An improved awareness of the anatomy of the cutaneous branches of the peroneal artery may result in more frequent use of this bone as an osteoseptocutaneous transfer.

The fibula was the first bone to be used successfully as a vascularized transfer. Taylor reported its use in 1975 for the repair of two large tibial defects. Since that time, the fibula has become the most commonly used bone for reconstruction of large long bone defects in the tibia, femur, humerus and radius. A vascularized fibula or iliac crest is indicated if a bony defect is too large for non vascularized bone grafting techniques to be successful. Although much thinner than the tibia or femur, when used for their reconstruction, the fibula will gradually hypertrophy in response to the stresses placed on it. For replacement of the radius and ulna, it is an excellent size match. In children, one of the most valuable applications of this transfer is the repair of congenital pseudarthrosis of the tibia.

Anatomy of the Fibula Bone Transfer

The fibula is the only expendable long straight bone in the body. It has a slender shaft with thick cortices. The shaft has four surfaces (anterior, posterior, medial and lateral), three borders (anterior, posterior and interosseous) and a prominent medial crest. These borders and surfaces vary in location at different levels in the bone.

Beginning 2 cm below the knee joint, the head of the fibula articulates with the tibia, and has attached to it the powerful biceps femoris and the lateral collateral ligament of the knee. Curving around the fibular neck and tightly adherent to it is the vulnerable peroneal nerve. In order to prevent injury to this nerve and maintain the integrity of the knee, approximately 8 cm of upper end of fibula is left attached to the leg. The lower part of the fibula forms the lateral malleolus, the lateral flange of the ankle mortise. At the lower end, approximately 8 cm is left to maintain the ankle mortise. As the adult fibula is up to 40 cm in length, approximately 24 cm is available for transfer.

Secondary centres of ossification are present in the head and lateral malleolus. These centres fuse at 18 and 20 years of age respectively. The upper end of the fibula has been used as a vascularized transfer in an attempt to preserve the live epiphyseal plate to maintain growth. The lateral inferior geniculate artery, a branch of the popliteal, has been used to maintain the circulation to the metaphysis. However, the branches from the anterior tibial artery may be the prime blood supply to the head of the fibula [4].

The anatomy of the muscles surrounding the fibula must be thoroughly understood by the surgeon (Fig. 9-1). On the anterior surface are the extensor digitorum longus, extensor hallucis longus and the peroneus tertius. Laterally are the peroneus longus and peroneus brevis. Applied to the posterior surface are the soleus proximally, the flexor hallucis longus centrally and the peroneus brevis distally. Medially to the crest of the fibula and posterior to the interosseous membrane is the tibialis posterior.

Vascular Anatomy

Fibular transfer depends upon the endosteal and periosteal blood supplies from the peroneal artery. The endosteal circulation is supplied through a nutrient artery, which usually enters the middle third of the fibula. McKee reports that 73% of the foramina are located in the upper half of the middle third [3]. Although the occasional bone has a second foramen, 4–6% of bones have no foramen. The nutrient

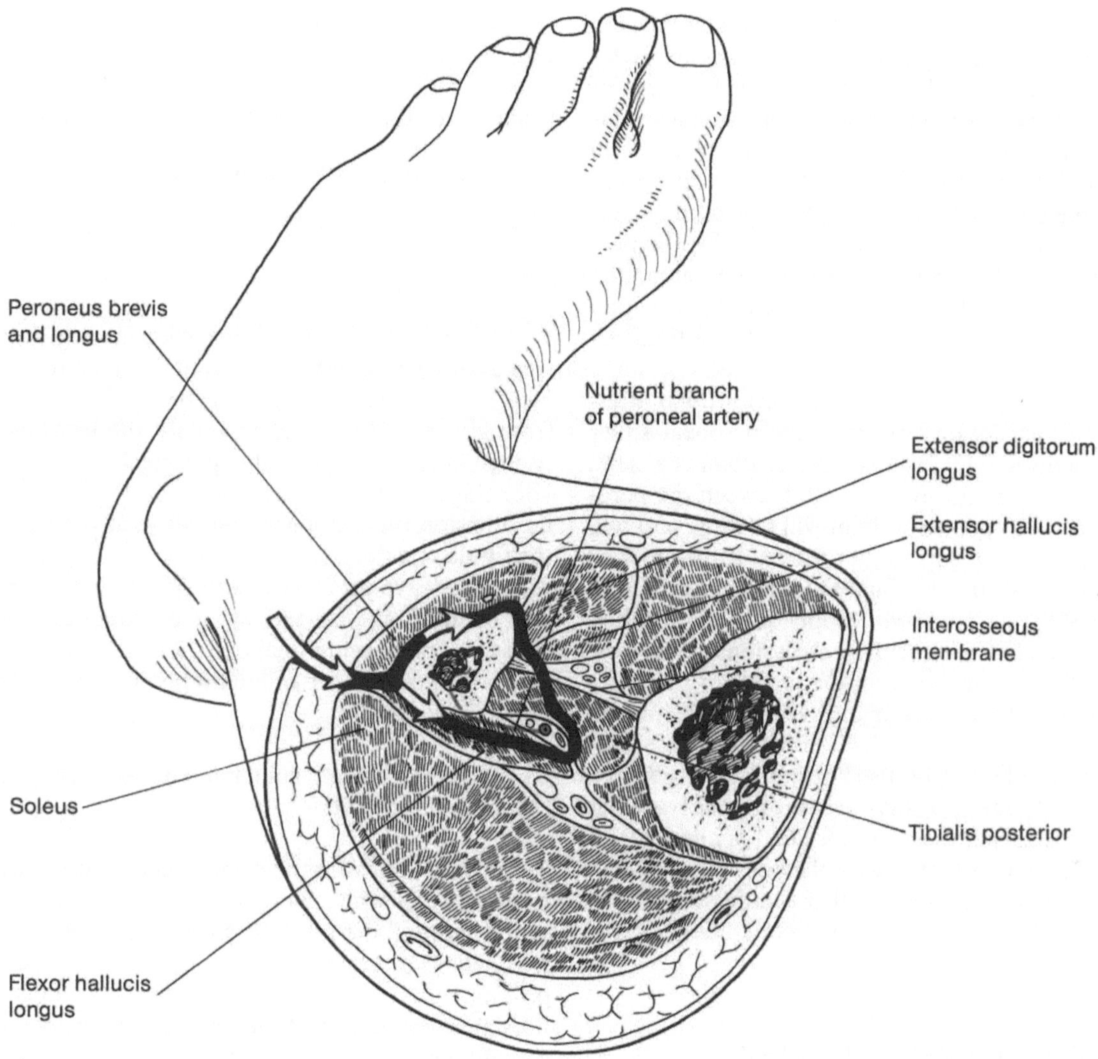

Fig. 9-1. Cross section of the mid calf. The arrows and heavy black line indicate the direction and plane of surgical dissection. The only muscle taken with the fibula is a portion of both the flexor hallucis longus and the tibialis posterior

artery enters the bone through a foramen located on the posterior or medial surface near the crest, and then divides into short ascending and long descending intramedullary branches [1].

The pedicle of the peroneal artery, although occasionally quite short, is usually at least 6 cm long, with a diameter of 1.8-3 mm. There are usually two venae comitantes. One of these is larger than the artery, measuring 3-4 mm in diameter. The peroneal artery is the largest branch of the posterior tibial, arising 2-4 cm below the origin of that vessel. It passes obliquely downwards and laterally across the posterior aspect of the tibialis posterior, and runs to the ankle in the fascia between the tibialis posterior and the flexor hallucis longus, just medial to the fibula. Occasionally, it runs within the muscle belly of the flexor hallucis longus. Along its course, it supplies periosteal, musculoperiosteal branches and a nutrient branch to the fibula. In order to preserve these branches, the musculature of the flexor hallucis longus and tibialis posterior, which lies between the artery and the bone, is taken with the transfer (Fig. 9-1).

In addition to the nutrient and periosteal vessels to the fibula, the peroneal artery gives off multiple branches to all of the surrounding muscles of the leg and to the lateral leg skin. There are 2-6 cutaneous perforating branches of the peroneal artery. They travel along the posterior crural septum and through the soleus and flexor hallucis longus muscle bellies [2, 7]. They supply a longitudinally oriented area of skin which can be raised as a septofasciocutaneous flap, centred over the mid portion of the fibula, with the axis along the posterior crural septum. Just proximal to the inferior tibiofibular joint, the peroneal artery gives off a transverse branch that joins the posterior tibial artery, and a perforating branch that passes forward between the fibula and tibia to join the lateral malleolar branch of the anterior tibial artery.

Although both anterior and posterior tibial arteries may be absent or very small, the peroneal artery is always present [5]. If the posterior tibial is absent, the distal communicating branch between the peroneal artery and posterior tibial will be large and will supply the plantar surface of the foot. If the anterior tibial is small or missing, the distal perforating branch of the peroneal will supply the anterior tibial and the dorsal foot structures. Occasionally, the peroneal artery originates from the anterior tibial, particularly when there is a high division of the popliteal artery. Since the peroneal artery is always present, the fibula can be used reliably as a transfer. However, its removal may jeopardize the vascular supply to the leg if the posterior tibial or anterior tibial is absent. In order to assess the possibility of anatomic variations which might preclude surgical resection of the peroneal artery, preoperative angiography is required.

Elevation of the Fibula Bone Transfer

An angiogram is done to locate the peroneal artery, identify its relationship to the fibula and to ensure that there are no anatomical abnormalities of the anterior tibial or posterior tibial arteries. The only other decisions to be made are what length of bone to remove and which leg to use. The orientation of the fibula in the recipient site is usually unimportant except for the location of the pedicle. The length of bone is estimated from preoperative x-rays of the defect and a final decision made at the time of the preparation of the recipient site.

Surgical Technique

The lateral exposure was described by Gilbert as a modification of Taylor's original posterior exposure [1, 6]. The lateral exposure, with early division and retraction of the fibula, provides easy exposure of the peroneal artery and greatly facilitates the dissection. Originally, the bone was taken with a large muscle cuff about the entire fibula to protect branches of the peroneal artery which surround the fibula. Experience has proven this cuff to be unnecessary for preservation of the periosteal blood supply.

A. Fibula Transfer

1. The patient is lying supine with the leg draped free and the hip and knee flexed. Palpate the thick biceps femoris tendon entering the head of the fibula from above and behind, and mark the head of the fibula. Below this, roll the peroneal nerve under your finger and mark its location on the skin. Place the incision on a straight line between the head of the fibula and the lateral malleolus. If a long fibula is required, leave an 8 cm length of upper and lower end of the fibula on the leg. If a short fibula (e.g. 10 cm) is taken, center it above the midpoint in order to increase the chance of including the nutrient foramen (Fig. 9-2a).

2. Incise the skin and subcutaneous tissue, exposing the muscular fascia.

3. Clear the fat from the deep fascia to allow visualization of the white line which marks the posterior crural septum, the intermuscular fascia between the peroneus musculature and the soleus. The soleus has oblique muscle fibres, while the peroneus longus fibres are longitudinal. This plane can be palpated as a cleft between the muscle bellies and is immediately posterior to the center line of the fibula. Incise along the anterior or posterior surface of the septum until the fibula is exposed. If a long fibula is removed, the lower portion is best exposed by dissection anterior to the peroneii.

4. Anterior Dissection – Remove the peroneal musculature from the antero-lateral part of the fibula, leaving 1 mm of muscle on the periosteum. Note and preserve the superficial peroneal nerve on the deep surface of the proximal part of the peroneus longus. Divide the septum between the lateral and anterior muscle compartments. Hugging the fibula, carry the dissection around the front of the fibula, detaching the extensor digitorum longus and extensor hallucis longus and exposing the interosseous membrane (Fig. 9-2b). The anterior tibial artery and deep peroneal nerve may now be seen on the deep surface of the tibialis anterior. Incise the interosseous mem-

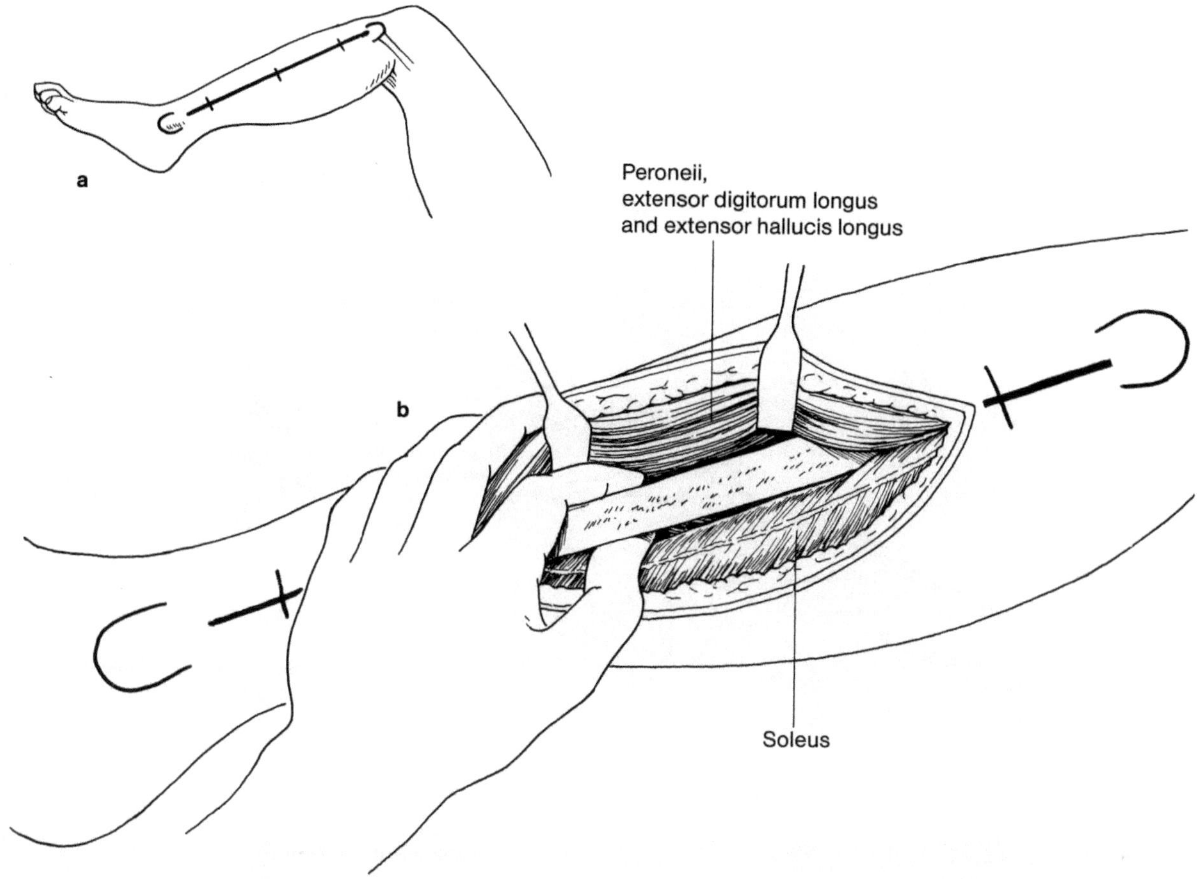

Fig. 9-2. **a** The surgical surface landmarks are the fibular head, with the attached biceps femoris tendon, and the lateral epicondyle. The incision is placed on a straight line between these two points. The upper and lower cross marks are drawn 8 cm from either end and represent the usual upper and lower maximum limits of fibular resection. The nutrient foramen usually lies proximal to the midportion of the fibula. **b** The fibula is exposed by elevation of the anterior and posterior musculature. Only periosteum is left on the fibula

brane adjacent to and along the full length of the bone to be removed.

5. Posterior Dissection - Leaving 1 mm of muscle on the periosteum, detach the soleus and expose the flexor hallucis longus. The peroneal artery is usually found on the medial side of the flexor hallucis longus. However, the artery may pass through this muscle. Do not detach the flexor hallucis longus until the peroneal artery is exposed.

6. After determining the maximum amount of fibula required, incise the periosteum beyond the intended bone cuts in order that extra periosteal cuff be left on the fibula transfer. Divide the fibula at both ends with a saw. It is not necessary to visualize the peroneal vessels prior to dividing the bone.

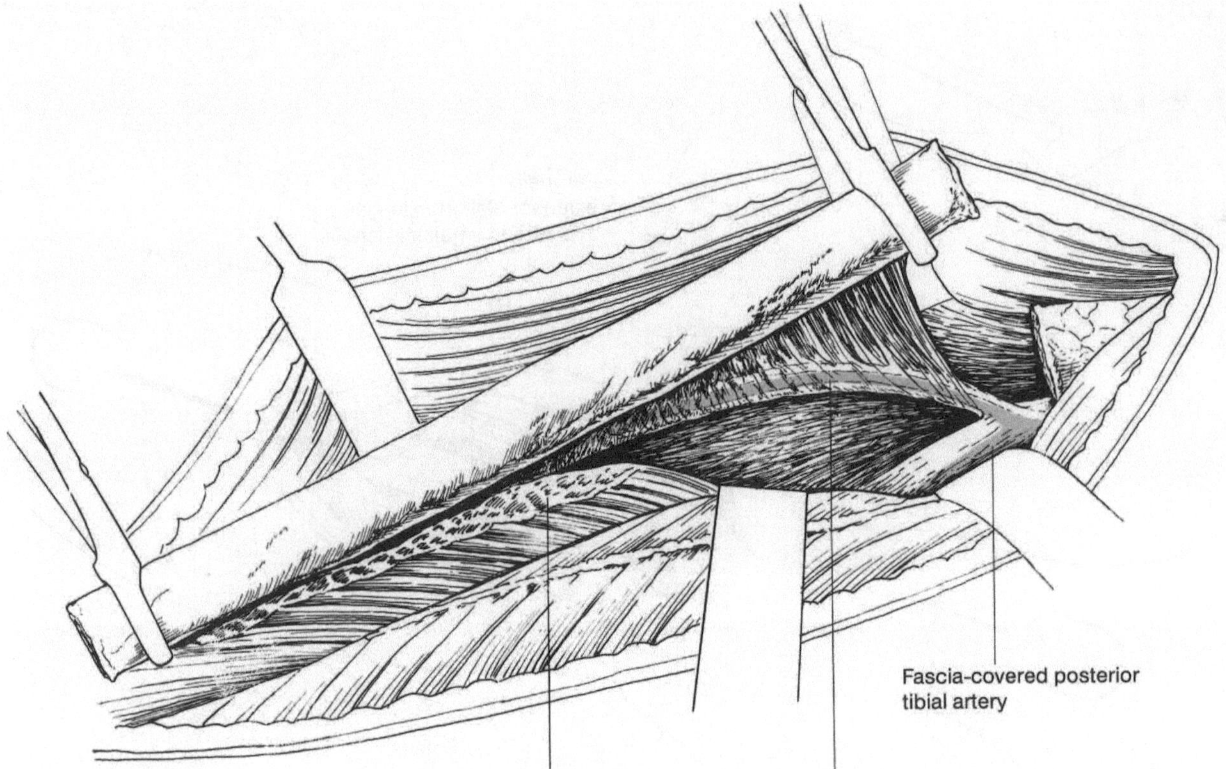

Fig. 9-3. The peroneal artery is easily exposed by dividing the fibula at both ends, and lifting and rotating the bone partly out of the way. The flexor hallucis longus and tibialis posterior muscles are divided parallel to and with direct visualization of the peroneal artery

7. Preparation of the Pedicle – Place small bone clamps on the fibula, and lift and rotate the bone anteriorly (Fig. 9-3). Follow the peroneal artery to the upper margin of the flexor hallucis longus. Divide the flexor hallucis longus longitudinally from above downwards, leaving on the bone any muscle which lies between the artery and bone. Retract and rotate the fibula posteriorly, dividing the tibialis posterior, leaving a half cm strip of muscle on the bone. Keep the peroneal artery in view until the lower end is reached. Ligate the peroneal artery at the lower end. After the bone is prepared, there will be only a small amount of flexor hallucis and tibialis posterior muscle on the bone (Fig. 9-4). Examine the transfer for bleeding from the periosteum and medullary cavity.

An alternative approach to the peroneal artery is to identify it at the distal bone end and trace the artery proximally, dividing the flexor hallucis longus and tibialis posterior from distal to proximal.

8. Closure – Close the leg in layers with a suction drain. A posterior slab will immobilize the ankle and allow muscle healing. Keep the patient in bed for 3–4 days before allowing ambulation.

B. Fibula Osteocutaneous Transfer

If a cutaneous flap is required, mark its axis over the posterior crural septum in the mid portion of the fibula. The skin flap is based on perforating vessels, most of which pass along the posterior crural septum. Include the underlying deep muscular fascia with the skin flap. Carry the dissection along the surface of the peroneii and soleus to converge on the

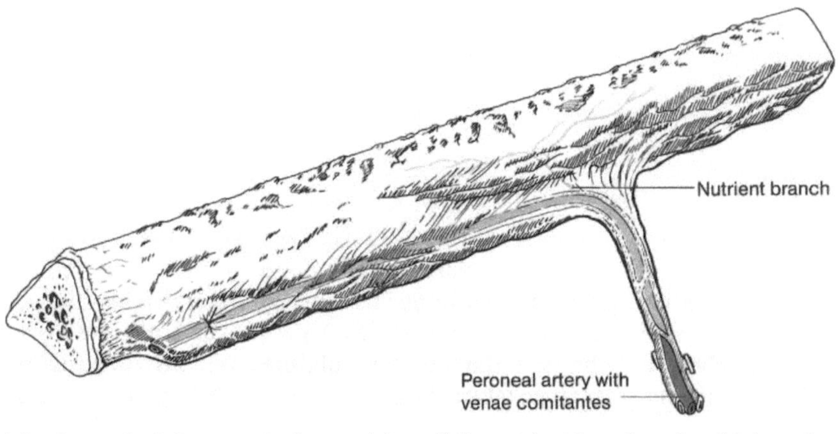

Fig. 9-4. The dissected fibula has minimal muscle left attached. The peroneal artery runs along the distal two-thirds of the bone, giving off the nutrient branch and multiple periosteal branches

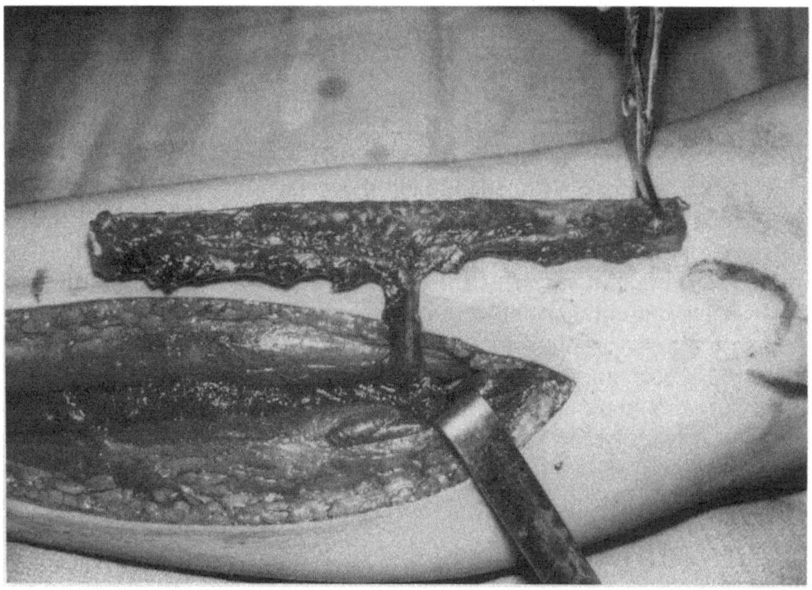

Fig. 9-5. Following its dissection, the fibula is still attached by its pedicle to the leg. There is good perfusion of the small muscle cuff and good perfusion of the bone and periosteum at both ends

posterior crural septum, and dissect down both sides of the septum to the fibula. Vessels will be seen on the septum and passing through the flexor hallucis longus to the skin. If there are no vessels on the septum, those passing through the muscle must be kept intact. From this point, the dissection is the same as for a bone only transfer.

References

1. Gilbert A (1979) Vascularized transfer of the fibular shaft. Int J Microsurg 1: 100
2. Hanel DP, Johnston G, Carmo J (1985) Further investigation of the vascularized osteocutaneous fibular graft. Presented at the Annual Meeting of the American Society for Reconstructive Microsurgery
3. McKee NH, Haw P, Vettese T (1983) Anatomic study of the nutrient foramen in the shaft of the fibula. Clin Orthop Rel Res. 184: 141
4. Restrepo J, Katz D, Gilbert A (1980) Arterial vascularization of the proximal epiphysis and the diaphysis of the fibula. Int J Microsurg 2: 49
5. Senior HD (1929) Abnormal branching of the human popliteal artery. J Anat 44: 111
6. Taylor GI (1975) The free vascularized bone graft. Plast Reconstr Surg 55: 533
7. Wei, Fu Chan Personal communication

Chapter 10. Iliac Crest

The iliac crest provides a well-vascularized bone graft which is rich in cancellous bone. Its arterial supply, the deep circumflex iliac artery (DCIA), provides branches to the bone, abdominal musculature and skin. This transfer can be taken in three different configurations: bone only, bone and abdominal musculature, and bone, abdominal musculature and skin. Although the iliac crest has been transferred based on the superficial circumflex iliac vessels, it was not until Taylor described the transfer of this flap based on the deep circumflex iliac artery that it became a reliable flap. However, it has enjoyed a mixed reception by some surgeons because it is a complex transfer to elevate and the multiple curves of the crest are a difficult shape to deal with in the recipient area. Elevation of this transfer can be done only with a thorough knowledge of the relevant anatomy. A study of the three dimensional curves of this bone will reveal that it can be ingeniously incorporated into many bony defects. For reconstruction of a massive mandibular defect that cannot be managed with a non-vascularized graft, this transfer has no peer. Also, when the problem is a large combined soft tissue and bone defect of the mandible or extremities, it is unique in its ability to supply a single stage recontruction.

Anatomy of the Iliac Crest Transfer

The portion of ileum which is available for microvascular transfer includes the anterior inferior iliac spine (AIIS), the entire iliac crest to a point a few centimetres lateral to the sacroiliac joint, and the upper portion of the wing of the ileum. Many muscles are attached to this bone. The three flat muscles of the abdominal wall are attached to the superior surface of the crest. The lateral surface gives origin to the tensor fascia lata anteriorly, the gluteus medius posteriorly, and the gluteus minimus inferiorly. The fan shaped iliacus arises on the inner surface from the iliac fossa, and passes anteriorly and medially beneath the inguinal ligament (Fig. 10-1 a).

The iliac crest is composed of cancellous bone sandwiched between two thin cortices. At the crest, the bone is at least 2 cm thick. It becomes thinner inferiorly towards the wing of the ileum. Because of the thickness and vascular connections, the most useful portion of the ileum for transfer is the crest and the 4 cm of ileum beneath the crest. The iliac crest can provide small or large pieces of vascularized bone from 6–16 cm in length (Fig. 10-2). However, when a large piece of bone is taken, its multiple curves can create problems in shaping it to fit bony defects. There are two curves in the crest, one in the sagittal plane and one in the horizontal plane. The curves often have an angular prominence at the tubercle which is located midway on the crest. There is considerable variability in the extent of bone curvature from patient to patient. When the mandible is being reconstructed, the curves may be incorporated into the mandibular shape. For long bone reconstruction, the curves are not helpful. If a large piece of crest is needed for extremity reconstruction, it must be straightened with osteotomies (Chap. 22). In view of its curved shape, it is useful to have models of the iliac crest available when planning a reconstruction.

There are three cutaneous nerves which pass through the area of dissection of this bone. The lateral cutaneous nerve of the thigh crosses superficial to the iliacus and runs under the inguinal ligament, adjacent to the anterior superior iliac spine (ASIS), and superficial to or through the sartorius, to supply an extensive area of lateral buttock and anterior lateral thigh skin. The anterior ramus of the 12th thoracic nerve provides a lateral cutaneous branch which pierces the abdominal musculature and exits over the crest about 4 cm behind the ASIS to innervate lateral buttock skin. Posterior to this nerve, a branch of the ilio hypogastric nerve pierces the abdominal musculature, and exits over the crest to supply skin on the lateral buttock. Usually, the lateral cutaneous nerve can be spared but the other nerve branches must be divided if they pass through the tissue to be transferred.

Vascular Anatomy

The relevant vascular anatomy was first described in detail by Taylor [1]. The deep circumflex iliac artery (DCIA) provides the pedicle for the iliac crest osteocutaneous transfer. This artery comes off the anterolateral aspect of the external iliac artery 1-2 cm superior to the inguinal ligament. It runs parallel to the ligament in a line of fusion of transversalis fascia and iliacus, and passes upwards and laterally towards the ASIS. From a position on the iliacus muscle 1-2 cm below the ASIS, it follows a curving path along this muscle and approaches the rim of the crest at a point 8-9 cm posterior to the ASIS. Here, it pierces the transversus abdominis, providing many large branches to the abdominal musculature and overlying skin (Fig. 10-1 a).

The first branch of the DCIA is an ascending artery which is given off before the ASIS. It pierces the transversus abdominis musculature and runs caudally between this muscle and the external oblique. A second branch in the same region comes off the deep surface of the DCIA and supplies the iliacus muscle. This latter branch is hidden from view and may be avulsed if its location is not anticipated. As the DCIA passes along the iliacus muscle, it gives off numerous branches which supply ilium and the overlying abdominal musculature and skin. Some

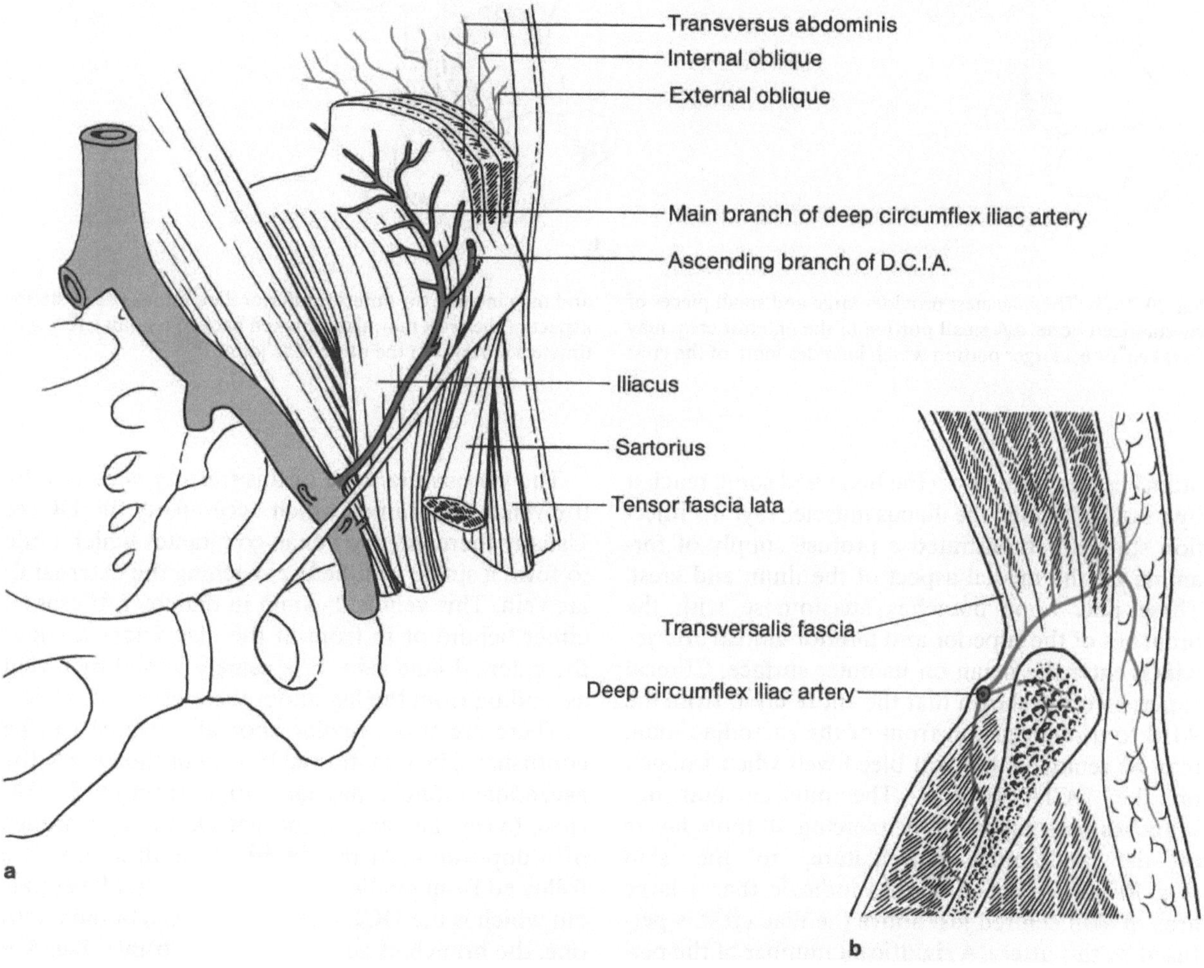

Fig. 10-1. **a** Antero-medial view of the left pelvis showing the anatomical relationships of the iliac crest to the seven muscles attached to it. The deep circumflex iliac artery (DCIA) takes origin from the external iliac artery and passes laterally to lie on the iliacus muscle. As it travels posteriorly on this muscle, it gradually approaches the upper margin of the iliac crest, giving off along its route the branches to the muscle, bone and skin which supply the transfer. **b** Cross section of the mid portion of iliac crest and surrounding structures. Abdominal wall musculature is seen above and attached to the crest. The DCIA lies on the medial surface of the crest, under the iliacus fascia. Branches supply the iliac crest, iliacus muscle, and the ilium. Branches to the skin pass to and through the abdominal wall musculature

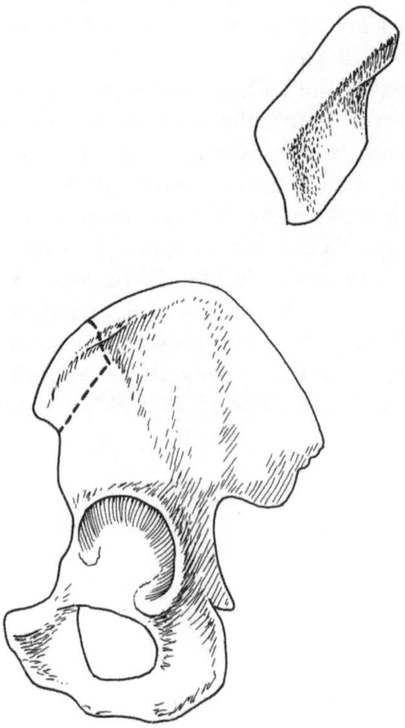

a

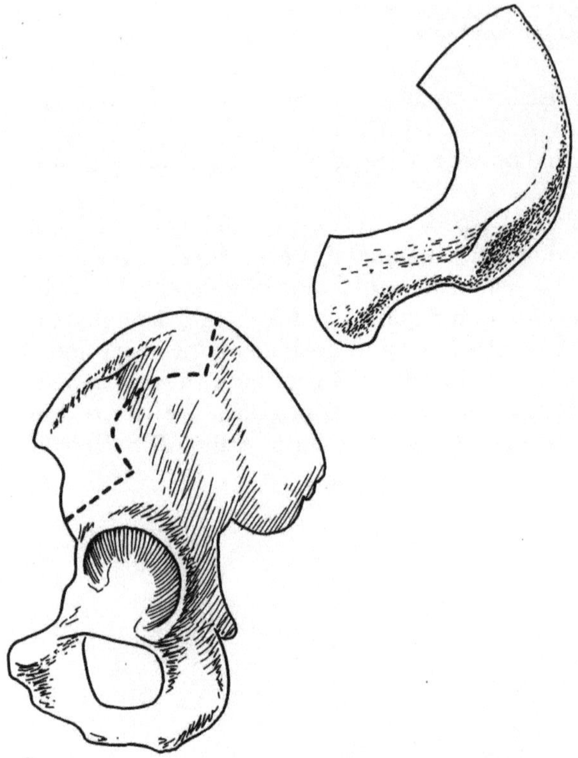

b

Fig. 10-2 a, b. The iliac crest provides large and small pieces of vascularized bone. **a** A small portion of the anterior crest may be taken, or **b** a larger portion which includes more of the crest and may include the anterior inferior iliac spine. The posterior aspect of the crest may also be taken back to a point a few centimeters anterior to the sacro iliac joint

branches pass directly to the bone and some reach it by passing through the iliacus muscle. Taylor's injection studies demonstrated a profuse supply of foramina on the medial aspect of the ilium and crest. These iliac bone branches anastomose with the branches of the superior and inferior gluteal arteries which enter the ileum on its outer surface. Clinical experience has shown that the entire crest, from the AIIS to a point just in front of the sacroiliac joint, may be removed and will bleed well when isolated on the DCIA pedicle. The musculocutaneous branches pass superficially, piercing all three layers of the abdominal musculature, to the skin (Fig. 10-1b). Injection studies indicate that a large area of skin centred just above the iliac crest is perfused by this artery. A significant number of the perforating branches emerge through the external oblique within 2 cm of the attachment of this muscle to the crest, beginning 6 cm posterior to the ASIS. The DCIA measures 1.5-3 mm in external diameter and provides a 6 cm pedicle length from the external iliac artery to the ASIS.

The venous drainage of this transfer is carried by the venae comitantes which accompany the DCIA. Usually there are two venae comitantes which unite to form a single vein before reaching the external iliac vein. This vein is 2-4 mm in diameter. It crosses either behind or in front of the iliac artery to enter the external iliac vein. It is usually joined by a vein ascending from the leg under the inguinal ligament.

There are two vascular anomalies which can be confusing. The first arterial branch of the DCIA, the ascending branch, may take origin from the DCIA, close to the iliac artery, and present the appearance of a duplication of the DCIA. As both arteries are followed from medial to lateral, it will not be apparent which is the DCIA and which is the branch until one, the branch, is seen piercing the transversus abdominis musculature and ascending caudally. We have experienced this anomally in two clinical cases. The other anomaly of the DCIA is even more confusing. In this vascular variation, the DCIA does pierce the transversus abdominis musculature, usually medial to the ASIS as if it were the first branch. It then lies in a plane between this muscle and the external oblique throughout its course adjacent to the iliac crest. This anomaly was identified in one clinical case. The procedure, which involved a large osteocutaneous transfer, was continued and the skin and bone were well-vascularized.

Elevating the Iliac Crest Osteocutaneous Transfer

Using clinical and radiological measurements, assess the size of both skin and bone defects and the relative position of each. Determine the best orientation of the transfer in the recipient site by the configuration of the bone and skin defect and the location of the recipient vessels. When the preferred orientation of the bone has been decided, the most suitable iliac crest will be apparent. As the bone and abdominal muscle are bulky, the skin flap must be wider than expected to provide coverage in extremity reconstruction. Preoperative arteriography is not routinely used to assess the DCIA. Previous abdominal surgery, such as a herniorraphy or appendectomy, may compromise the pedicle and injure the perforating branches, and thereby affect the selection of the side for transfer.

Surgical Technique

1. The patient is supine on the operating table. If a large skin flap is required, it is helpful to elevate the buttock on the side of the transfer. However, this rotation of the pelvis makes the preparation of the pedicle more awkward.

Palpate and mark the pubis, femoral artery, (ASIS), iliac crest and inguinal ligament. Mark the perforators parallel to and 1-2 cm above the iliac crest. They begin 6 cm lateral to the anterior superior iliac spine and continue laterally.

Place gentle traction on the skin towards the umbilicus and mark the axis of the flap. The axis of the skin flap is a line drawn from the ASIS to the inferior angle of the scapula. Thus, the axis of optimum vascularity gradually moves above the iliac crest. Outline the skin flap as needed, close to this axis, but relative to the anticipated bone graft. The flap does not need to be centred on this axis as long as the perforators are included in the flap (Fig. 10-3).

2. Incise the skin flap circumferentially. If you wish to minimize the bulk of the flap, carry the incision through the first layer of fat to Camper's fascia and undermine beneath this layer until you get closer to the iliac crest. Then go through the second layer of fat to the abdominal musculature. Lift the skin flap from the abdominal musculature, keeping the areolar tissue layer which lies on the musculature with the flap, and undermine to within 3-4 cm of the crest.

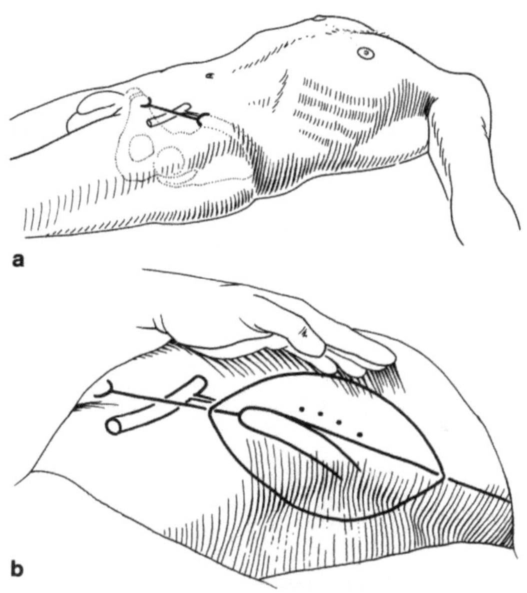

Fig. 10-3. **a** The surface landmarks are the pubic tubercle, the anterior superior iliac spine, the iliac crest, and the femoral artery. **b** The axis of the cutaneous flap is a straight line which passes from the ASIS to the inferior angle of the scapula. In an older person, the redundant abdominal musculature often rolls over the iliac crest when in the reclining position. The skin and muscle must be gently retracted toward the umbilicus before drawing the skin flap to identify the undistorted position of the abdominal wall with respect to the iliac crest. The flap is drawn symmetrically about the axis, which lies close to the cutaneous perforators, marked by dots on the illustration

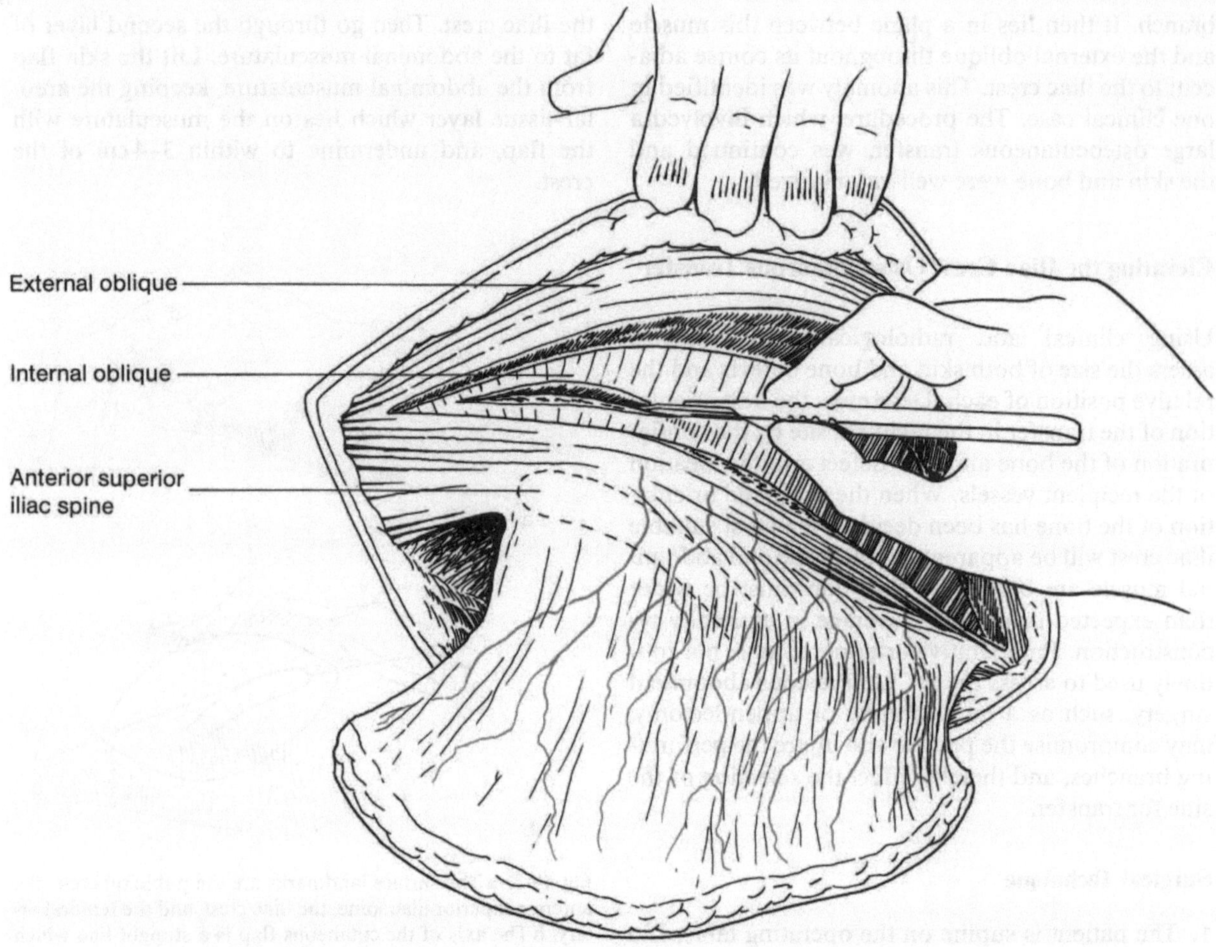

Fig. 10-4. Lateral view of the dissection of the left iliac crest. The cutaneous flap is incised and is hanging from the external oblique muscle. The external oblique has been divided 3-4 cm above and parallel to the iliac crest, to incorporate the cutaneous perforators of the DCIA. An incision is being placed through the internal oblique. Traction by the surgical assistant on the redundant abdominal musculature allows the correct amount of muscle to be left on the crest

3. When the patient is reclining, the abdominal musculature will roll over the iliac crest. To determine the location for the muscle incision, the assistant must place traction on the musculature towards the umbilicus. While traction is exerted, incise the external oblique, internal oblique, and transversus abdominis along a line parallel to and 3-4 cm above the iliac crest. This strip of abdominal musculature will carry the perforators of the DCIA which supply the skin. Except for the initial few cms opposite the ASIS, this cuff of muscle should extend the full length of the bone being removed. At the posterior portion of the muscle cuff, there are branches of the DCIA which must be divided.

Incise the transversalis fascia and retract the extra peritoneal fat, exposing the junction of the fascia of the iliacus and transversalis. The DCIA can be palpated beneath the iliacus fascia at its junction with the transversalis fascia (Fig. 10-5).

4. Incise the inferior margin of the skin flap down to tensor fascia lata. If a fascial attachment is required on the transfer, a strip of tensor fascia can be left on the bone. Otherwise, incise the fascia at its origin to the bone. Leaving the periosteum on the lateral surface of the ilium, remove the tensor fascia lata, gluteus minimus and medius from the portion of bone to be removed.

5. The pedicle is prepared after the skin and muscle dissection in order that it not be harmed inadvertently during subsequent parts of the dissection.

Incise the skin parallel to and above the inguinal ligament. Identify the ligament and place an incision

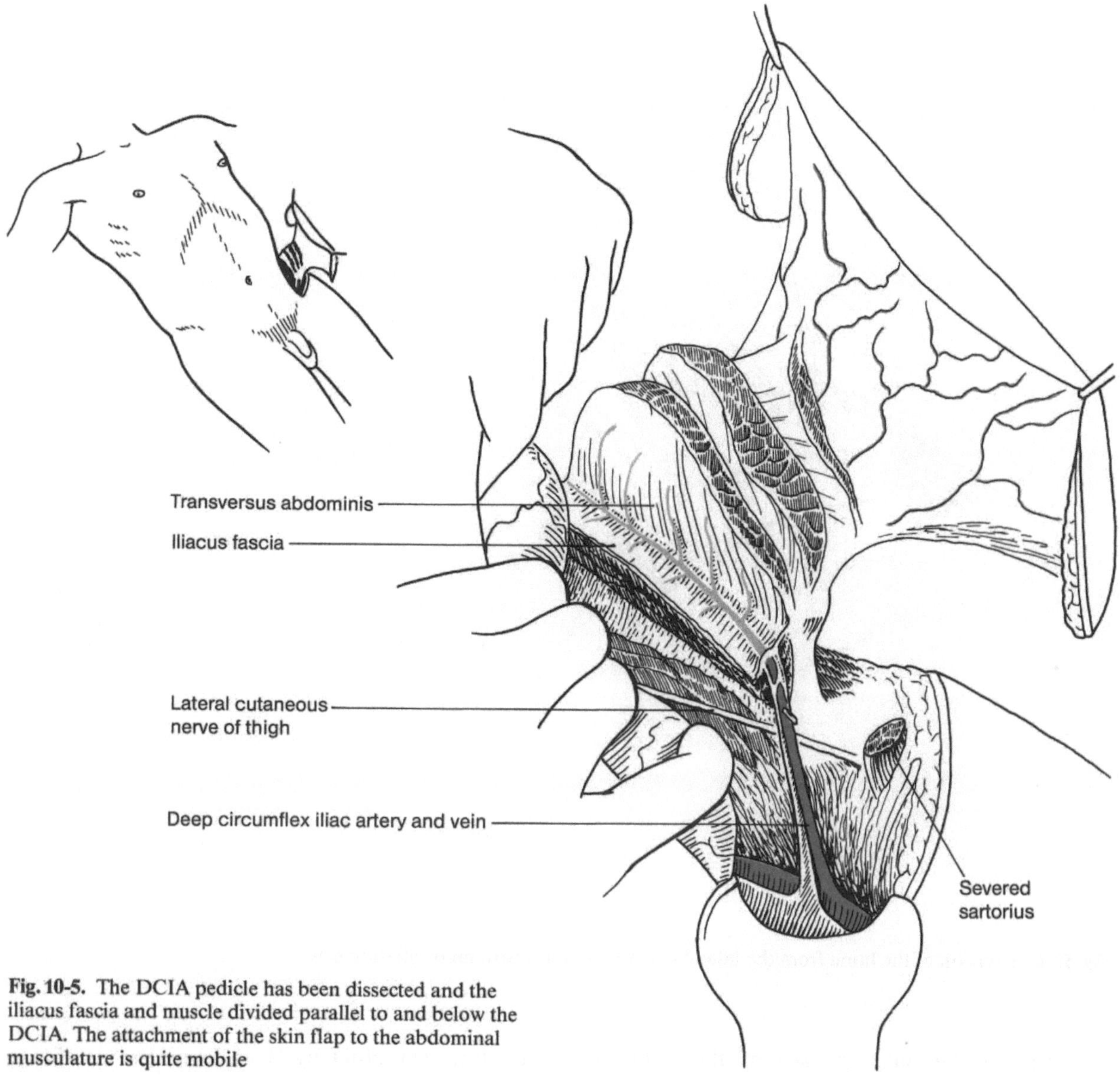

Fig. 10-5. The DCIA pedicle has been dissected and the iliacus fascia and muscle divided parallel to and below the DCIA. The attachment of the skin flap to the abdominal musculature is quite mobile

through all layers of the abdominal wall, parallel to and 1 cm above the ligament. Retract the layers of the abdominal wall and clear the fibro fatty tissue anterior to the external iliac artery. First identify the external iliac artery. The DCIA will readily be seen 1-2 cm above the inguinal ligament on the anterolateral surface of the iliac artery. Identify the vena comitans. This single vein may pass anterior or posterior to the iliac artery on its course to the iliac vein. The vena comitans is very thin and can be torn easily. Follow the DCIA and the vein laterally, separating them from the transversalis and iliacus fascia and the lateral cutaneous nerve of the thigh. Identify and divide the two branches which are given off before the ASIS: the ascending branch and the muscular branch coming off the vessel's deep surface. Isolate the pedicle to a point on the iliacus opposite the ASIS.

6. Retract the abdominal contents and expose the iliacus. Divide the iliacus parallel to the crest and 1-2 cm below the course of the DCIA. Sweep the remaining iliacus inferiorly to expose the iliac fossa. Cauterize vessels passing on the surface, within, and deep to the iliacus in its posterior portion. Divide the sartorius at its origin and the iliacus at the same level (Fig. 10-5).

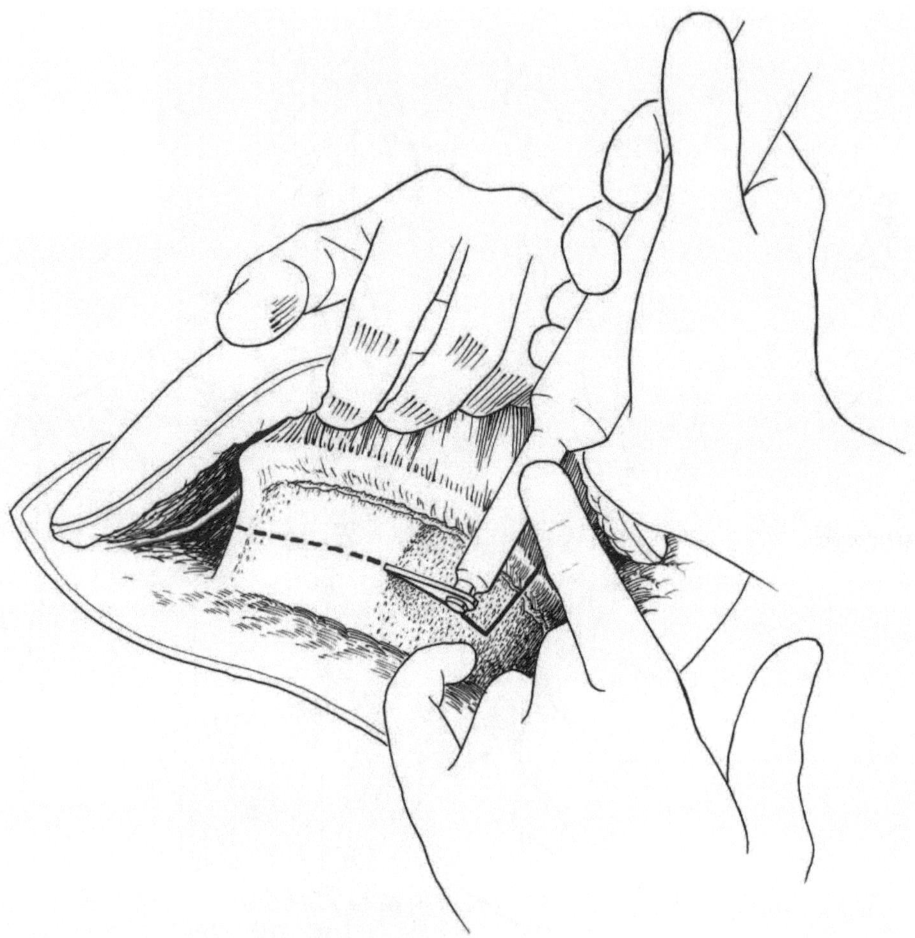

Fig. 10-6. Division of the bone from the lateral side of the ilium with an oscillating saw

7. Mark on the outer surface of the ilium the amount of bone that will be needed for the reconstruction. It is useful to remove a larger piece of bone than you anticipate needing in order that you have some to spare when doing the final shaping of the bone.

Cut the crest from the lateral side while the assistant observes the medial bone surface for the penetration of the saw blade. An oscillating saw held upside down is useful (Fig. 10-6). Leave the transfer attached to the DCIA for a few minutes and observe the cut edges of bone and the skin flap. The crest will ooze from the cancellous margins and the dermis should bleed when the pedicle is intact.

8. Place a double suture ligature through the origin of the DCIA and the vena comitans, and divide them and remove the transfer (Fig. 10-7).

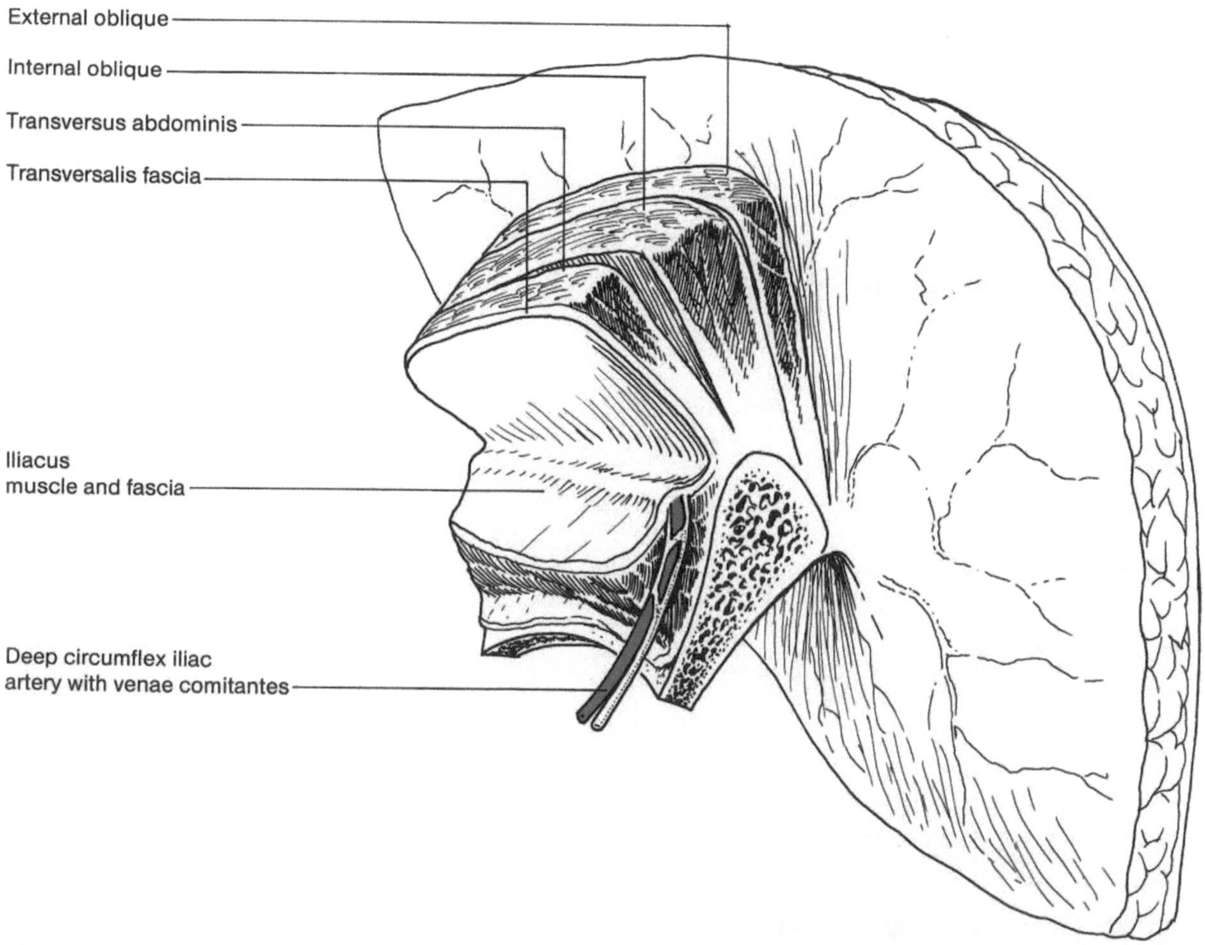

Fig. 10-7. The separated transfer showing all tissue structures: bone, muscle and skin and their relationship to the pedicle and its branches

Fig. 10-7. The separated transfer showing all tissue structures: bone, muscle and skin and their relationship to the pedicle and its branches

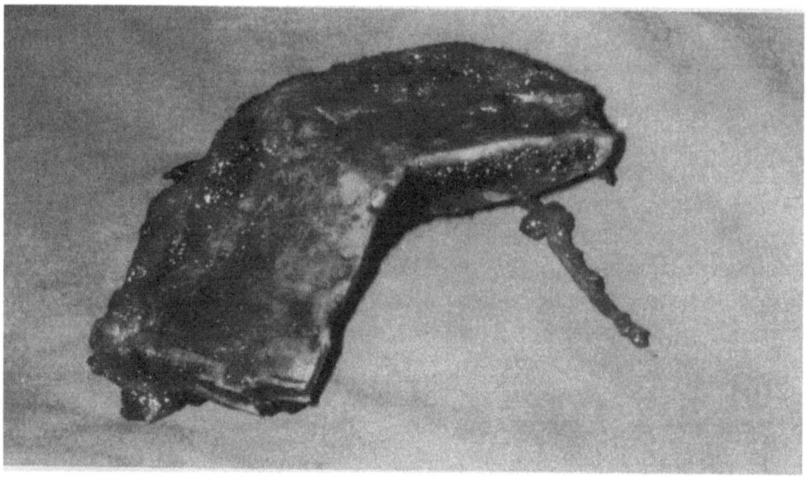

Fig. 10-8. View of the external and cut inferior surface of the iliac crest as a bone only transfer. Note changing thickness of the cut surface from the anterior crest by the pedicle to the posterior crest on the left

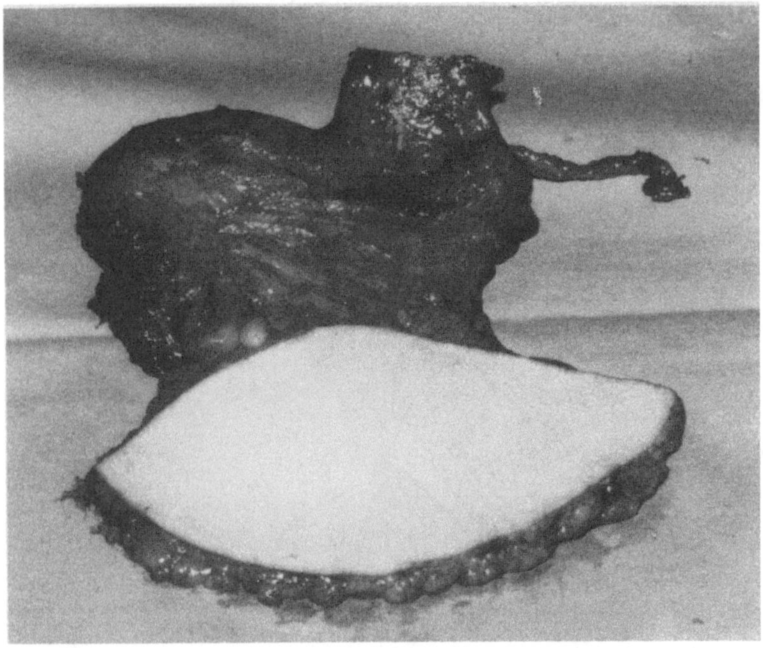

Fig. 10-9. Osteocutaneous iliac crest transfer. The large skin flap is attached to a mobile cuff of abdominal muscle wall. The pedicle is seen emerging from the ASIS on the right

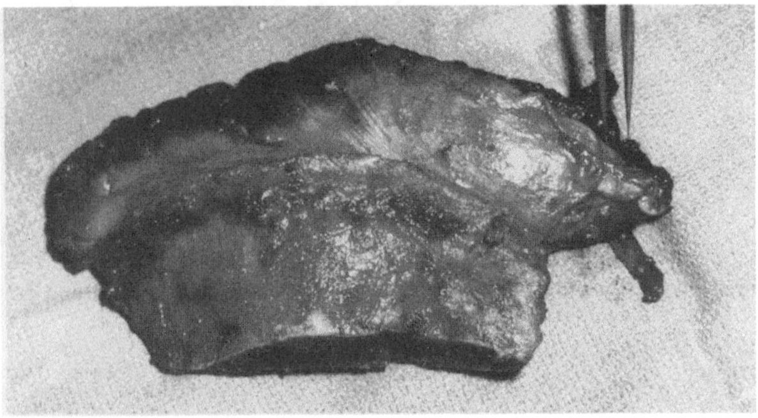

Fig. 10-10. External surface of an iliac crest transfer taken with a large cuff of abdominal musculature. Forceps point to the DCIA

Closing the Iliac Crest Donor Site

1. Control bleeding before closure. Common sites of bleeding are the abdominal musculature, the tensor fascia lata, the medullary cavity of the ilium and the large veins at the posterior portion of the iliacus.

2. Suture the transversalis fascia to the iliacus fascia. This must be a careful closure in order to prevent herniation of the abdominal contents. Insert a suction drain on top of this closure.

3. Suture all three layers of abdominal musculature to the tensor fascia lata and the gluteus medius.

4. Reconstitute all layers of the abdominal wall above the inguinal ligament in their normal anatomic layers and close the skin directly. A surprisingly large ellipse of skin may be taken and still allow direct skin closure because of the decreased prominence of the ilium following bone removal. Closure may be facilitated by flexing the hip.

References

1. Taylor GI, Townsend P, Corlett R (1979) Superiority of the deep circumflex iliac vessels as the supply for free groin flaps: experimental work. Plast Recon Surg 64: 595
2. Taylor GI, Townsend P, Corlett R (1979) Superiority of the deep circumflex iliac vessels as the supply for free groin flaps: clinical work. Plast Recon Surg 64: 745
3. Taylor GI (1982) Reconstruction of the mandible with free composite iliac bone grafts. Ann Plast Surg 9: 361

Chapter 11. Metatarsal

The surgeon who develops skill in using this bone transfer will be favourably impressed by it. The particular advantages of the metatarsal are that it is a very well-vascularized bone graft and can be taken with a thin flexible skin flap. Whereas the fibula is available for long defects and the iliac crest for medium length defects, the metatarsal is suitable for the shorter defect. In short bony defects, non-vascularized bone grafts will often be suitable. However, when the bone graft bed is not well-vascularized, as in a previously infected or radiated bed, the metatarsal will prove very useful. Its most common application has been reconstruction of the mandible, particularly following anterior arch resection. With the dorsal foot skin attached, it provides excellent intra oral coverage of the mandibular reconstruction [3, 4]. With a wedge osteotomy in the mid shaft, an anterior mandibular arch shape may be created without compromising the circulation. Both ends of the bone are well-vascularized cancellous bone. These bone ends, when fitted into a bony defect, provide an excellent healing surface for rapid bony union - an advantage over the radius and fibula transfers. An advantage of this flap's remote location is that it may be raised simultaneously with the head and neck tumor excision, without interfering with the exterpative surgeon. A long vascular pedicle is available for anastomosis to the neck, with a reliable vessel size for anastomosis. It is occasionally useful in the extremities for metacarpal reconstruction, particularly when a metacarpal defect is accompanied by a dorsal skin loss.

The disadvantages of the flap are the difficulties in elevating it and in obtaining primary healing of the foot. After 10 days of complete bed rest, patients are ambulated gradually. It usually takes a number of months before they are walking normally and they may have prolonged foot discomfort. This flap should be used cautiously in the young and physically active person.

Anatomy of the Metatarsal Transfer

The 2nd metatarsal is 6-7 cm in length in the adult. The shaft, which is 1 cm in diameter, is strong cortical bone. The base of the bone, which is 2-2½ cm in depth, is well-vascularized cancellous bone. The head of the metatarsal is about 1½-2 cm in diameter and also well-vascularized cancellous bone. In this transfer, the arterial supply to the metatarsal is the first dorsal metatarsal artery (FDMA). Arterial branches of the FDMA pass through and around the first dorsal interosseous musculature to the metatarsal periosteal network. Branches in this periosteal network penetrate the 1-2 nutrient foramina which are located at each end of the bone, adjacent to the neck and base of the metatarsal [1]. The vessels passing through these foramina provide a rich intramedullary blood supply. The detailed blood supply to the foot is described in Chapter 3.

Elevating the Metatarsal Osteocutaneous Transfer

Evaluate the circulation to the foot by checking the patency of both the anterior tibial and posterior tibial arteries. Compress each one separately at the ankle and palpate the pulse in the other artery. If one or the other pulse is not present with compression of the opposite pulse, a proximal obstruction may be present and arteriography is necessary. A Doppler pulse pressure study may be helpful in assessing the adequacy of circulation to the foot. The dorsalis pedis cannot be taken if neither the posterior tibial nor peroneal artery is patent and able to supply the foot. An understanding of the vasculature of the dorsal foot skin flap is helpful in understanding the osteocutaneous transfer (Chap. 3).

When an attached skin flap is being taken, its size, shape and orientation on the metatarsal are determined by the size, shape and position of the soft tissue loss relative to the bony defect in the recipient area. Usually the skin flap is centred over the bone

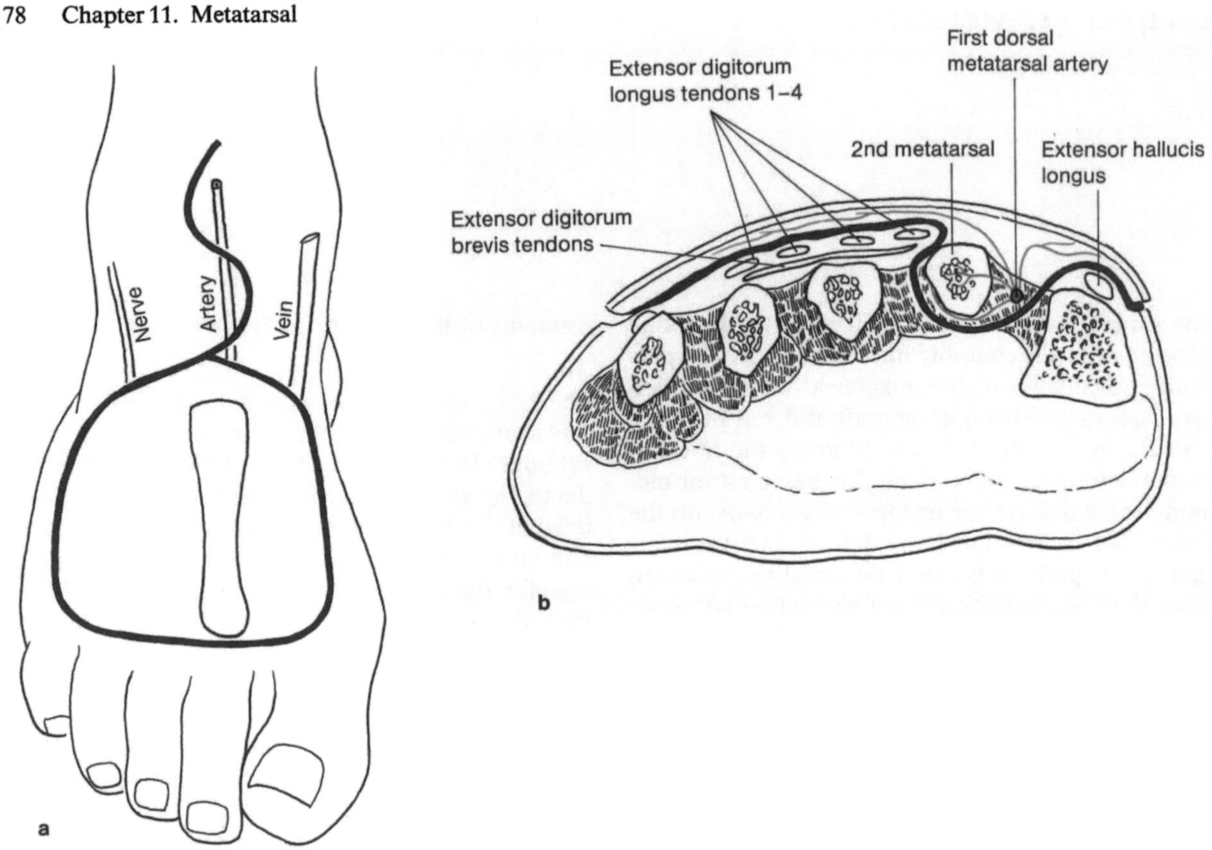

Fig. 11-1. **a** The dorsal skin flap is outlined over the second metatarsal. The expected position of the superficial peroneal nerve, dorsalis pedis artery, and saphenous vein is marked. **b** Cross section through the mid shaft of the metatarsals. The osteocutaneous transfer includes all of the tissue which is superficial to the heavy black line. The transfer includes all of the first dorsal interosseous musculature which is lateral and dorsal to the FDMA

(Fig. 11-1 a). However, if the estimation of flap position is misjudged, it can be moved, as the flap is moderately mobile on the bone. Medial and lateral positions of the flap on the bone are easier to adjust than proximal distal movements.

Surgical Technique

1. The skin flap is raised as described for the dorsal foot skin flap steps 1-4. pgs 19, 20. The lateral margin of the skin flap is undermined to the extensor digitorum longus of the second toe and the medial margin to the extensor hallucis longus.

Usually, the entire 2nd metatarsal is taken, and then appropriately shortened to fit the defect. For a shorter bone, the base of the metatarsal may be left in the foot. However, division of the bone at this level may damage some of the nutrient arteries to the proximal end of the metatarsal.

2. With the tourniquet down, identify the first dorsal metatarsal artery (FDMA) at the distal margin of the flap. If it does not pulsate, divide the vessel to be sure that it spurts. It is easy to mistake the artery for a thick walled superficial vein. Remember that the artery may be found on the surface of the interosseous muscle or at any level within the muscle. Divide the artery and suture it to the edge of the skin flap (Fig. 11-2).

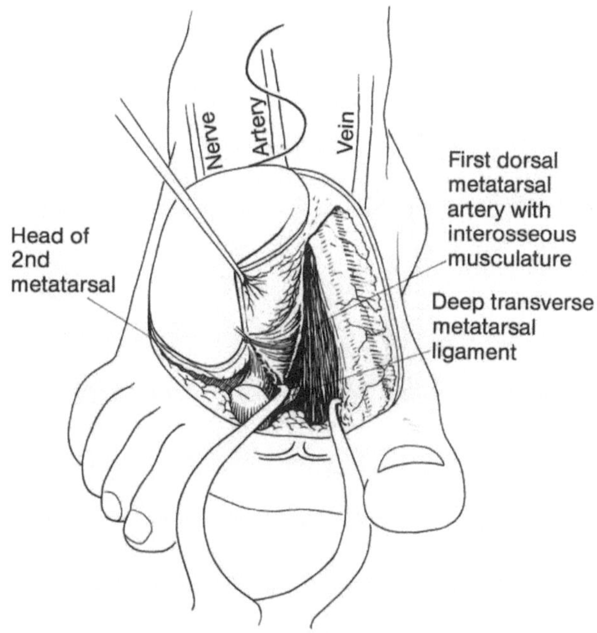

Fig. 11-2. The FDMA is divided at the distal margin of the skin flap and sutured to the flap to aid in visualization of the vessel. The first and second metatarsals are spread apart to aid in the proximal dissection of the FDMA and plantar communicating branch of the dorsalis pedis artery

3. Beginning at the distal flap margin, develop a plane of dissection medial and deep to the FDMA. This plane will be on the opposite side of the FDMA from its branches to the skin and bone (Fig. 11-1 b).

Proximal dissection along the FDMA is facilitated by dividing the deep transverse metatarsal ligament, spreading the metatarsals apart with a self retaining retractor and dividing the extensor digitorum brevis tendon (Fig. 11-2). If the pulsating FDMA is visualized on the deep and medial surface of the flap during the proximal dissection, it will not be injured.

4. When the dissection along the FDMA reaches its origin on the plantar communicating branch of the dorsalis pedis, clean this branch and its two venae comitantes and follow the dorsalis pedis into the communicating branch. Always keep the dissection on the medial side of the vessels to prevent injury to the cutaneous and muscular branches.

5. When you have clearly identified the origin of the FDMA from the communicating branch, divide the communicating branch and its venae comitantes below the take off of the FDMA. This is a tight spot with little room to work. If you do not clearly identify the arteries, you may inadvertently divide an FDMA if it has a low origin on the communicating branch.

Occasionally, the plantar metatarsal artery to the big toe has an origin immediately adjacent to the FDMA. Division of the communicating branch between the dorsal and plantar metatarsal arteries is then difficult. Nevertheless, if the plantar metatarsal artery is the main vascular supply to the big toe, it is preferable to leave it. This evaluation can be made by cross clamping the plantar artery and observing the circulation to the big toe.

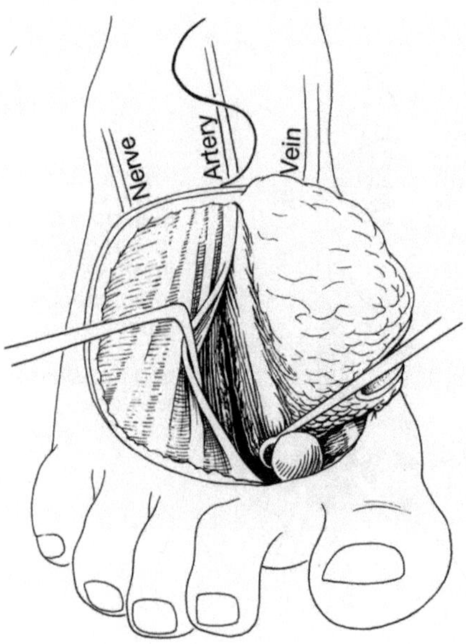

Fig. 11-3. The second extensor tendon is retracted and the metatarsal head is separated from the MP collateral ligaments, volar plate and transverse metatarsal ligament. With medial retraction of the metatarsal, the second dorsal interosseous muscle is separated from the bone

6. By dividing the collateral ligaments and volar plate at their attachment to the metacarpal head, disarticulate the 2nd toe at the MT joint. Retract the second toe extensor digitorum longus laterally, carefully preserving the paratenon. Develop a plane of dissection along the lateral surface of the 2nd metatarsal, leaving a thin layer of interosseous muscle on the bone to preserve the periosteal vessels (Fig. 11-3).

7. The only attachments left are the tarsal metatarsal ligaments. To identify the joint spaces, wiggle the metatarsal and palpate the dorsal joint spaces between the second metatarsal and the three cuniforms and first metatarsal, and incise these ligaments. The plantar ligaments are at least 2 cm beneath the dorsal surface and their division can be awkward. Slide a thin straight osteotome or a sharp periosteal elevator into each joint space, and use it with a pushing, slicing motion to divide the volar ligaments.

8. When the metatarsal is attached only by its pedicle, replace it in the foot and observe the circulation to the skin, muscle and periosteum before removal of the transfer (Fig. 11-4).

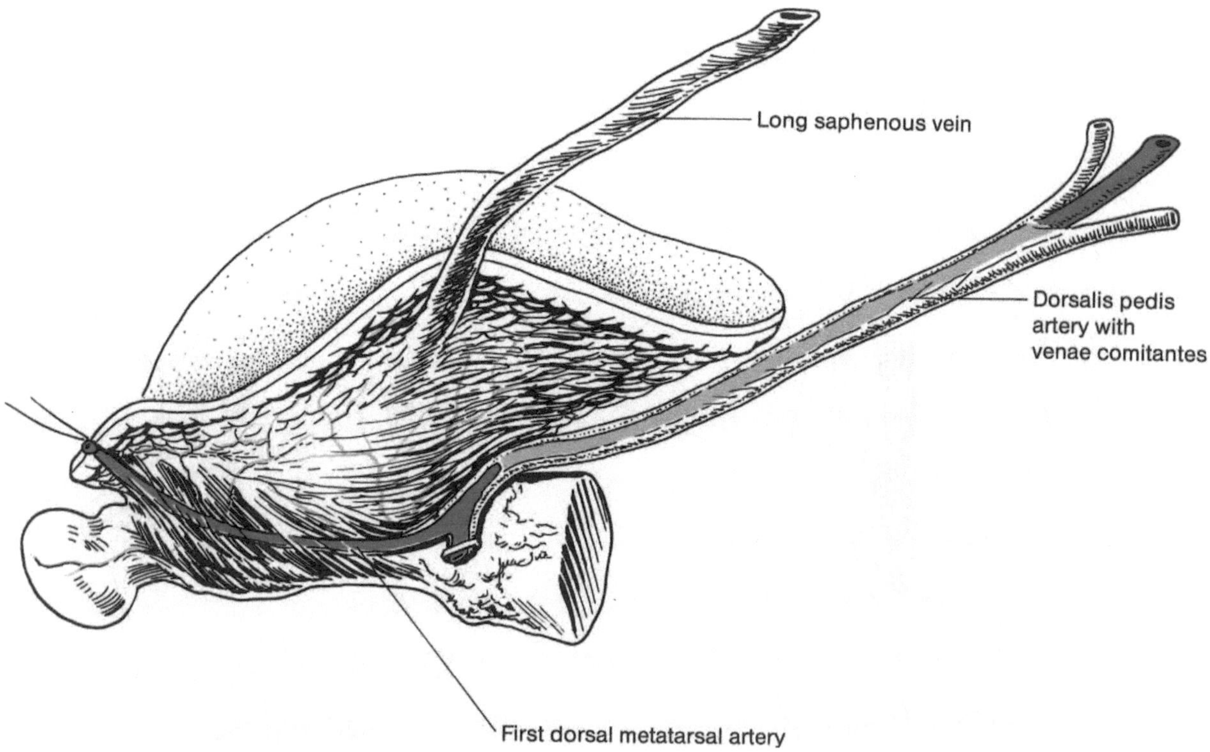

Fig. 11-4. The transfer, completely separated, demonstrating the relationship between the dorsal skin, metatarsal, intervening interosseous musculature and the vascular pedicle. The FDMA takes origin from the plantar communicating branch of the dorsalis pedis

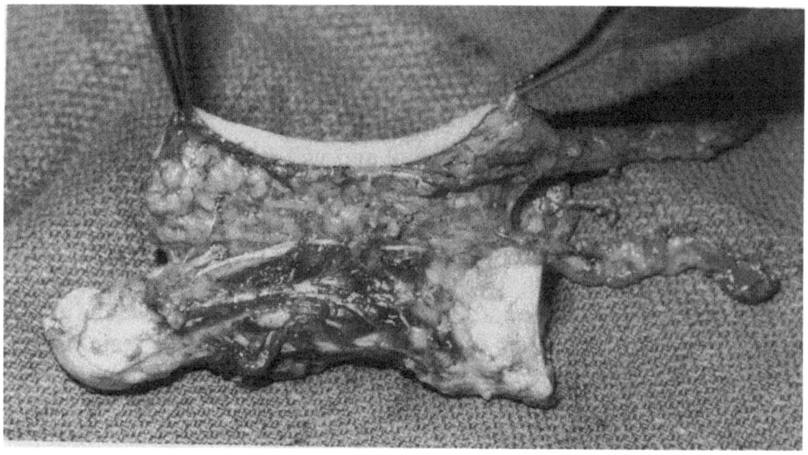

Fig. 11-5. The completed transfer, showing the medial side of the second metatarsal with the mobile skin flap elevated to show the interosseous musculature, saphenous vein *(upper)* and dorsalis pedis *(lower)* entering transfer

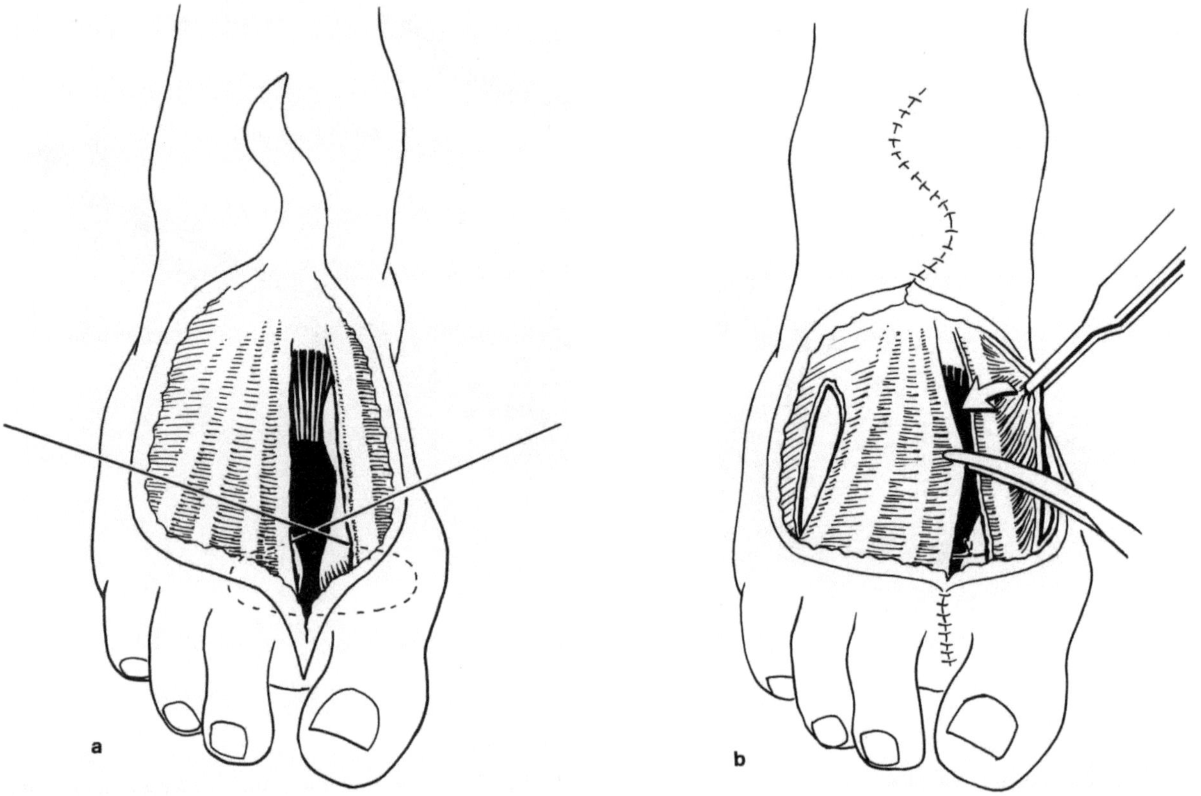

Fig. 11-6. **a** Approximation of the first and third metatarsals. A heavy suture about the metatarsal necks partially closes the defect. **b** To provide a skin graft bed, the second to fifth extensor tendons are brought medially, and the fascia medial to the extensor hallucis longus is brought laterally, to join the second extensor tendon. The layer of fascia flipped over the extensor hallucis longus provides a good surface for a skin graft bed

Donor Site Closure

1. Remove the second toe as it is flail and will prevent approximation of the first and third metatarsals. Filleting the toe does not provide useful cover for the dorsum of the foot.

2. Approximate the first and third metatarsal heads with a heavy suture which encircles both of their necks and lies deep to the extensor tendons. This suture will close the distal portion of the foot defect and approximate the 1st and 3rd toes (Fig. 11-6a).

3. Cover the proximal portion of the defect with the extensor tendons and their paratenon. Place an incision lateral and parallel to the extensor tendons to the fifth toe. Using a blunt instrument, separate the second to fifth extensor tendons from the underlying structures and move them medially as a bi-pedicled flap. Place an incision 1.5 cm medial and parallel to the extensor hallucis longus again through the fascia which is continuous with the paratenon. Undermine this fascia and the extensor hallucis longus. Take this fascia, turn it over the extensor hallucis longus tendon and sew it to the extensor digitorum longus to the second toe (Fig. 11-6b). Bringing these tendons and their paratenon together covers the metatarsal defect with a vascularized layer of tissue which will accept a skin graft. If the tourniquet was not used except for short periods and the paratenon was irrigated frequently during the dissection, it will not have dried or been damaged and will provide a viable bed for skin grafting. Repair the extensor retinaculum and tears in the paratenon over the extensor tendons (Fig. 11-7).

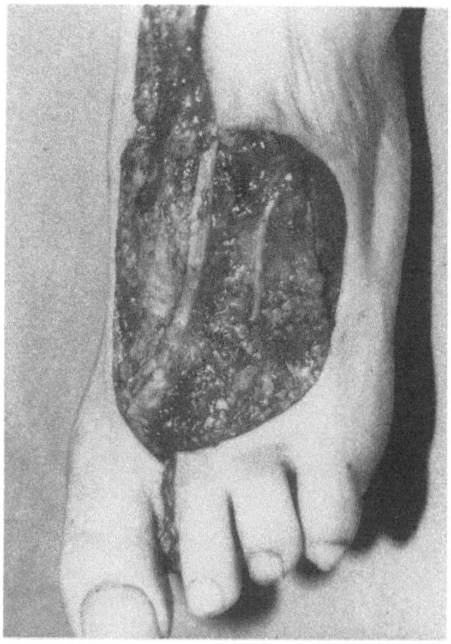

Fig. 11-7. The extensor tendon flaps have been brought together, providing a well-vascularized bed for the skin graft. The second toe is removed

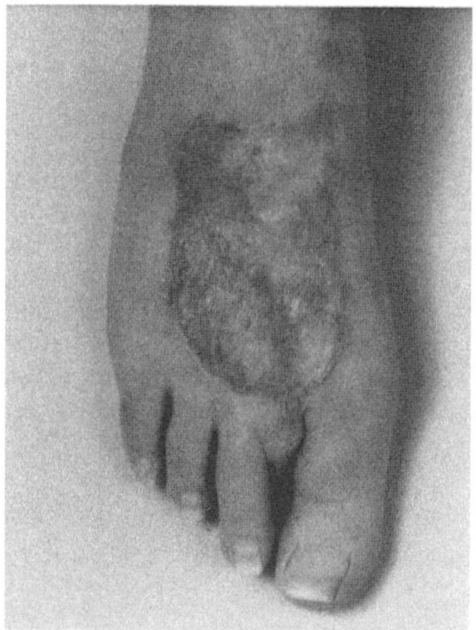

Fig. 11-8. Appearance of the foot 3 months after removal of the transfer

4. Apply a medium thickness split thickness skin graft and a very gentle tie over dressing on the graft.

Splint the ankle, foot and toes. Postoperative toe movements are not allowed as they will move the extensor tendons under the skin graft and may decrease graft take.

5. Elevate the foot and confine the patient to bed for 10 days. There may be small areas of skin graft loss which will heal secondarily. However, with care, a 100% skin graft take can be obtained (Fig. 11-8).

References

1. Crock HV (1967) The Blood Supply of the Lower Limb Bones in Man, Livingstone Ltd. Edinburgh
2. Duncan MJ, Manktelow RT, Zuker RM, Rosen I (1985) Mandibular Reconstruction in the Radiated Patient - The Role of Osteocutaneous Free Tissue Transfer. Plast Reconstr Surg 76: 829
3. Macleod AM, O'Brien BMcC, Morrison WA (1979) Microvascular techniques in reconstruction following major resections for cancer of the head and neck. Aust & New Zealand J of Surg 49: 648
4. Macleod AM, Robinson DW (1982) Reconstruction of defects involving the mandible and floor of mouth by free osteocutaneous flaps derived from the foot. Br J Plast Surg 35: 239

Part II
Microvascular Reconstructions

Head and Neck Reconstruction

Reconstructive microsurgery has made a major contribution to reconstruction in head and neck problems. In some situations, such as soft tissue coverage of the face or intra-oral area, it has provided another alternative to accepted pedicle techniques. In other situations, microsurgery has provided a unique solution to problems such as facial paralysis and major mandibular defects which previously did not have satisfactory reconstructions.

The advantages of a microsurgical free tissue transfer are many. It provides a well-vascularized transfer which is capable of healing, despite its lying in a poorly-vascularized bed which may have had previous radiation, infection, or scar tissue. One-stage reconstructions are now available for procedures such as contour reconstruction, which used to required a 3- or 4-stage procedure, bringing tissue from the abdomen, through a wrist carrier, to insert into the face.

The vasculature in the neck and face is quite reliable for microvascular anastomosis. The facial artery, superior thyroid artery, and superficial and deep veins are not prone to vascular spasm. In the elderly, these vessels have a low incidence of arterial sclerosis, and in the radiated patient, the vessels can still be used for microanastomosis.

When a free flap is compared with pedicled flaps such as the pectoralis major, which must remain attached to the chest, the surgeon has more flexibility in positioning the flap.

Most of the transfers which are used in the face come from a site distant to the head and neck. They can be prepared simultaneously with the face to diminish the operating time. The only disadvantage to a microvascular transfer is the time which is required for the microanastomoses and the potential that an anastomosis can fail with complete loss of the transfer.

Chapter 12. Head and Neck Coverage

Facial Coverage

One of the unsolved problems in dealing with the patient who has a major skin loss in the face is providing a skin replacement which is a good color match with the remaining skin. Facial skin defects are best replaced with skin flaps which are taken from above the clavicle. However, when a large soft tissue coverage is required, it is necessary to obtain the flap from below this region and a less suitable color match can be expected. The options are pedicled flaps such as the delto pectoral and acromiothoracic flap, and free flaps such as the groin, scapular, forearm or delto pectoral flap.

The free delto pectoral flap, which has been proposed by Harii, may provide the best color match of the free flaps available. This flap is based on the small 2nd or 3rd perforating artery of the internal mammary and drained by a vena comitans. The transverse flap axis passes laterally from the sternum through the 2nd or 3rd interspace towards the shoulder. Unfortunately, the venae comitantes are small and may be inadequate for flap drainage. The donor site scar is a significant disadvantage in this flap. For the very large defect, the groin flap will provide reliable coverage. However, in Caucasians, the color match is not ideal, often pale and yellowish - a significant drawback. However, the color of the flap tends to improve over time with exposure to sun and wind (Fig. 12-3 a, b).

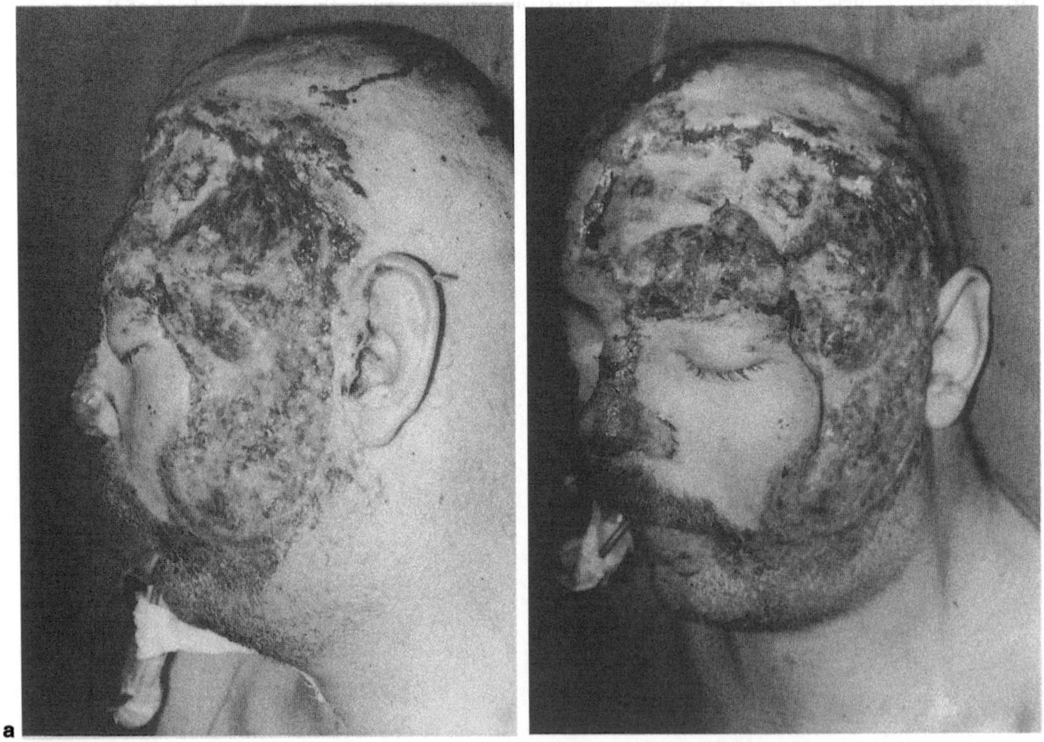

a b

Fig. 12-1 a, b. During a motor vehicle accident, this man lost the skin and subcutaneous tissue from 2/3rds of his forehead, the left temple, and left cheek. The frontal bone and body of zygoma are exposed

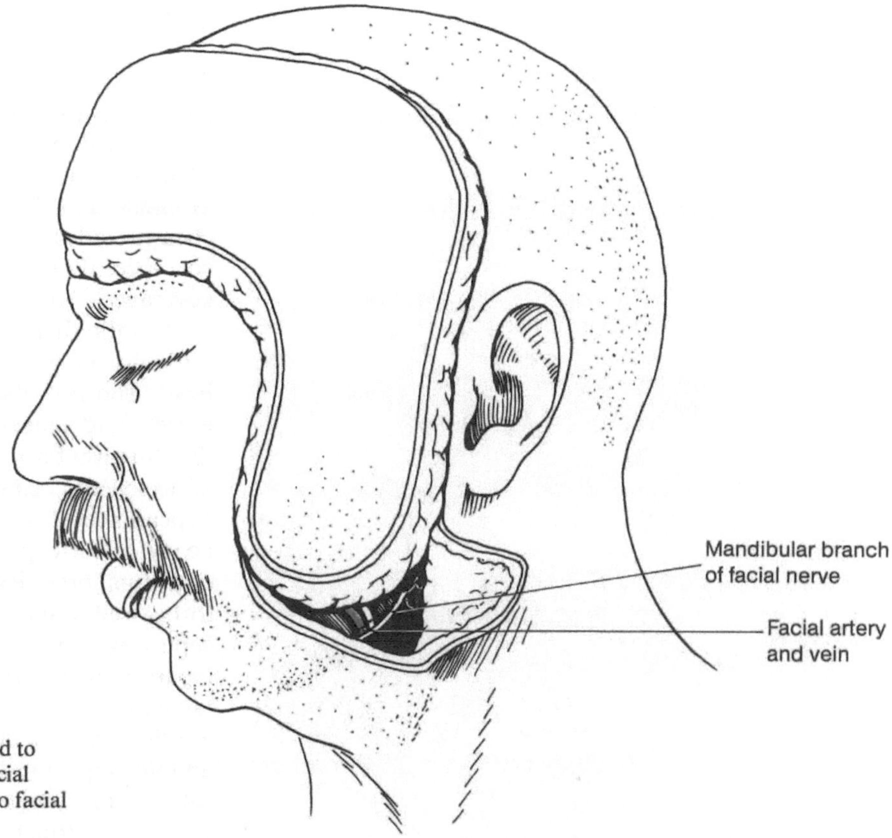

Fig. 12-2. Groin flap transplanted to face with anastomosis of superficial circumflex iliac artery and vein to facial artery and vein

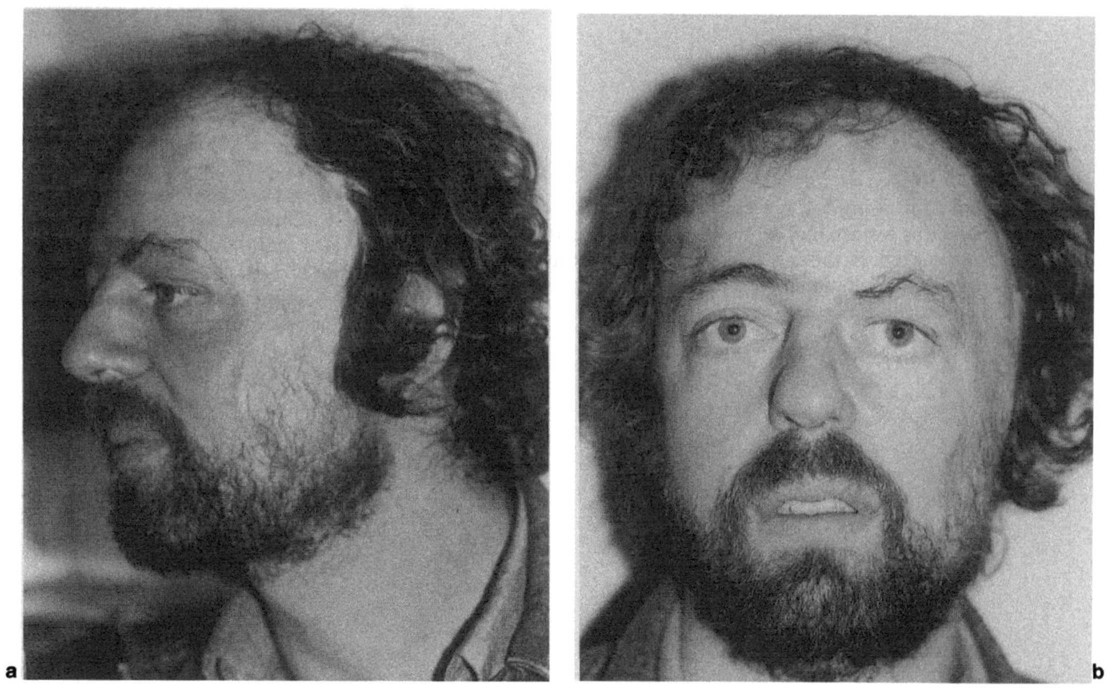

Fig. 12-3 a, b. Patient's appearance after cheek defatting, eyebrow reconstruction with hair transplantation, and a sideburn reconstruction with postauricular scalp flap. After suntanning the flap, the color is acceptable but still not as pink as normal cheek skin

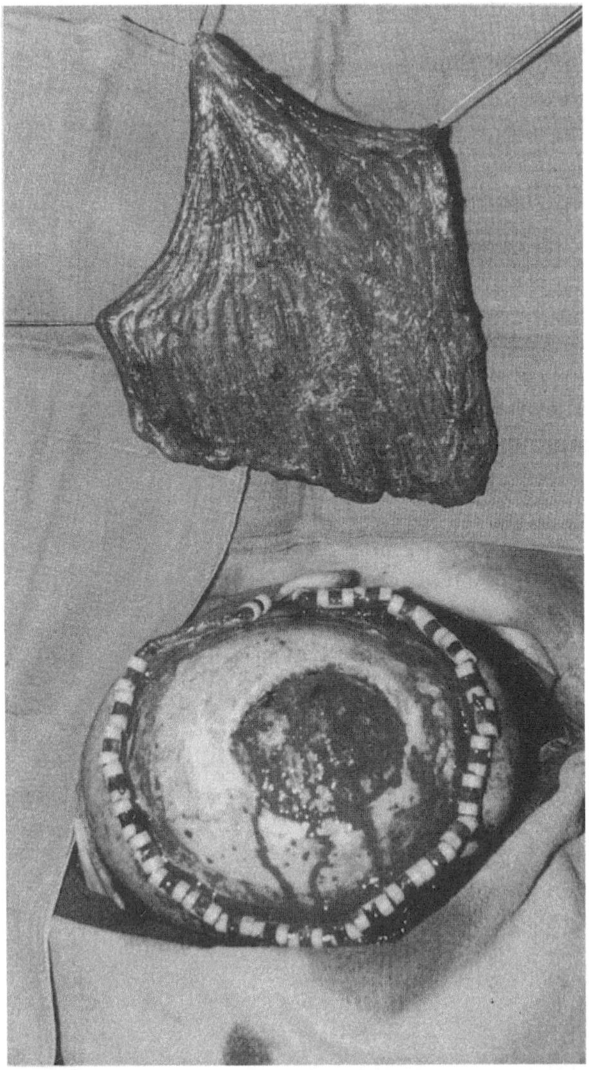

Fig. 12-4. Following a recurrent eccrine adenocarcinoma of the scalp, this woman had a 16 × 16 cm area of scalp and periosteum resected. In the central area, the outer cortex of skull was removed. A latissimus dorsi muscle has been prepared for scalp coverage

Scalp Coverage

The first choice for flap coverage of scalp defects is the adjacent scalp itself. Considerable coverage can be obtained by undermining, incising the galea, and designing the flaps for maximum sharing of the available skin. The banana flap procedure of Orticochea provides a surprisingly large amount of scalp coverage. When local skin is not available, and flap coverage is required, a free flap should be considered as the first choice for coverage because of the difficulty in getting distant pedicled flaps to the head. The free flaps which are available are skin, muscle and omentum [2, 4]. Of the skin flaps, the thin forearm flap provides the largest coverage with an excellent cosmetic reconstruction. However, the appearance of the skin grafted donor forearm is a heavy price to pay for a good looking scalp. The omentum provides a large thin scalp which conforms well to the convex shape of the skull, and accepts a skin graft. The disadvantage is the need for a laparotomy. A surprisingly large thin flap can be obtained by using the latissimus dorsi muscle and skin grafting the surface. As the donor defect is minimal and the appearance of the reconstructed scalp is excellent, this is my preferred free tissue transfer for scalp reconstruction (Fig. 12-7).

References

1. Arnold PG, Rangerathnam CS (1982) Multiple flap scalp reconstruction: Orticochea revisited. Plast Reconstr Surg 69: 605
2. Gordon L, Buncke HJ, Alpert BS (1982) Free latissimus dorsi muscle flap with split thickness skin graft cover: a report of 16 cases. Plast Reconstr Surg 70: 173
3. Harii K, Ohmori K, Ohmori S (1974) Free delto pectoral skin flaps Br J Plast Surg 27: 231
4. McLean DH, Buncke HJ Jr (1972) Autotransplant of omentum to a large scalp defect with microsurgical revascularization. Plast Reconstr Surg 49: 268
5. Orticochea M (1971) New 3-flap reconstructive technique. Br J Plast Surg 24: 184

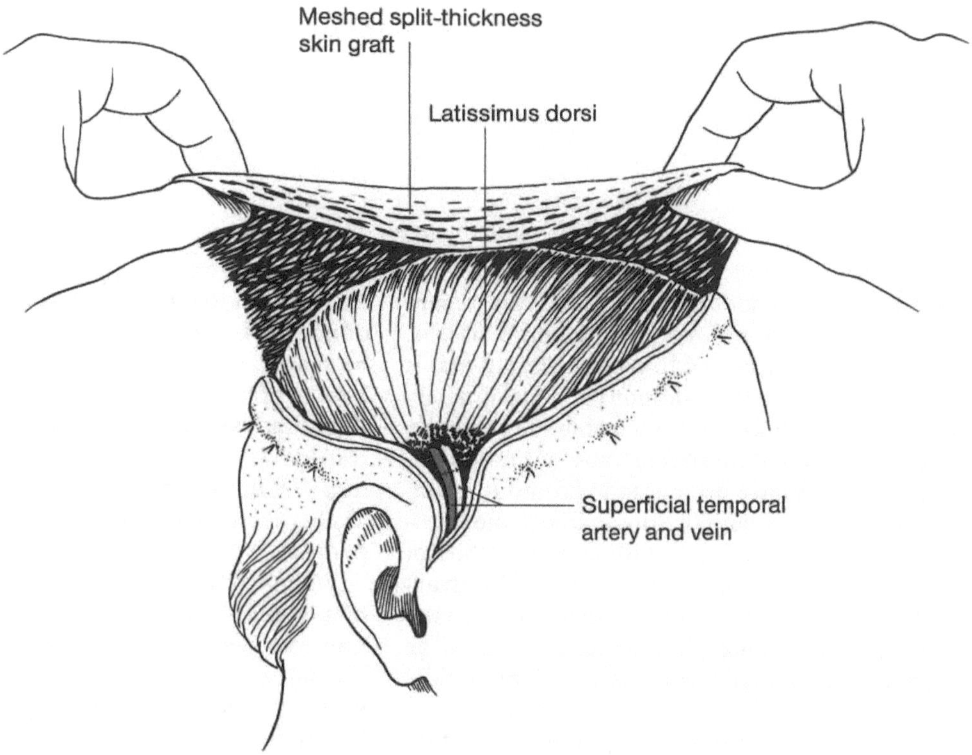

Fig. 12-5. The latissimus dorsi has been placed in the scalp defect with repair of the thoraco dorsal artery and vena comitans to the superficial temporal artery and vein. The edge of the muscle is placed beneath the undermined scalp to prevent marginal dehiscence. A sheet or meshed skin graft can be placed on the muscle

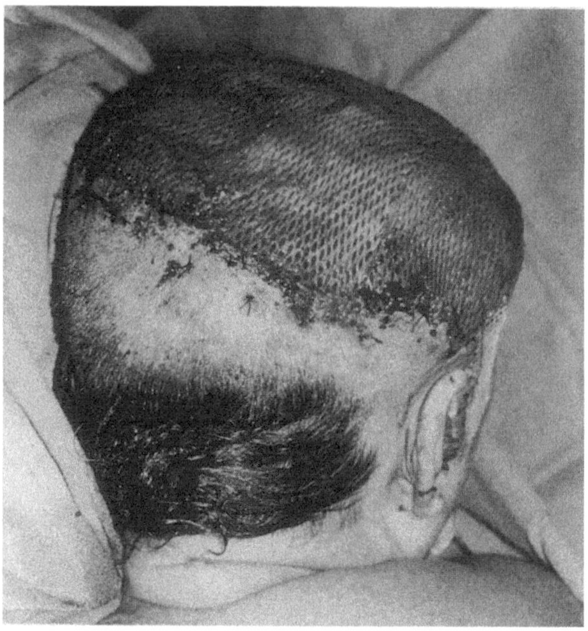

Fig. 12-6. Immediate postoperative appearance of a meshed skin graft on the latissimus dorsi transfer

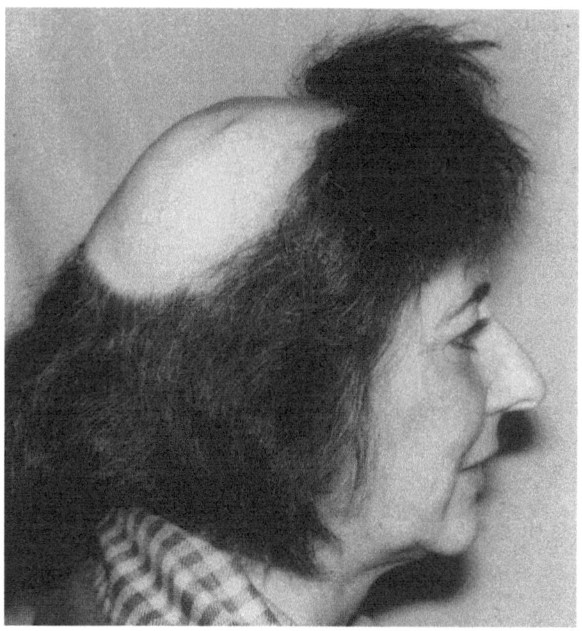

Fig. 12-7. Appearance of the scalp reconstruction one year postoperative. The flap is now approximately ½ cm thick, and has a durable skin graft cover which can easily accept a wig

Chapter 13. Facial Contour Reconstruction

Contour restoration of the face usually requires the addition of soft tissue and sometimes the reconstruction of bone. To reconstruct Romberg's disease, lateral facial dysplasia, and lipodystrophy, all that is usually required is the addition of appropriately placed soft tissue bulk. The best technique to supply soft tissue is a buried free tissue transfer. De-epithelialized skin flaps have been used for contour reconstruction for many years [3]. Prior to free tissue transfer, the awkward waltzing or wrist carrier method of getting the flap into the face was a major disadvantage. With the techniques of microvascular anastomoses, the flap is placed in the face in a one stage procedure. A second procedure is necessary for final contouring.

Different tissues have been employed for contour reconstruction including the omentum, muscle, and skin flaps. The de-epithelialized groin skin flap has certain advantages which make it my preferred choice over other transfers. It can be cut to fit the shape and size of the facial defect, and the presence of dermis allows secure fixation of each finger of the flap into each recess in the facial pocket. The final result is a soft smooth reconstruction which does not droop, and gives the patient a near normal texture and contour to the face. The defect from a groin flap donor site is minimal. Muscle and omentum cannot be shaped easily to fit the facial pocket. Unpredictable atrophy and the need for a laparotomy are further disadvantages of muscle and omental transfers respectively. However, both muscle and omental transfers have large reliable pedicles which are more easily prepared and anastomosed than the groin flap pedicle.

When a buried groin flap is used, a medial ellipse of skin is left on the flap. This skin provides a window to observe the postoperative vascular supply to the flap and prevents a too tight closure of the cheek skin. At a second operative sitting, 2–4 months after the transfer, the ellipse of flap skin and excess submandibular fat is excised. In Romberg's disease, it may be best if the condition has burnt out before the reconstruction is done. The appropriate time is usually in the late second or early third decade. This procedure has been used for children with facial lipodystrophy with the expectation that the flap will grow with the child.

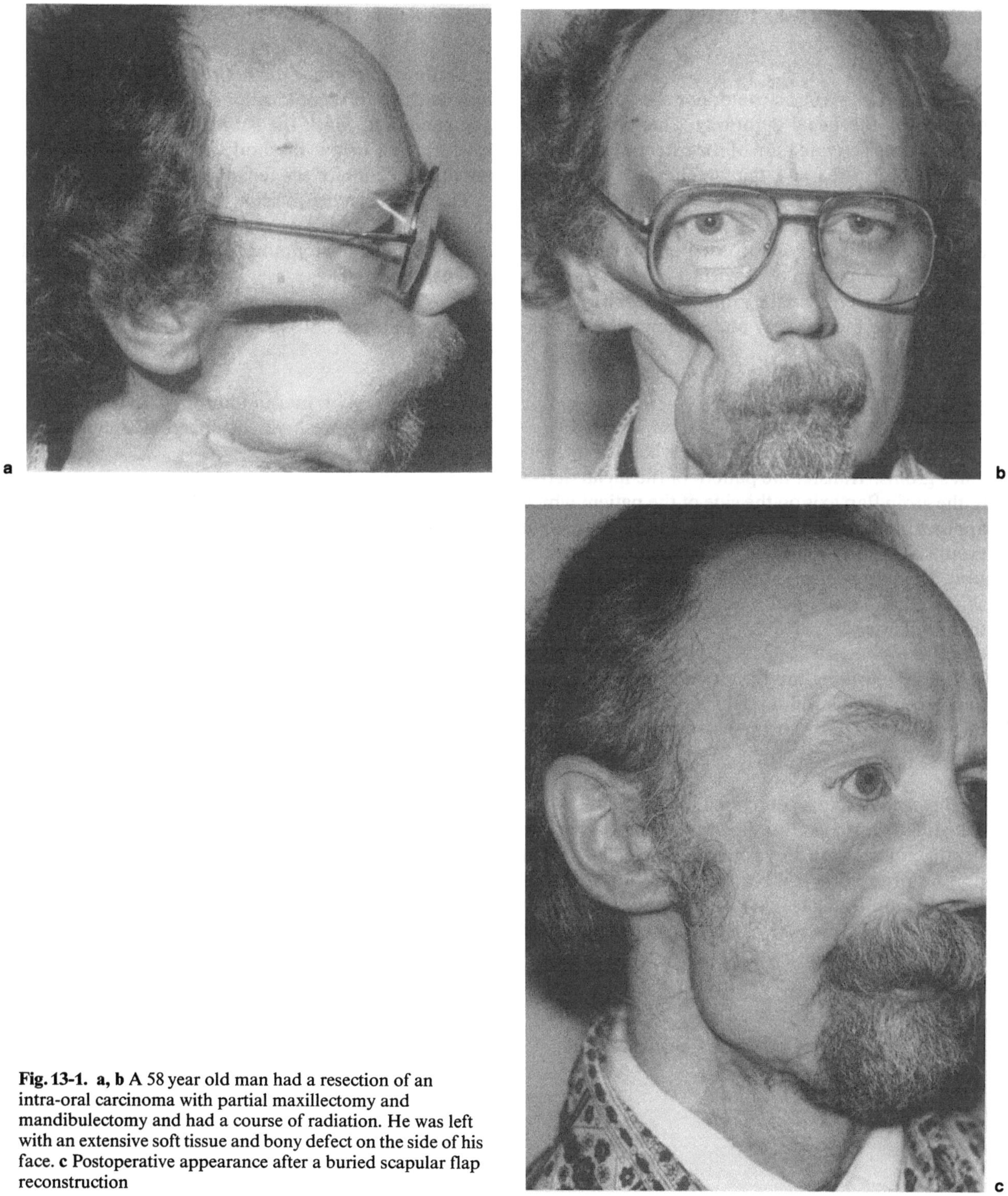

Fig. 13-1. a, b A 58 year old man had a resection of an intra-oral carcinoma with partial maxillectomy and mandibulectomy and had a course of radiation. He was left with an extensive soft tissue and bony defect on the side of his face. **c** Postoperative appearance after a buried scapular flap reconstruction

Technique of Soft Tissue Facial Contour Reconstruction

The groin flap is cut on the donor site to the shape dictated by the facial deformity. This objective requires a precise evaluation of the extent of the deformity, in both area and depth. The face is viewed from cephalad and caudad to assist in depth determination, and the desired depth of augmentation in each area of the face is recorded on the facial skin (Fig. 13-2a). A pattern of the defect is taken from the face and transferred to the groin (Fig. 13-2b). The location of the facial artery and submandibular incision are marked.

Elevation of Groin Flap

1. Mark the axis of the groin flap on each of the patient's groins. Transfer the pattern of the facial defect to the groin flap axis on the side of the patient which appears more suitable. Plan an ellipse of medial groin skin which will lie in the submandibular incision. The flap pedicle should lie under this ellipse of skin so that it will be in a position to be sutured to the facial artery.

2. Before elevating the flap, remove the epidermis and upper dermis with a scalpel in the area that will be buried, leaving the medial ellipse of skin untouched.

3. Elevate the flap as described in Chapter 2. When elevating from lateral to medial, lift the flap at the depth indicated on the pattern. When the medial portion of the flap is elevated, the full thickness of the flap must be taken in order to include the pedicle (Fig. 13-3a, b). This excess of fat may be debulked at the second operation.

Preparation of the Face

1. Outline on the face the desired area of augmentation, and, at different locations, the desired depth of augmentation. Mark the submandibular incision at least 1-2 cm below the body of the mandible and note the location of the facial artery.

The preauricular incision is preferred if only a cheek augmentation is required. However, usually the lower eyelid, circumoral and chin area will need augmentation. These areas are the most difficult ones to augment precisely and are too distant from a preauricular incision to be visualized adequately (Fig. 13-2a).

2. Carry the skin incision through the platysma. Watch for and preserve the marginal mandibular branch of the facial nerve.

3. Identify and prepare the facial artery and vein for anastomoses.

4. Develop a plane of dissection immediately superficial to the masseter fascia. Note the major branches of the facial nerve which exit from the medial margin of the parotid gland, and keep them on the deep surface of the dissection. Using blunt scissor dissection, long thin right angle retractors, and a headlight, develop a pocket which extends 1 cm beyond the area of desired augmentation. Observe and preserve the buccal branches of the facial nerve passing from a deep to a superficial plane near the corner of the mouth. Careful hemostasis is necessary throughout the dissection.

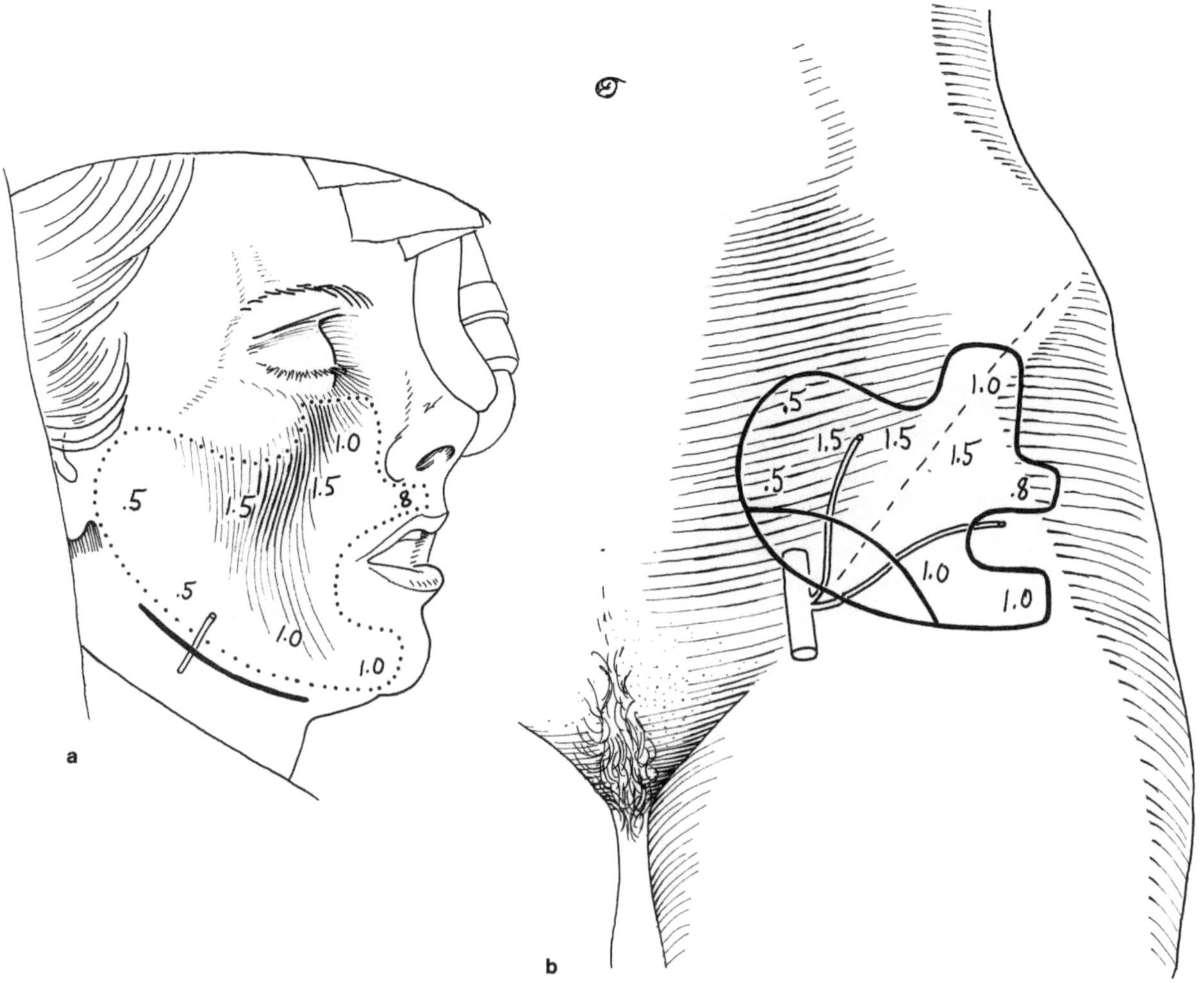

Fig. 13-2. a This patient, with Romberg's disease, has marked atrophy of the subcutaneous tissues on the right side of the face, including the lips, chin, cheek and lower eyelid. The area which requires augmentation is outlined by a dotted line. The estimated depth in centimeters which is required to augment each area is marked on the face. The submandibular incision is placed at least 1 cm below the margin of the mandible. A pattern of these facial markings is taken and transferred to the groin. **b** The pattern from the face is transferred to the left groin and centred on the groin flap axis (dashed line). Either the DCIA or SEA will be used as the pedicle, depending on which vessel is larger. An ellipse of skin is marked on the infero medial aspect of the flap to fit into the submandibular incision

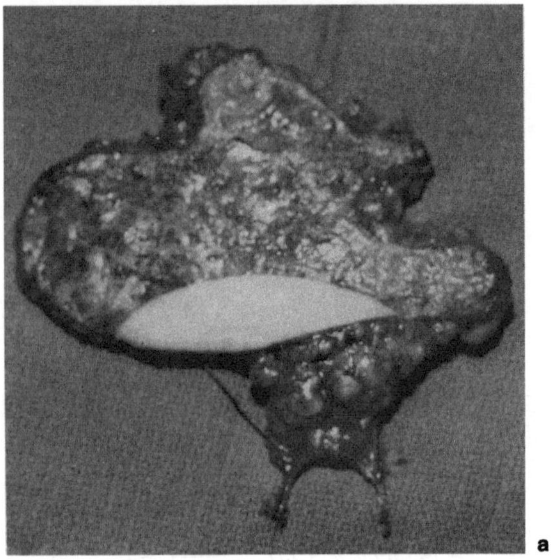

a

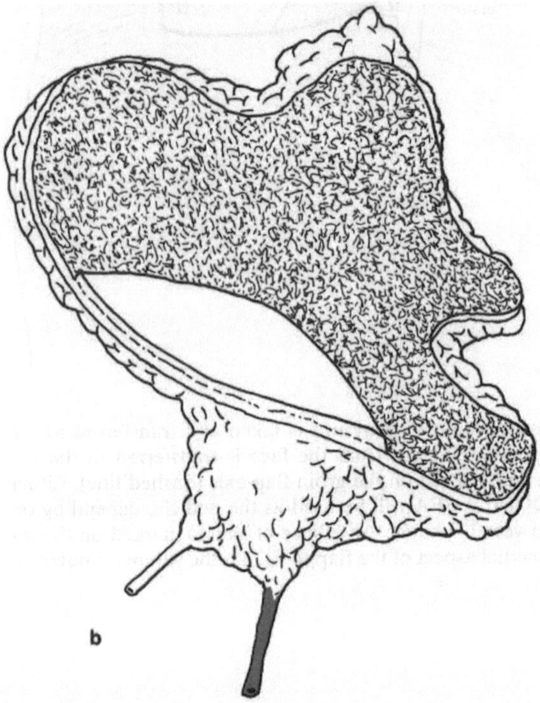

b

Fig. 13-3 a, b. Groin flap, cut to the shape of the pattern and prepared for transfer. The elliptical skin window is seen inferiorly and the rest of the skin has been de-epithelialized

Transfer of Groin Flap

1. Place the flap on the defect on the patient's face and evaluate the size and thickness. Trim it further, if necessary, except in the area of the pedicle.

2. At the completion of the procedure, the flap will be held into the facial pocket with long stay sutures. Insert the stay sutures now with a long Keith needle and place them through the skin 1-2 cm beyond the limits of the pocket. Draw the flap into the pocket for a trial fit. With the flap in the pocket, evaluate the appearance of the reconstruction in each area of the face. Remove the flap and trim it further if necessary.

The area in and beneath the lower eyelid is the most difficult to augment adequately. The force of gravity results in some postoperative drooping in this location. Therefore, make the pocket generous, insert more bulk than you think necessary, and place the stay sutures on either side of the eye above the level of the canthi (Fig. 13-4 a).

3. Remove the flap from the pocket, leaving the stay sutures still attached, and lay the flap on the patient's neck with the fat side up. This position allows excellent exposure for the anastomoses which are usually end to end repairs between the artery and vein of the groin flap and the facial artery and vein, and usually have an excellent size match.

4. Following the anastomoses, observe the flap for perfusion and obtain final hemostasis of the flap margins. Gently slip it into the pocket like the page of a book, and pull the margins of the flap snugly into place by suturing the stay sutures over gauze boluses on the skin (Fig. 13-4 a-c). Lift the inferior part of the flap and observe the position of the vessels. If they were left too long at the time of anastomosis, they may be kinked. This possible problem should be anticipated prior to the anastomosis.

5. Insert drains at positions distant from the flap vessels and suture the skin island into the submandibular incision.

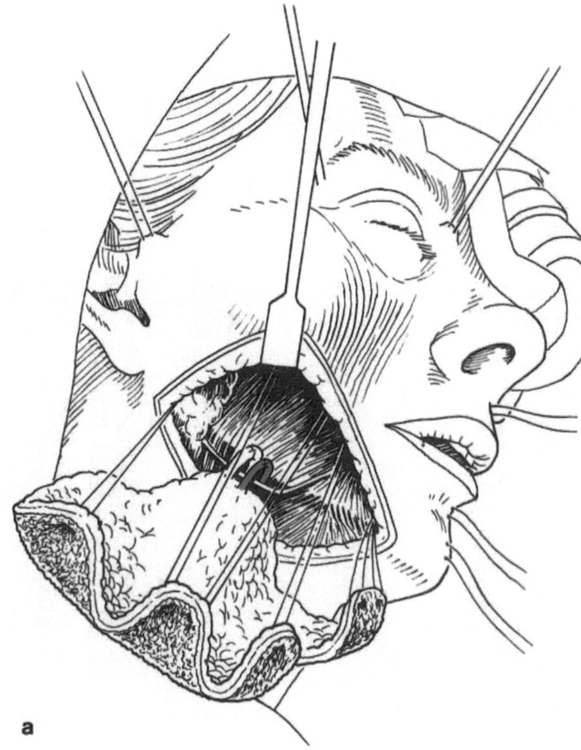

a

Fig. 13-4. a, b Following the microanastomoses, the flap, which has been lying on the patient's neck, is turned and slipped into the facial pocket. It is held in place with long stay sutures which were placed prior to the anastomoses and positioned well beyond the margins of the facial pocket c The stay sutures are tied over pads and the ellipse of skin is set into the submandibular incision.

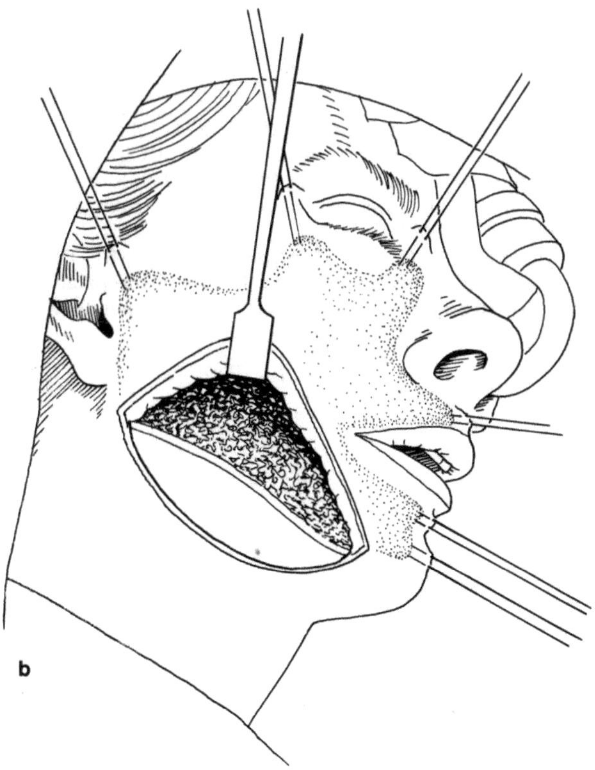

b

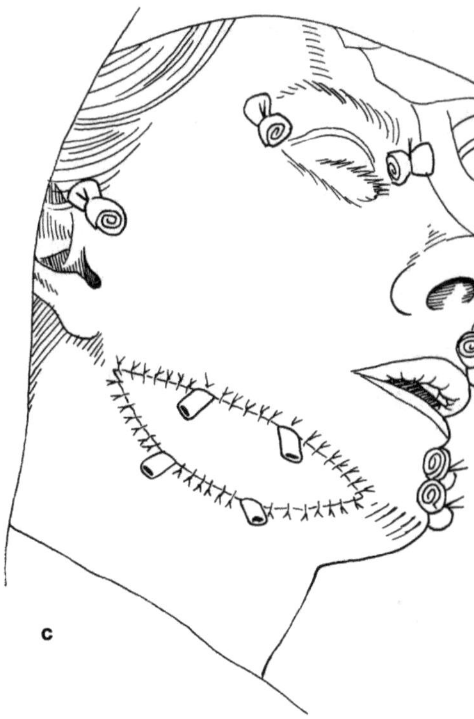

c

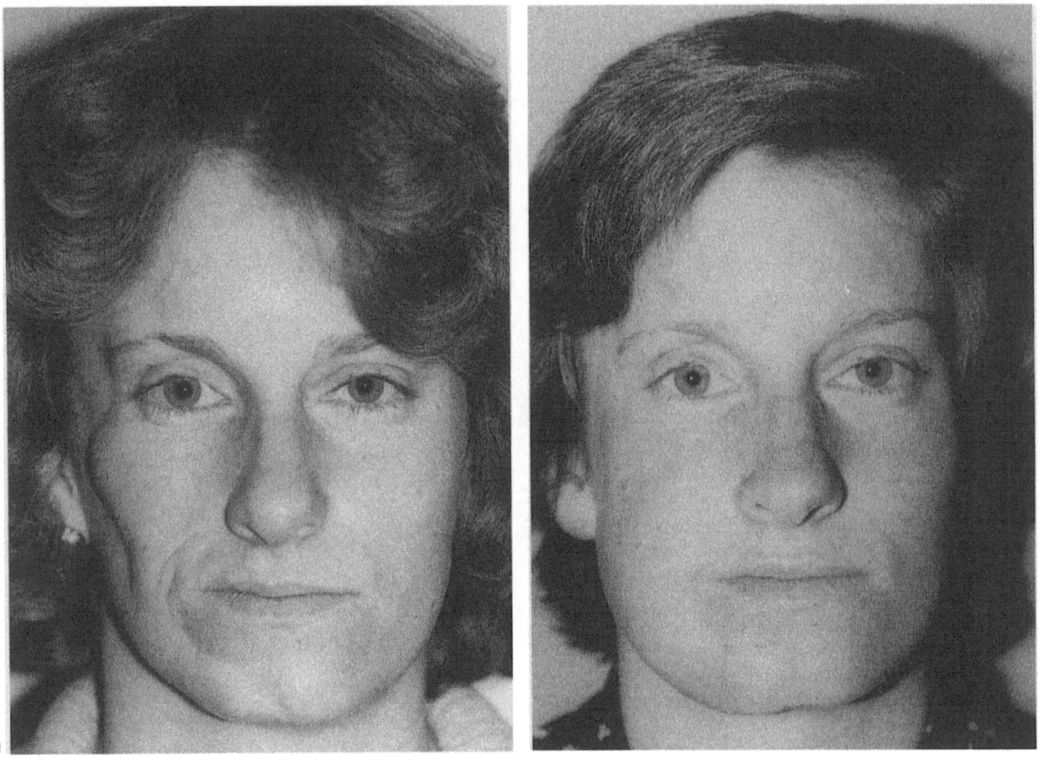

a b

Fig. 13-5. **a** A 26 year old woman, with stable Romberg's disease, has marked soft tissue atrophy of the temple, cheek, lower eyelid, lips and chin. **b** Postoperative appearance after a buried groin flap reconstruction and second stage skin ellipse and fat removal

References

1. Harashima T, Nakajima T, Yoshimura Y (1977) A free groin flap reconstruction in progressive facial hemiatrophy. Br J Plast Surg 30: 14
2. Jurkiewicz MJ (1980) Discussion Restoration of Facial Contour Using Free Vascularized Omental Transfer Plast Reconstr Surg 66: 568
3. Newmann CG (1952) The use of large buried pedicled flaps of dermis and fat. Clinical and pathological evaluation in the treatment of progressive facial hemiatrophy. Plast Reconstr Surg 11: 315
4. Tweed AEJ, Manktelow RT, Zuker RM (1984) Facial contour reconstruction with free flaps Ann Plast Surg 12: 313
5. Upton J, Milliken JB, Hicks, PD et al. (1980) Restoration of facial contour using free vascularized omentum Plast Reconstr Surg 66: 560
6. Vasconez LO, Mathes SJ, Alpert BS et al. (1981) The contouring of soft tissue defects in the face: a comparative retrospective study utilizing dermis grafts and muscle as pedicled or free flaps Plast Surg Forum 4: 220

Chapter 14. Intra-Oral Reconstruction

The reconstruction of intra-oral lining is commonly required after tumor resection. For major defects, the choice is between a pedicled flap such as the pectoralis major, latissimus dorsi, trapezius or delto pectoral flap and a free tissue transfer. When a lateral mandibulectomy has been done, a pedicled myocutaneous flap often provides a good reconstruction with the bulk of the muscle filling out the side of the face in the region of the mandible. However, if a portion of the mandible has not been resected, the muscle bulk of these flaps is often excessive and a free tissue transfer may be preferable.

A trend in head and neck tumor surgery is to have a two team approach. One team does the exterpation and the other carries out the transfer. In this way, the microvascular team can prepare the transfer while the exterpation is taking place and be prepared to begin the reconstruction immediately following tumor removal. With this type of simultaneous team work, the exterpative surgeon estimates the maximum size of tumor which will be removed in order that the reconstructive team may begin elevating a flap that will be large enough for the maximum defect created. A large tumor may require excision of multiple structures, including the external facial skin, buccal mucosa, maxilla, mandible, roof and floor of mouth, tongue and palate. The exterpative surgeon is at ease knowing that as much tissue as necessary can be removed to provide a good tumor cure operation without having to worry about the problems of closing and reconstructing the defect.

Selection of Appropriate Free Tissue Transfer

The choice of free tissue transfers for replacement of intra- oral lining is between cutaneous flaps from the groin, forearm or dorsal foot and an opened segment of jejunum.

The groin flap is frequently bulky, has a short pedicle and is not commonly used in this location. The dorsal foot flap provides a thin, malleable piece of skin which conforms well to the intra-oral cavity. However, the need to keep the patient in bed for 10 days to obtain a skin graft take on the foot is a disadvantage of this flap. The forearm can yield a larger piece of skin than the dorsal foot flap. It is particularly thin if taken from the distal forearm and fatter when taken proximally. There is a long reliable pedicle which will reach vessels in the neck. However, the visible donor site is often objectionable to women. When the radial volar forearm is particularly hairy, the flap may be based on the ulnar artery where the overlying skin is less hirsute.

The jejunum has a reliable pedicle, is well-vascularized and provides an unusually pliable piece of tissue which conforms well to the irregularly shaped defects which are often produced by intra-oral tumor resection. The jejunum will produce mucous which may be helpful in the patient who has a dry mouth from previous radiation and there is often a persistence of jejunal folds.

Technique of Intra-Oral Lining with a Free Tissue Transfer

Preparation of the Oral Cavity

The most common arteries used are the facial, the superior thyroid, and the external carotid. Unless a radical neck dissection with removal of the internal jugular has been done, there are usually many veins available, including the facial, superior thyroid and external jugular. If the internal jugular vein has been removed, prepare an anterior jugular vein or a vein on the other side of the neck. Evaluate the intended recipient vessels under magnification to be sure that they are undamaged. The artery should provide a vigorous spurt if it is suitable for microvascular repair.

Free Tissue Transfer to Oral Cavity

1. After removing the tissue transfer [forearm skin - Chap. 4, dorsal foot skin - Chap. 3, or jejunum - Chap. 15], tack it loosely in place. By placing the flap in its correct location before doing the anastomoses, you can ensure that the pedicle will be neither too tight nor too redundant.

If vessels on the face, such as the facial artery and vein, are used, movements of the head will not produce traction on the pedicle. However, if the pedicle is brought down from the oral cavity for anastomosis to a neck vein, rotation movements of the neck postoperatively may produce traction on the pedicle if it is too short. Evaluate this possibility by rotating the head from side to side while observing the pedicle.

2. Select the best route for the pedicle. There are two routes for pedicle placement to neck vessels, such as the superior thyroid artery and vein: lateral to the mandible or down through the floor of the mouth, medial to the mandible. The latter is the more direct route. However, postoperative edema of the tongue may produce compression of the pedicle against the unyielding mandible and result in venous engorgement. If the pedicle is brought over the outside of the mandible, this problem will not occur.

3. Do the anastomoses in the usual manner, usually as end to end repairs.

4. Following the successful completion of the anastomoses, evaluate the transfer and be sure that the entire transfer is perfusing well. Any tissue that does not have good perfusion should be removed prior to being inserted in the oral cavity.

5. Begin suturing the flap at the posterior and medial margins of the defect. Do the final trimming of the flap as you insert it. Replace the cheek flaps while suturing the lateral and anterior portions of the flap in place. Use a two-layered closure as it is more reliable in protecting the wound from breakdown. The area most sensitive to breakdown is the suture line over the mandible.

6. Close the neck flaps, and insert suction drains with care to ensure that they cannot slide onto the pedicle and obstruct it. If a tracheostomy is used, sew the flanges of the tracheostomy tube to the neck. Tie tapes placed around the neck may produce venous obstruction. Elevate the head of the bed to minimize postoperative edema.

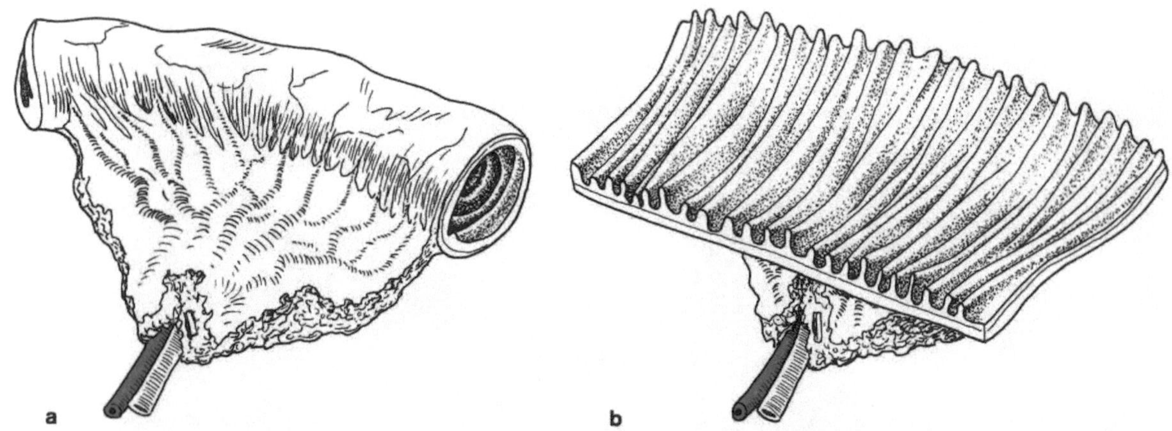

Fig. 14-1 a, b. The jejunum, when opened on its antimesenteric border, provides a large piece of supple, well-vascularized tissue which is suitable for intra-oral lining

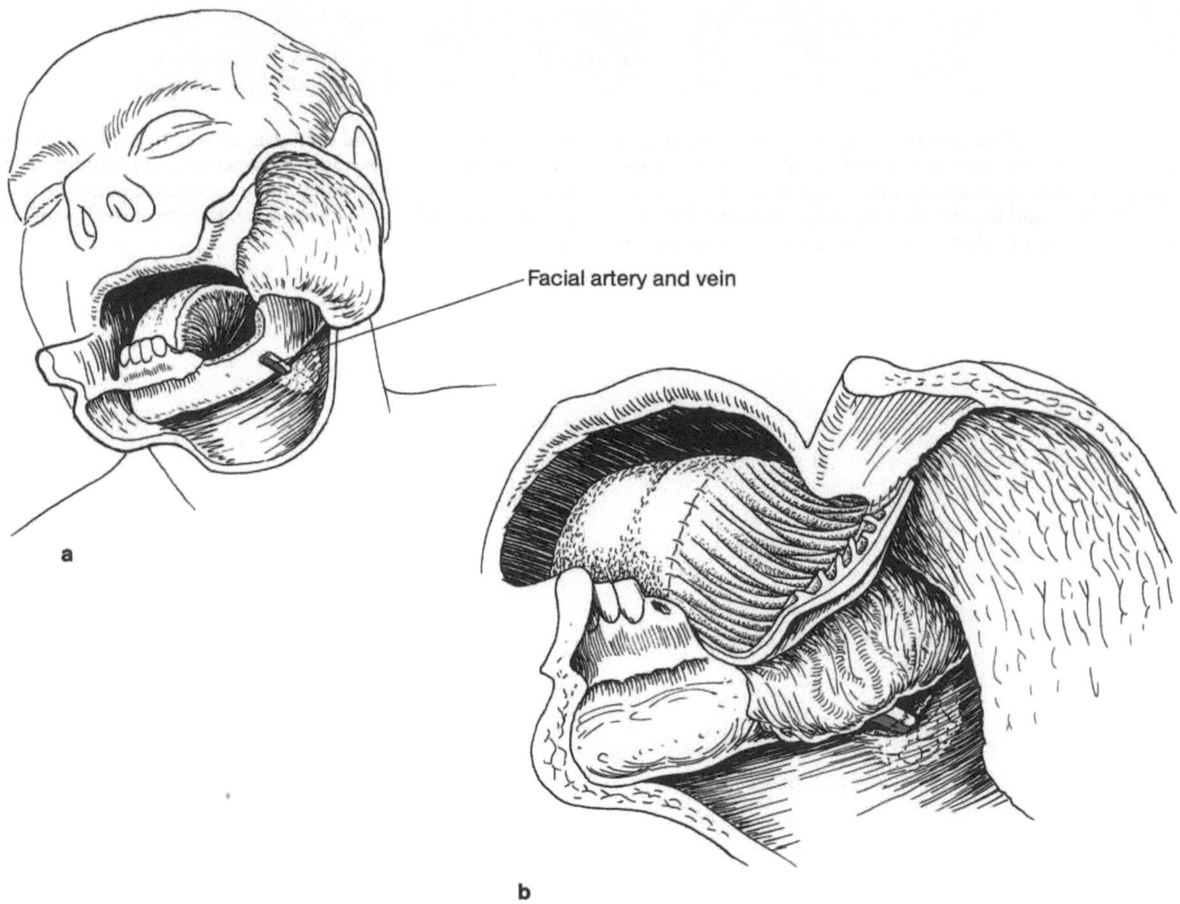

Fig. 14-2. **a** The patient had a tumor of the left alveolar margin which required marginal mandibular resection and resection of the left floor of mouth, margin of tongue and left buccal mucosa. The facial artery and vein will be used as recipient vessels. **b** The opened jejunum has been set into the floor of mouth and sutured to the tongue and buccal mucosa. Anastomoses between the mesenteric and facial vessels are seen beneath the mesenteric fat

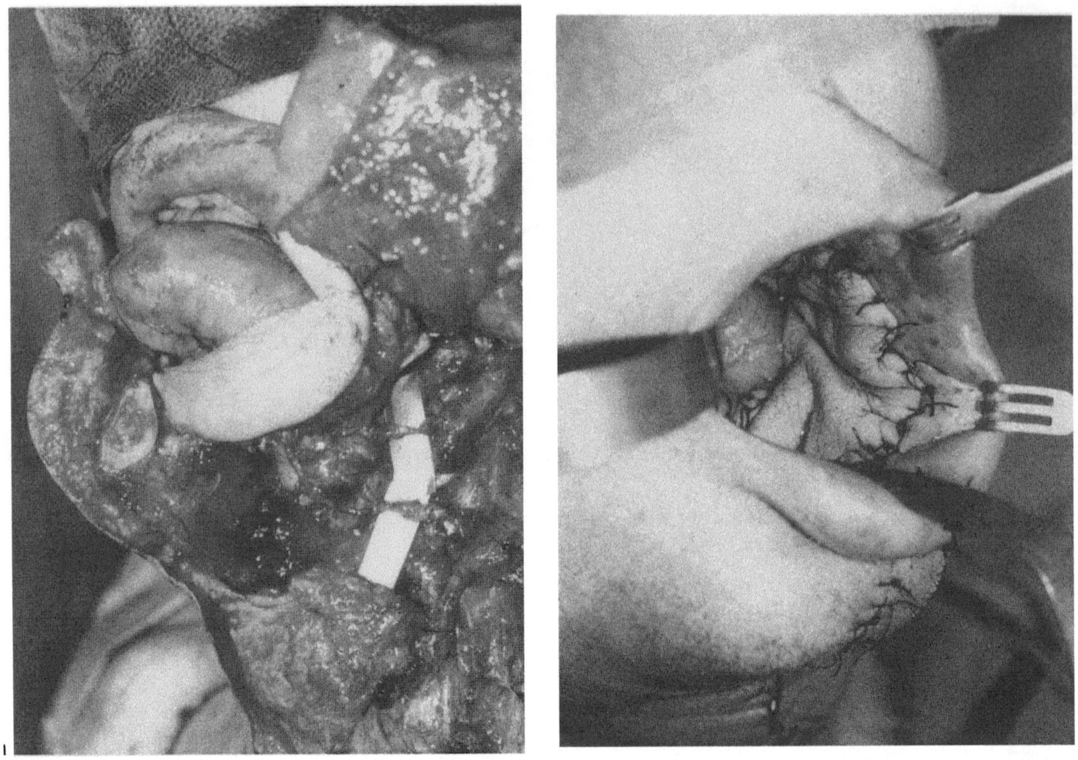

Fig. 14-3. a This patient is seen immediately following a tumor resection of the left floor of mouth and left mandible. A soft tissue reconstruction has been done to provide lining for the floor of mouth and buccal mucosa, using the dorsal foot skin flap, which is now in place. Anastomoses are seen between the dorsalis pedis artery and the facial artery, the saphenous vein and facial vein. **b** Immediate postoperative appearance of the dorsal foot flap after completion of its insertion into the floor of the mouth and buccal mucosa and closure of the lip-split incision

Chapter 15. Esophagus Reconstruction

Portions of the gastrointestinal tract may be used as microvascular transfers for reconstruction of the hypopharynx and esophagus. The colon, jejunum and portions of the stomach have been successfully used. For most reconstructive problems, the jejunum provides the most suitable tissue. Its vascularity is reliable and it can be removed with minimal morbidity. It provides a tubular transfer which is the right size for esophageal reconstruction (Fig. 15-1).

Intestinal transfer by revascularization was reported by Seidenberg in 1959, long before the development of other free tissue transfers [10]. Although repeated by others, the technique of free intestinal transfer did not become popular until microvascular techniques were available to ensure the reliability of the procedure [1-9].

Anatomy of the Jejunum

When an appropriate piece of jejunum is being selected for transfer, the important considerations are its shape and its vascular supply. Because of the multiple curves of the jejunum, it is difficult to obtain a straight length which is longer than 12-15 cm without separating it from its mesentery at both ends. A useful method of straightening the curvature of the selected segment of jejunum is to place multiple incisions through the peritoneum tangential to the bowel. If a longer piece of bowel is needed, two vascular pedicles may be necessary.

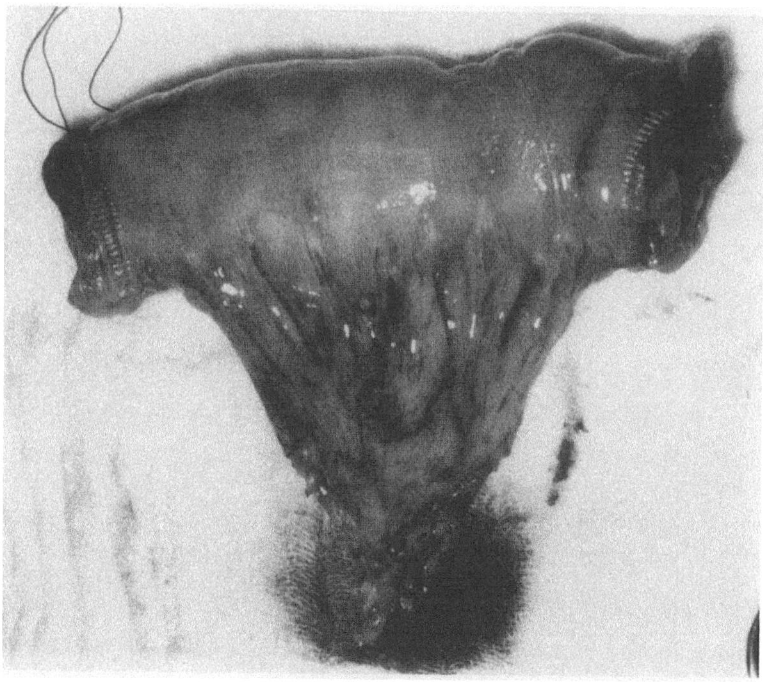

Fig. 15-1. A 12 cm length of jejunum, prepared for transplantation - the ideal replacement for a segment of GI tract

The vessels supplying the jejunum are branches of the superior mesenteric artery. These branches join peripherally to form vascular arches. Each arch gives off branches which join to form a more peripheral group of arches. This system of arches and multiple branches ends with many parallel branches which enter the bowel at right angles (Fig. 15-2). The pattern of branching most suitable for transfer on a single pedicle is usually found in the proximal jejunum. In this region, there are many groups of arteries running in the mesentery at right angles to the jejunum for a distance of 3-5 cm and originating from a common arch. A single artery can readily be found which feeds this arch. This vessel is used as the pedicle. The venous system is an exact parallel of the arterial system.

Technique of Esophageal Reconstruction with Jejunum

1. Do a laparotomy and identify the small bowel.

2. If the vascular pattern is partially obscured by mesenteric fat, lift the jejunum out of the abdomen and transilluminate it with an operating room light (Fig. 15-3,4). With transillumination, it is possible to ensure that the vessel to be anastomosed will supply the entire piece of jejunum to be transferred.

3. Select a straight piece of jejunum with a suitable vascular pattern. Take a pie shaped sector of mesentery which includes the desired vascular network, with the pedicle at the apex. Cross clamp the jejunum with rubber shod clamps on each side of the segment selected and divide the jejunum.

4. Leave the jejunal segment sitting in the abdomen, attached by only its vascular pedicle, in order that its perfusion can be observed. Suture the bowel with a double-layered closure and suture the rent in the mesentery to prevent herniation of the bowel. After evaluating the perfusion of the jejunal segment, divide the pedicle.

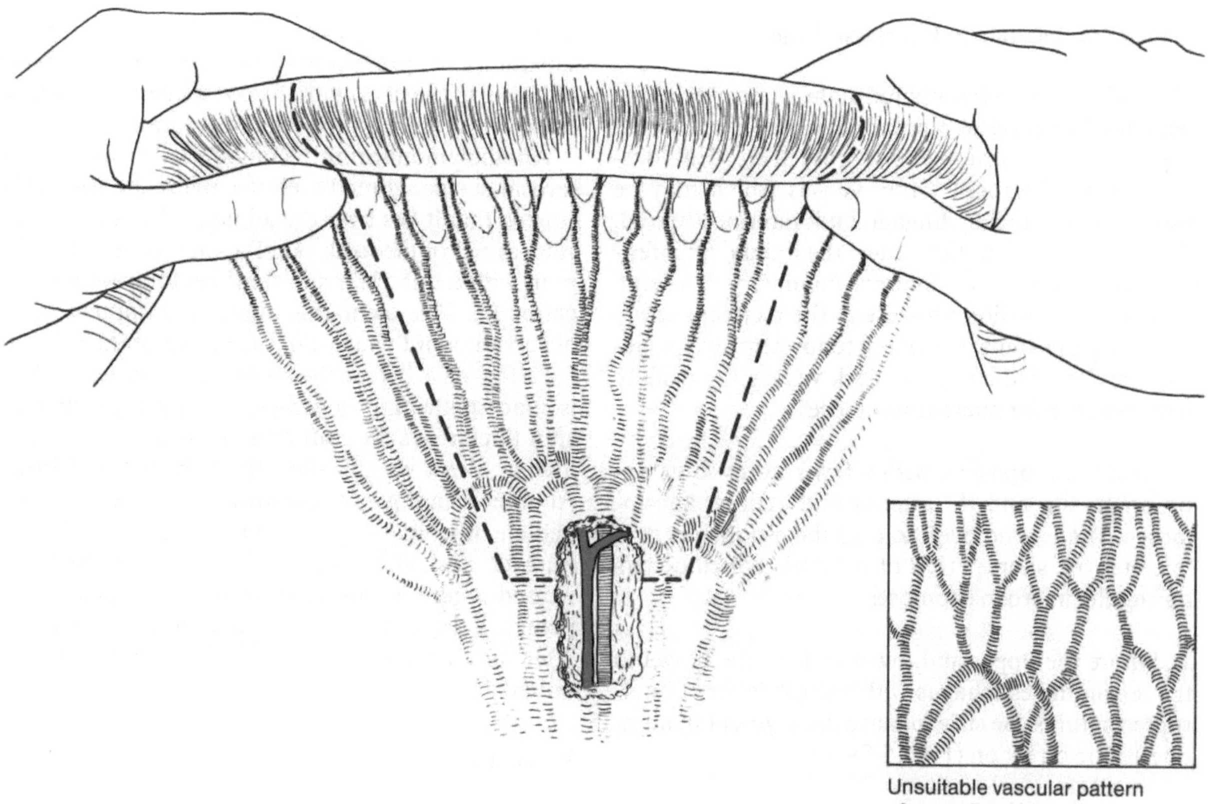

Fig. 15-2. When the proximal intact jejunum is lifted from the abdomen, the vascular pattern becomes apparent. The dotted line indicates the area of resection. The vascular pattern seen in the box illustrates the less suitable pattern found in the mesentery of the distal jejunum

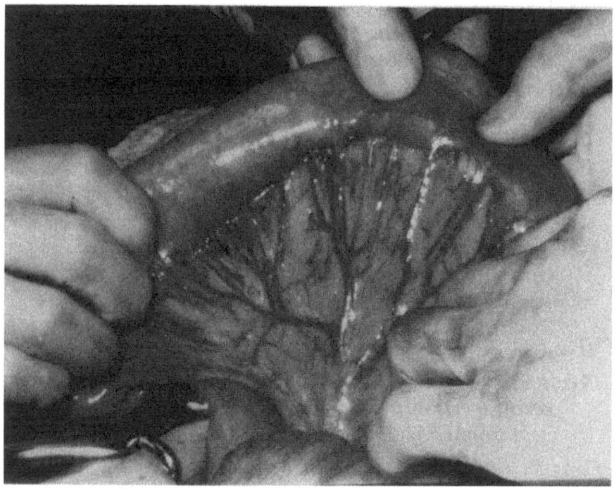

Fig. 15-3. The intact jejunum is examined for a suitable segment for transplantation.

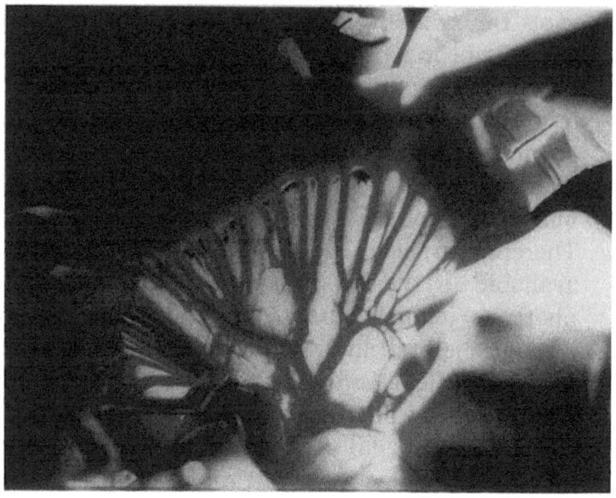

Fig. 15-4. Trans-illumination of the mesentery aids in visualizing the vascular pattern

Transfer of Jejunum to Pharyngo Esophagus

The recipient area is prepared at the same time as the jejunum. For cervical esophageal reconstruction, the superior thyroid artery and vein lie in an ideal location for anastomoses. Other vessels which may be used are the facial, lingual and inferior thyroid. When the reconstruction enters the thorax, an inferior vessel such as the internal mammary is useful. Assess the perfusion pressure in the recipient artery by testing the spurt. Despite arteriosclerotic changes and previous radiation, the neck vessels are usually quite reliable for microanastomoses.

1. Tack the esophagus with a few sutures to its appropriate site and do arterial and venous anastomoses. There is no need to cool the esophagus as it tolerates the short period of ischemia which occurs during the microanastomoses.

2. Suture the upper and lower ends of the bowel to the remaining esophagus with a single layer of interrupted sutures. Be sure to place the segment in an isoperistolic direction (Fig. 15-5 a, b).

3. When closing the skin, insert suction drains, keeping them away from the anastomoses.

Postoperative Care

Considerable mucous is produced by the transfer in the first few postoperative days. When the edema has settled down and the patient is swallowing fluids well, oral intake can gradually be increased to full fluids and eventually a regular diet. However, there may be significant edema for some time which prevents the swallowing of solid food. Late strictures have not been a problem with the jejunum.

It is important to monitor the jejunum following its transfer. Anastomosis thrombosis and an unrecognized gangrenous jejunum will cause a serious neck infection. If in the thorax, a gangrenous jejunum may produce a life threatening mediastinitis. Therefore, a technique of flap monitoring must be available. If the repair is sufficiently high in the pharynx, jejunal mucosa may be seen directly through the oral cavity. Otherwise, it may be visualized with a flexible fibre optic scope passed through the oral cavity once or twice a day to examine the transfer. Twice daily observation does not allow identification of a vascular problem and its correction in time to salvage the transfer. However, this observation does prevent the leaving of a necrotic piece of bowel in the neck with the consequences of subsequent wound breakdown and infection.

Another monitoring technique is to observe the serosal surface directly. Hester plans the neck incision so that it lies over the jejunum. He leaves a few sutures out of the neck skin flap and covers the jejunum with a thin clear silastic sheet to prevent desiccation [3]. This technique allows intermittent direct observation of the color of the serosa of the jejunum for a few days before the silastic is removed. If there is inadequate flap coverage, he applies a meshed split thickness skin graft directly to the jejunum, allowing direct visualization through the graft mesh. Another technique of monitoring is to create a small pedicle of jejunal mucosa attached to one end of the transfer and allow this to protrude through the wound where it can be observed. The base of the pedicle is ligated and the wound closed a few days after the transfer, when monitoring is no longer required.

References

1. Flynn MB, Acland RD (1979) Free intestinal autografts for reconstruction following pharyngo-laryngo esophagectomy. Surg Gyn Obs 149: 858
2. Germain M, Gremilet C, Patricio J (1979) Replacement of the esophagus by a jejunal loop revascularized by vascular microanastomoses. Intl J Microsurg 1: 60
3. Hester TR, McConnel FMS, Nahai F, Jurkiewicz MJ, Brown RG (1980) Reconstruction of cervical esophagus, hypopharynx and oral cavity using free jejunal transfer. Am J Surg 140: 487
4. Hiebert CA, Cummings GO (1961) Successful replacement of cervical esophagus by transplantation and revascularization of a free graft of gastric antrum. Ann Surg 51: 103
5. Jurkiewicz MJ (1965) Vascularized intestinal graft for reconstruction of the cervical esophagus and pharynx. Plast Reconstr Surg 36: 509
6. Nakayama K, Tamai T, Yamamoto K et al. (1962) A simple new apparatus for small vessel anastomoses. Surgery 52: 918
7. Peters CR, McKee DM, Barry BE (1971) Pharyngo-esophageal reconstruction with revascularized jejunal transplants. Ann Surg 121: 675
8. Roberts RE, Douglas FM (1961) Replacement of the cervical esophagus and hypopharynx by a revascularized free jejunal autograft. N Engl J Med 264: 343
9. Robinson DW, MacLeod A (1982) Microvascular free jejunum transfer Br J Plast Surg 35: 258
10. Seidenberg B, Rosemak S, Hurwitt ES (1959) Immediate reconstruction of the cervical esophagus by a revascularized isolated jejunal segment. Ann Surg 149: 162

a

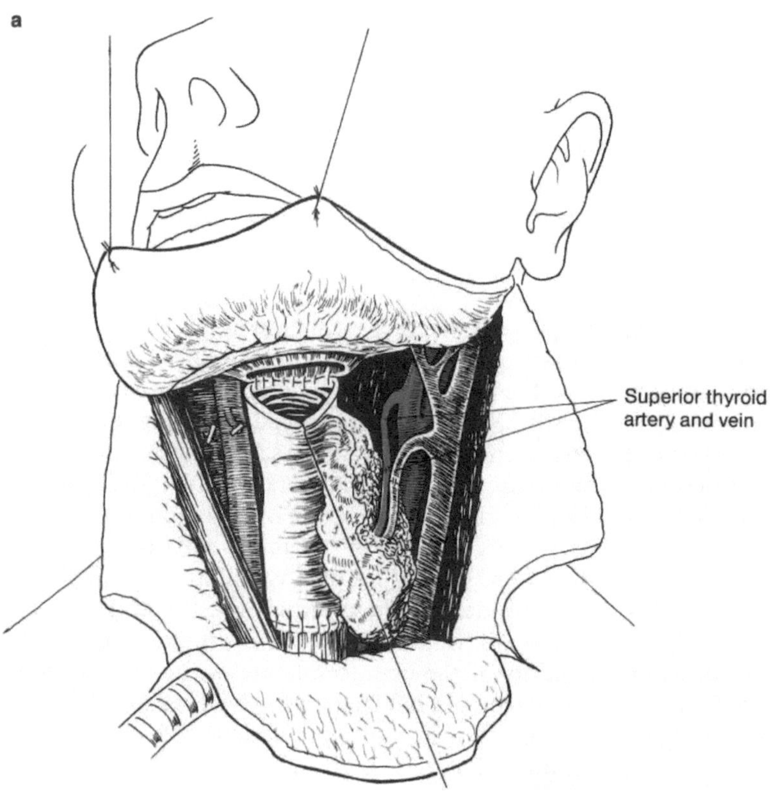

Fig. 15-5 a, b. Left antero lateral view of the neck, after a laryngopharyngectomy and cervical esophagectomy. A 12 cm length of jejunum was used to reconstruct the esophagus. The suction drain in the photo is carefully placed so that it cannot lie on the anastomoses

b

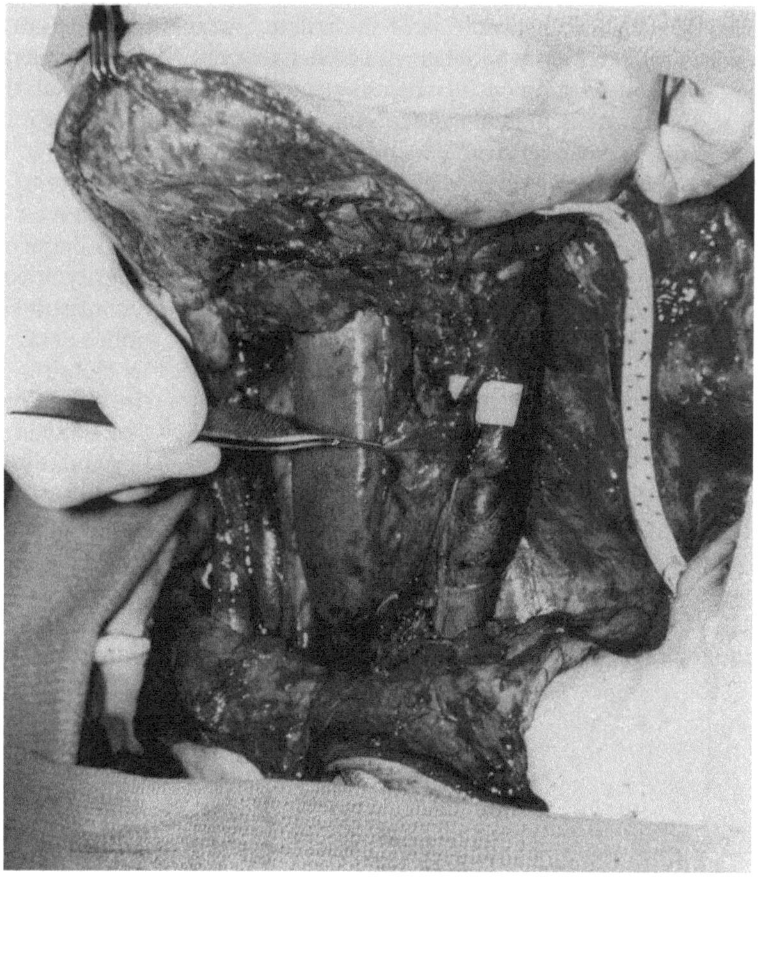

Chapter 16. Mandibular Reconstruction

Accurate reconstruction of large mandibular defects is difficult because of the mandible's complex bony shape and the usual association with intra- and extra-oral soft tissue defects. The management of the soft tissue losses is one of the biggest problems in many mandibular reconstructions. Reconstruction is commonly required following severe trauma and tumour exterpation. In these situations, the vascularity of the tissue bed in which the bone will be placed may be compromised by previous radiation, infection and scar tissue.

The objective of mandibular reconstruction should be to restore facial contour and function. With loss of the mandible, the patient has a problem with mastication, swallowing, retention of saliva, and speech. These functional problems are compounded by associated defects of the palate, pharynx and tongue. Many patients who have had mandibular reconstruction wish to be able to wear dentures. They pose a particularly difficult challenge to the reconstructive surgeon and dental prosthetist. Prior to commencing surgery, the surgeon should establish with the patient a realistic set of reconstructive goals with reasonable functional expectations.

The reconstruction of a mandibular defect may be achieved with a foreign material or an autogenous substance. The foreign materials which are available include the unsophisticated but useful k-wire, various acrylic and silastic reconstructions, and sophisticated pre-formed metallic carbon and plastic prostheses. Although many of these materials have a place in mandibular reconstruction, their usefulness is often short term as they have a high incidence of extrusion or exposure of the prosthesis and infection. If bony reconstruction is possible, it will provide the most satisfactory long term solution. Techniques of bone reconstruction utilize either non-vascularized or vascularized bone grafts. The iliac crest and the rib are commonly used for non-vascularized grafts. When the tissue bed receiving the reconstruction is healthy and the size of the defect is small, non-vascularized bone works well [2, 3]. If the bed has had previous infection or radiation, is a particularly large area, or requires soft tissue reconstruction, the virtues of a vascularized graft should be considered. These virtues are the ability of the vascularized graft to survive irrespective of the vascularity of the bed, to tolerate contamination without becoming infected and to heal reliably to the remaining portions of the mandible. As an additional bonus, all of these grafts may carry a skin flap which can be used for intra-oral or extra-oral soft tissue reconstruction, or both. The vascularized bone grafts which are available include the iliac crest, the second metatarsal, the rib, the lateral margin of the scapula and a portion of the radius.

For large bony defects, the iliac crest is the preferred transfer [5, 6, 7]. A massive piece of bone can be removed which can be sculptured to the approximate shape of the mandible without affecting its vascularity. It can carry a large island of skin which can reconstruct huge soft tissue defects. It is available for both lateral mandibular defects and central defects. In fact, it is possible to reconstruct virtually the entire mandible with one vascularized iliac transfer. For smaller defects of 7 cm or less, the metatarsal is particularly well suited [1, 4]. Its primary application has been for anterior mandibular defects. The skin flap which is carried with the metatarsal provides an excellent intra-oral soft tissue cover. For small to medium large defects, the margin of the scapula, and the radius are available. Both of these have reliable skin flaps.

Mandibular Reconstruction with the Iliac Crest

The iliac crest is used when a large vascularized bone graft is required. It is particularly useful when there is an associated large soft tissue defect involving intra-oral and extra-oral tissues.

Mandibular defects requiring iliac crest reconstruction can be classified into central mandibular defects and lateral mandibular defects. As an osteocutaneous transfer, the skin can be used to reconstruct external cheek, chin and submental skin, and intra-oral soft tissues. However, the skin flap tends to be bulky and paler than the facial skin. Obesity is a relative contraindication to the use of this flap because of the thick subcutaneous fat on the skin flap. We have used this bone for mandibular reconstruction 26 times with survival of the bone 25 times. Of these procedures, 21 were osteocutaneous flaps with complete flap survival in 16 cases, flap tip necrosis in 4, and complete flap loss with survival of the bone in one. In the surviving bone grafts, union occurred at the osteosyntheses in all cases.

Operative Planning

For tumour resections, the maximum size of the portion of the mandible to be removed can be estimated from the clinical and radiological assessment of the disease. The surgeon doing the reconstruction can then prepare the iliac crest transfer while the tumour is being exterpated.

In most reconstructions, the ileum is placed upside down so that the superior margin of the crest forms the inferior margin of the mandible. For lateral mandibular reconstruction, the natural transverse curve of the crest approximates the curve of the body of the mandible. If a central reconstruction is required, an osteotomy is needed to provide sufficient curvature to the reconstruction. As the deep circumflex iliac artery lies on the iliacus, the vessel will lie on the medial surface of the mandibular reconstruction. It must be positioned so that it will not be compressed between the reconstruction and the tongue. In practice, this compression has not been a problem, as it has with the metatarsal, perhaps because the iliacus provides padding for the vessels. The preferred side for the iliac crest donor site depends upon the design of the reconstruction and the location of the recipient vessels.

If the reconstruction is done at the same time as the tumour excision, the exact size and shape of the desired mandible can be determined by measuring the removed piece of mandible. Creating a sterile full size sketch or template provides a model for the reconstruction.

When an established mandibular defect is being treated, it is more difficult to determine the correct size and shape of the bone reconstruction as it is an estimate. It is difficult to determine precisely the size and shape of a missing bone when the positions of the remaining mandibular fragments and soft tissues are distorted. Make a silastic reconstruction of the missing portion of mandible using a 1 cm thick silastic block and temporarily fit it in place. Loosely close the skin flaps over the reconstruction and evaluate the appearance of the reconstructed jaw. Adjust the size and shape of the silastic mandible as necessary until the reconstruction looks right.

Surgical Technique

A. Preparation of the Face

1. Elevate the mucosa and periosteum from the mandibular ends to allow wire fixation. Examine the cut bone ends to see if they are healthy and there is good medullary bleeding. If necessary, trim them back to a level which will result in a successful osteosynthesis. Identify the recipient vessels and prepare them for microanastomoses. Because of their location and size, the preferred recipient vessels are the superior thyroid artery and vein. The facial artery may also be used. However, unless a long vessel length is mobilized, this artery usually lies too far under the mandible for comfortable exposure for the microanastomosis.

Vascular repairs using irradiated vessels in the head and neck have a high success rate. In our experience with over 50 cases of head and neck free tissue transfer, using vessels which had previously received tumourcidal doses of radiation, we have not had an arterial or venous thrombosis resulting from previous radiation.

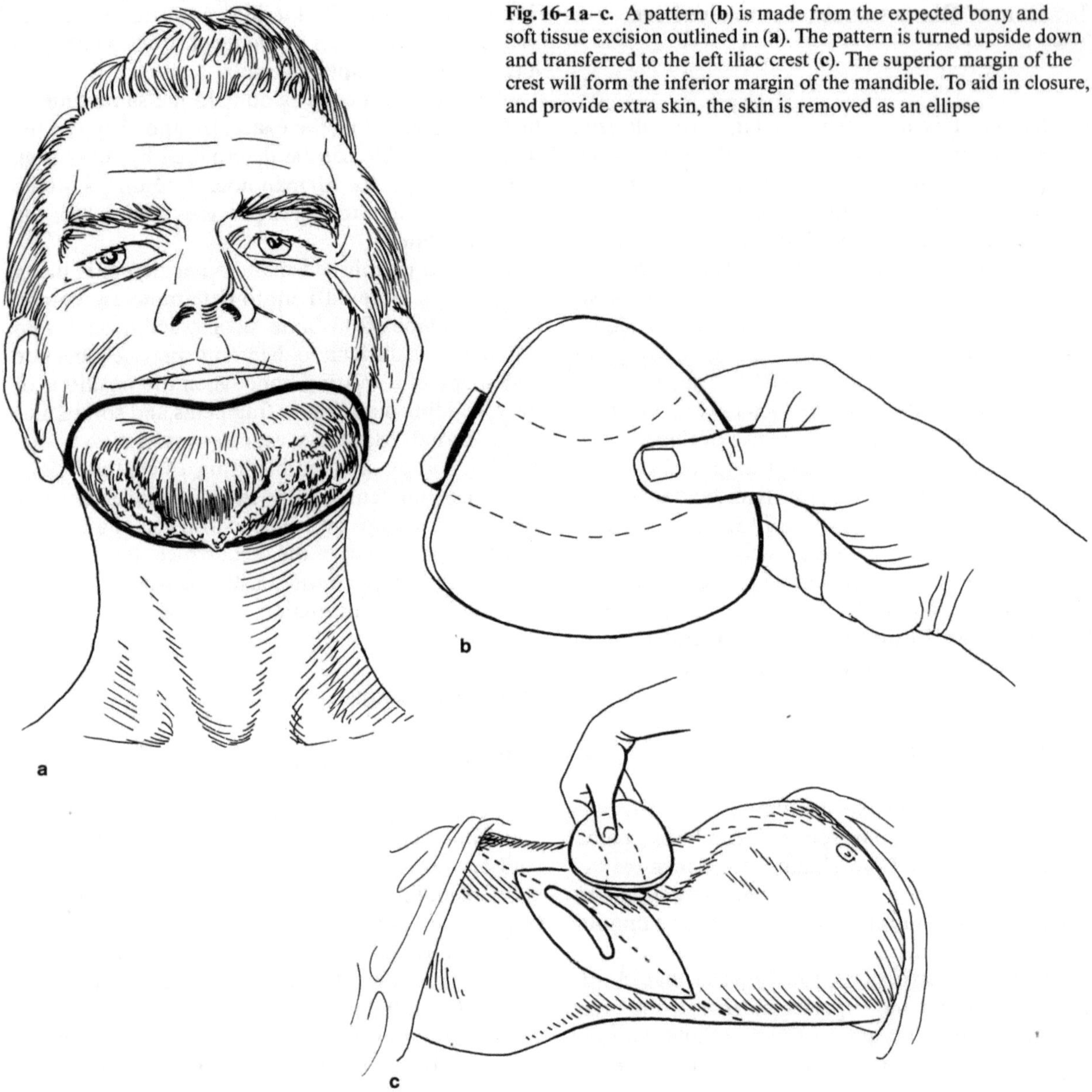

Fig. 16-1 a–c. A pattern (**b**) is made from the expected bony and soft tissue excision outlined in (**a**). The pattern is turned upside down and transferred to the left iliac crest (**c**). The superior margin of the crest will form the inferior margin of the mandible. To aid in closure, and provide extra skin, the skin is removed as an ellipse

B. Reconstruction of the Central Mandible

A reconstruction of the central mandible includes the anterior portion of both bodies of the mandible. The iliac crest graft is taken from the same side of the body as the recipient vessels (Fig. 16-1).

The special problems in central mandibular reconstruction include positioning the reconstructed mandible so that there will be neither an open nor a closed bite deformity, obtaining the correct amount of anterior mandibular projection, and reconstructing the angle at the mental process such that the width of the reconstructed mandible will be normal.

The technique of removing the iliac crest is described in chapter 10.

For an angle to angle reconstruction, 12–15 cm of iliac crest are usually required. A vertical height of 2.5 cm of crest forms a mechanically stable, cosmetically pleasing height for the mandibular body.

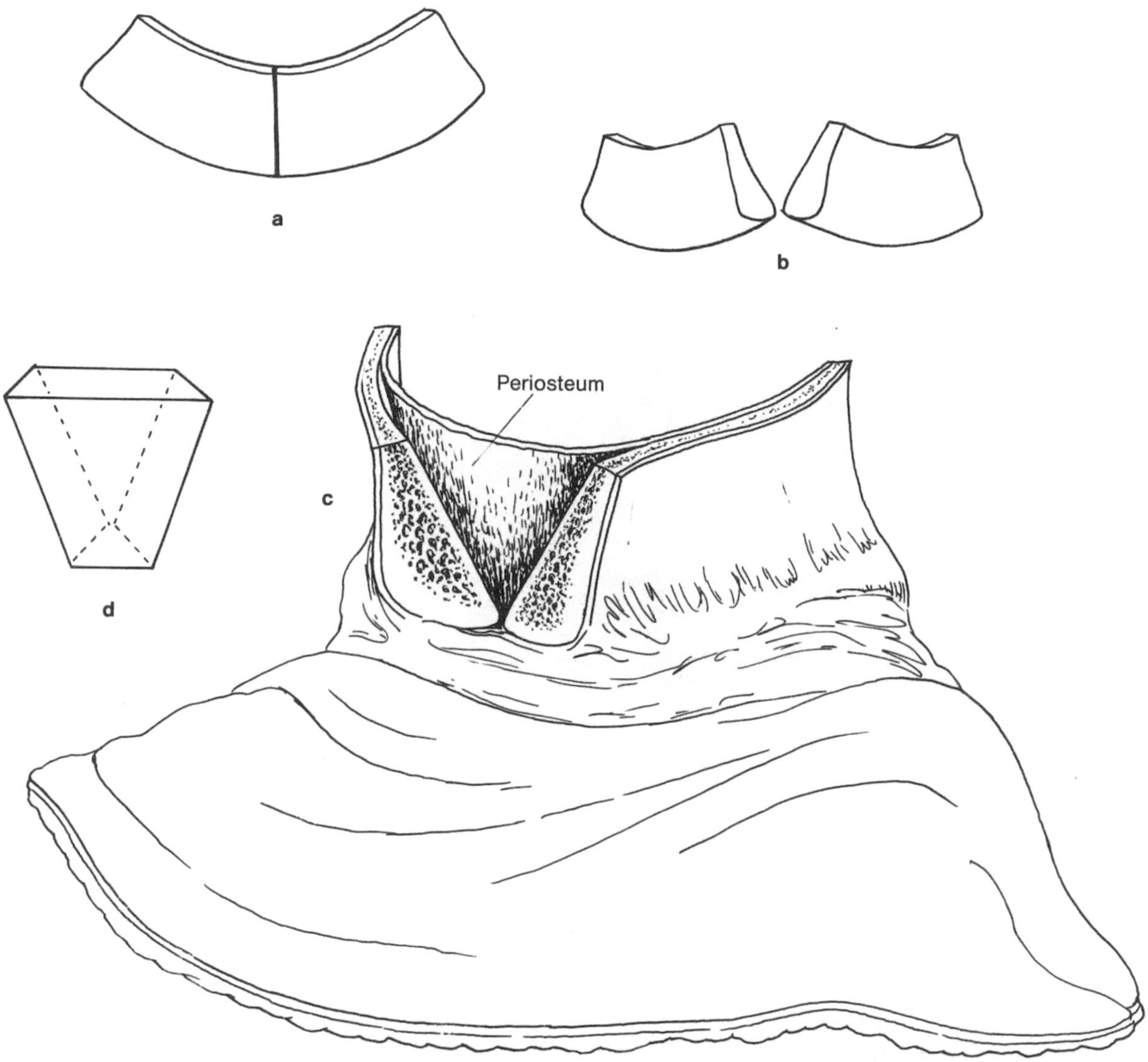

Fig. 16-2. **a** An osteotomy is placed through the inverted crest at the intended site of the mental prominence. **b** After the osteotomy, the two bone fragments are folded medially and inferiorly to simulate the position of the bodies of the mandible. **c** The periosteum and iliacus on the medial surface carry vessels which supply each fragment. **d** The opening which is created at the osteotomy is filled with a bone block which is shaped to the defect and wired in place

1. Turn the removed iliac crest upside down so that the crest forms the inferior border of the mandible. Using the intraoperative sketch or the silastic reconstruction, cut the crest to the desired shape and size. Create the mental angle by placing an osteotomy through the crest at the site of the intended mental process. Strip the periosteum and iliacus from the inner surface at the site of the osteotomy in order that it not be divided when the bone is cut. Bend the two bone fragments, opening the osteotomy on the anterior and superior surface of the reconstruction. The crest's natural curve in the sagittal plane will produce an open bite deformity if the osteotomy is not opened on its superior surface (Fig. 16-2a–c). The angle between the fragments determines the width of the mandible. Cut a block of cancellous bone from the remainder of the iliac crest to fit precisely the shape of the opening at the osteotomy site, and wire this firmly into place with interosseous wires (Fig. 16-2d). Trim the upper margins of the reconstruction to create a smooth, rounded simulation of the alveolar ridge.

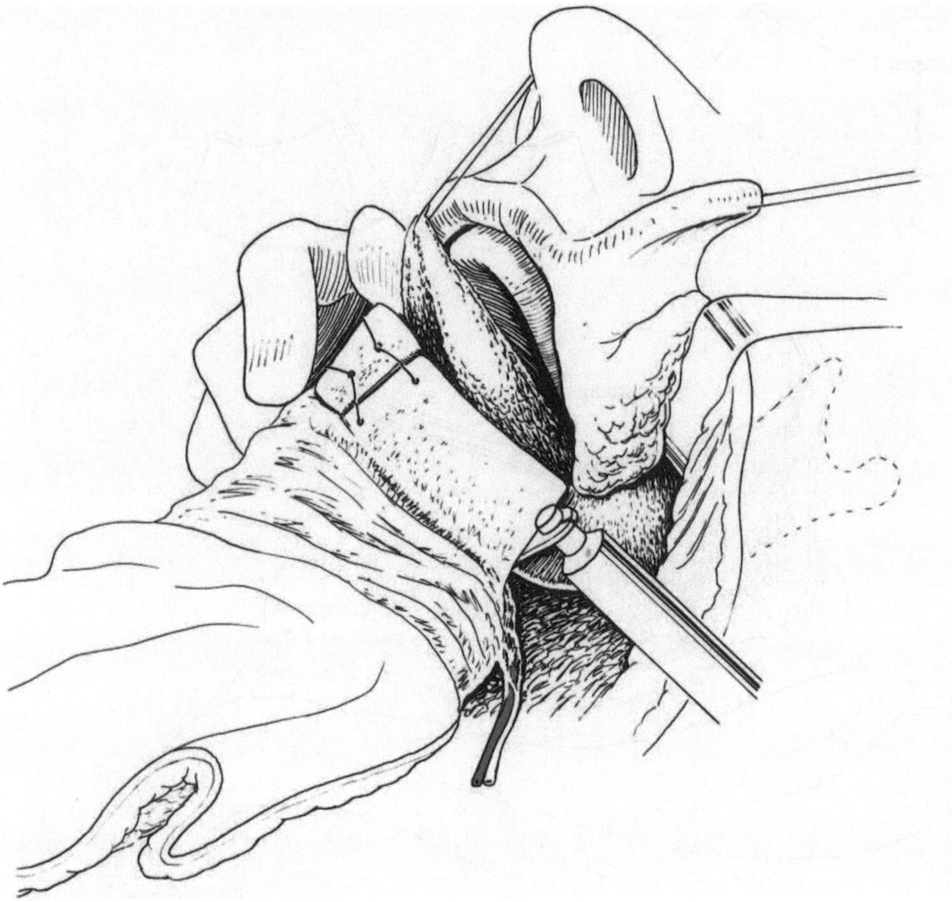

Fig. 16-3. The mandibular reconstruction is held in the face in the desired location in order that the correct plane for the graft saw cut can be visualized. This cut will match the cut surface of the mandible

2. Use a butt joint between the adjacent surfaces of the graft and mandible, and apply double wire loop fixation. The adjacent surfaces of the butt joints must fit flush. Otherwise, the reconstruction will not sit in the correct position in the face after interosseous wire compression of the joints. In order to visualize the correct plane for the saw cut, place the mandibular reconstruction into the face in the desired location, and cut the graft while observing the plane of the mandibular cut surface (Fig. 16-3). The reconstruction can be likened to a bucket handle which can pivot up and down at its posterior attachments. If the position of fixation is not correct, either an open or a closed mouth deformity or an asymmetric reconstruction will be produced. When the mandibular reconstruction is complete and the skin and intra-oral tissues are closed, the mandible should lie in its normal relaxed position. In this position, there is a 2–3 cm gap anteriorly between the maxillary alveolus and the reconstructed mandible.

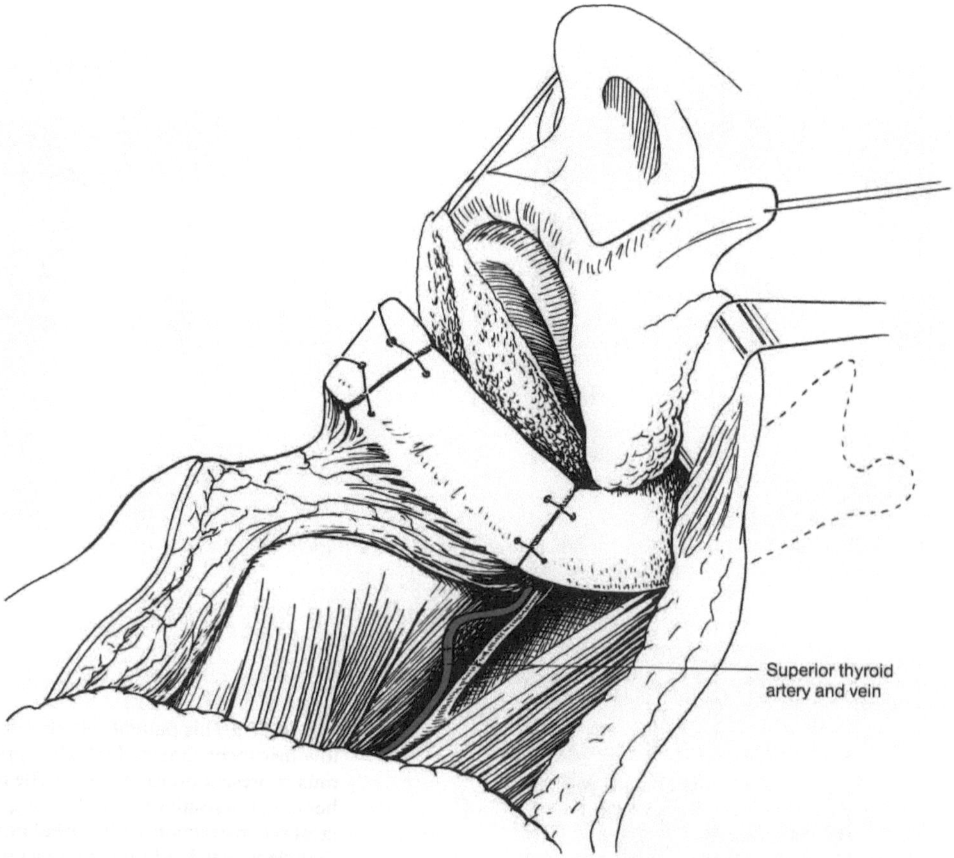

Fig. 16-4. Reconstructed mandible, wired in place, with the attached skin flap lying on the anterior neck

3. Do end to end microvascular repairs between the DCIA and its vena comitans and the recipient vessels in the neck. Prior to doing the vascular anastomosis, turn the head from side to side to evaluate the effect of movement on the position of the pedicle. Postoperatively, when the patient makes a head movement, there should be no traction on the repair (Fig. 16-4).

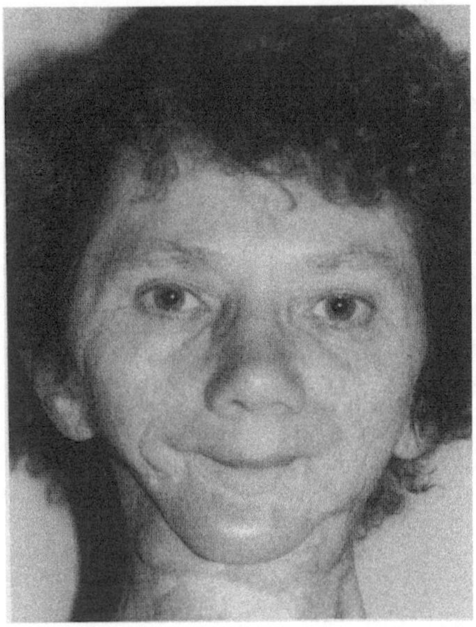
a

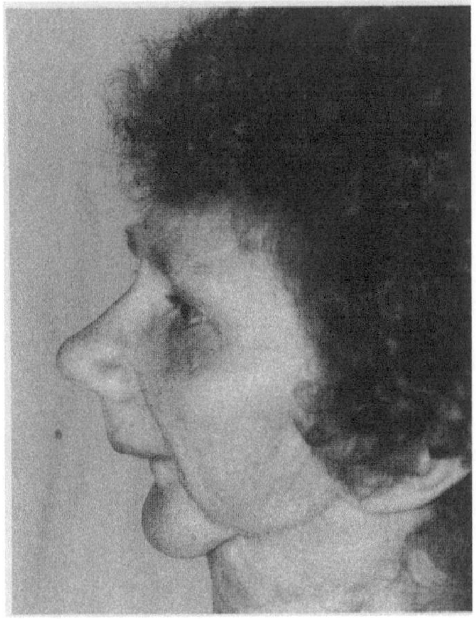
b

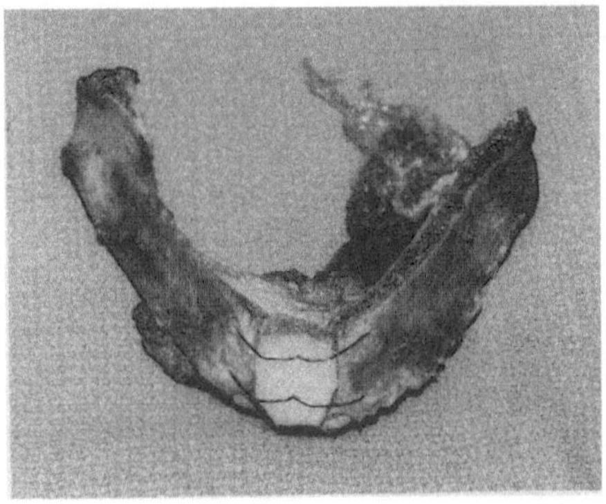
c

Fig. 16-5. **a** This patient lost almost her entire mandible following cancer surgery. Only the upper half of the ascending ramus is present on each side. **b** The remaining prominence of her chin is a result of a free floating silastic mentoplasty. **c** Iliac crest reconstruction with central bone block wired in place. Pedicle is seen leading from iliacus muscle on inside of left body of mandible. **d, e** Postoperative appearance after insertion of mandibular reconstruction

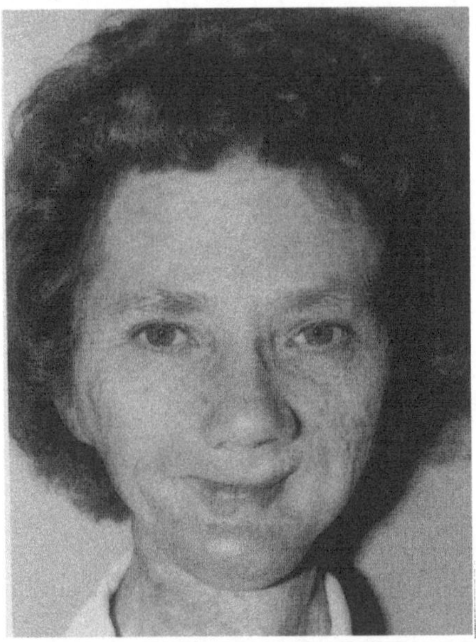
d

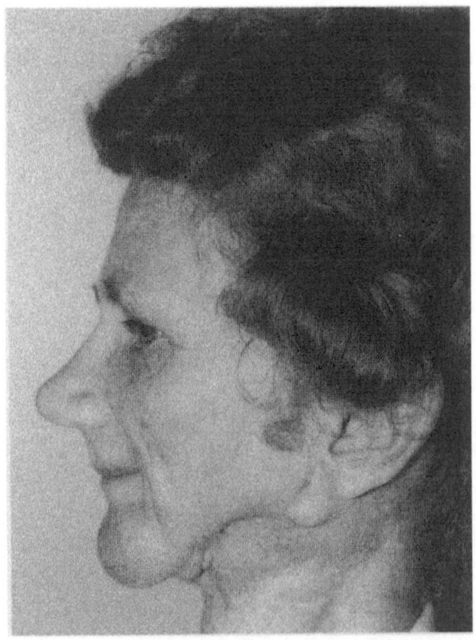
e

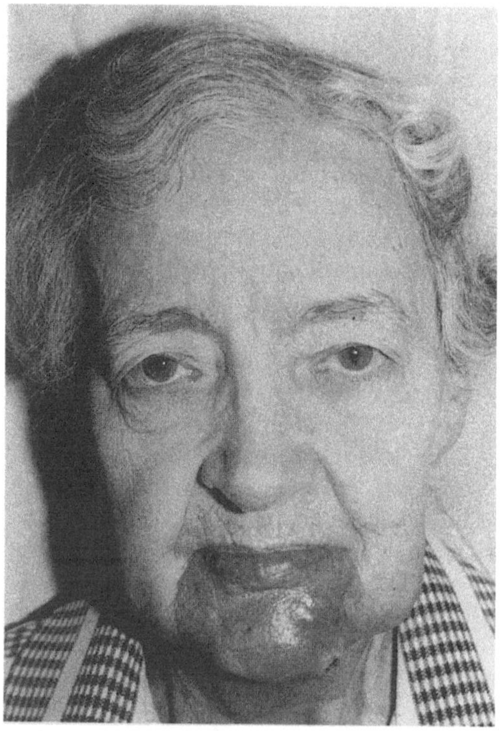

a

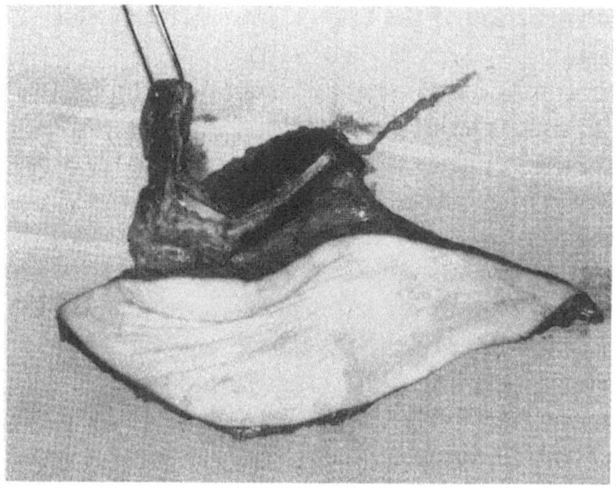

b

Fig. 16-6. **a** This patient had extensive carcinoma of the floor of the mouth invading both bodies of the mandible and the external chin skin. **b** Iliac crest osteocutaneous transfer. A bone block has been placed in the central osteotomy to create the shape of the mandibular arch for reconstruction of the mandible. Reconstruction will be from angle to angle. The skin flap will be turned counter clockwise 90 degrees and used for intra-oral and extra-oral soft tissue coverage. **c, d** Following reconstruction with iliac crest osteocutaneous transfer, the skin flap is seen covering the anterior and inferior chin

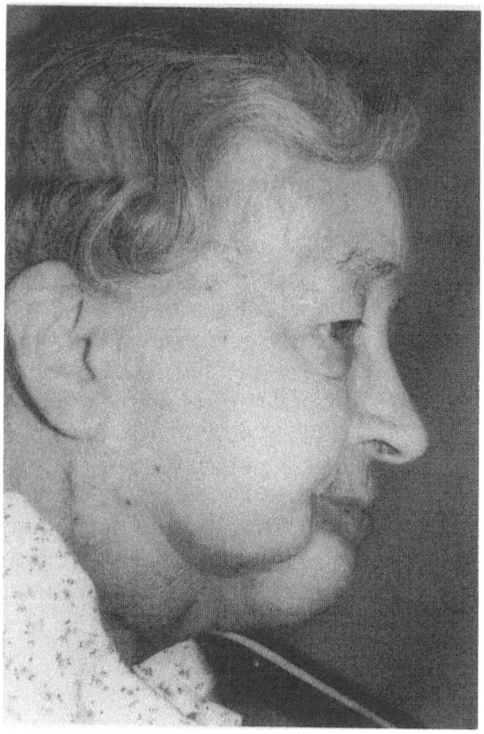

c

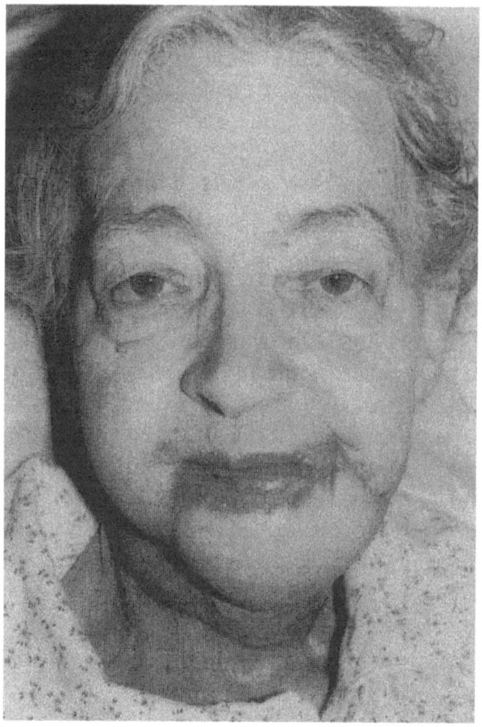

d

C. Reconstruction of the Lateral (Hemi) Mandible

For lateral mandibular reconstruction, there are two possible placements for the mandibular pattern. Both use the superior surface of the crest as the inferior margin of the mandible.

i) (Fig. 16-7 a) Place the ascending ramus towards the anterior portion of the ileum as described by Taylor. The anterior superior iliac spine (ASIS) forms the angle of the mandible and the anterior inferior iliac spine (AIIS) the condylar head. The posterior part of the crest forms the mental process. This design requires that the graft be placed in the same side of the face as the donor site in order that the natural curvature of the crest be in the right direction for the reconstruction. The pedicle will lie at the angle of the mandible, which is a particularly good location for repair to the facial or superior thyroid arteries.

ii) (Fig. 16-7 b). Place the ascending ramus on the posterior part of the iliac crest and the ASIS near the mental process. The graft will be taken from the side of the body opposite to the mandibular defect and the pedicle will lie near the mental process.

1. Before removing the bone, draw an outline of the desired mandibular shape on the lateral surface of the ileum. Use the sketch of the resected specimen or the silastic reconstruction as pattern. Remove the bone with an oscillating saw or side cutting burrs on a drill.

2. Hold the removed crest next to the sketch or the silastic reconstruction and evaluate the shape of the curve. If the curvature of the intact crest is not sufficient, place a vertical osteotomy in the bone where additional curvature is required. Separate the periosteum from the inner cortex at the intended site of the osteotomy in order that it will not be accidentally divided. The osteotomy allows the bone to be hinged on the periosteum to create the mandibular curvature. Fill the triangular opening at the osteotomy site with a wedge of cancellous bone as described for central mandibular reconstruction, and firmly wire it in place. As long as the periosteum and iliacus span the osteotomy, a blood supply will be provided to both segments of bone.

3. Prepare the muscles of mastication for insertion in the bone graft. Using heavy sutures, anchor the temporalis, pterygoid and masseter in the appropriate locations in the reconstructed mandible. The sutures for their attachment should be placed in these muscles prior to inserting the mandible in its location.

4. Do the mandibular fixation prior to vascular repairs. Use butt joints between the bone graft and the mandible. These are most easily cut in the correct position by placing the mandibular reconstruction into its desired position in the face. With the bony end of the reconstruction lying adjacent to the cut end of the mandible, cut the graft end in precisely the same plane as the cut mandibular surface. Considerable time must be spent in estimating where the reconstructed mandible should be sitting in order that there will be no deformity postoperatively. If the plane of the cuts is not correct when they are wired together, the mandible may deviate to one side or the other.

The use of butt joints is the simplest carpentry technique and, because of its simplicity, is preferable to trying to create step cuts or mortice and tenons. Fixation is obtained with interosseous wire loops between the mandible and the reconstruction. Usually two wires placed obliquely to each other provide firm stability. Occasionally, a longitudinal k-wire is added. If there is viable bone on both joint surfaces, and secure fixation, bone union can be expected even in a heavily radiated site. Intermaxillary fixation is not desirable. If the mandible is allowed to float free, there are minimal stresses on the osteotomy sites.

If doing an entire hemimandibular reconstruction, place the new condylar process in a cavity in the area of the glenoid fossa. Place a hole in the condylar neck of the reconstructed mandible and, using an awl, pass a suture over the zygomatic arch, anchoring the mandible in the fossa.

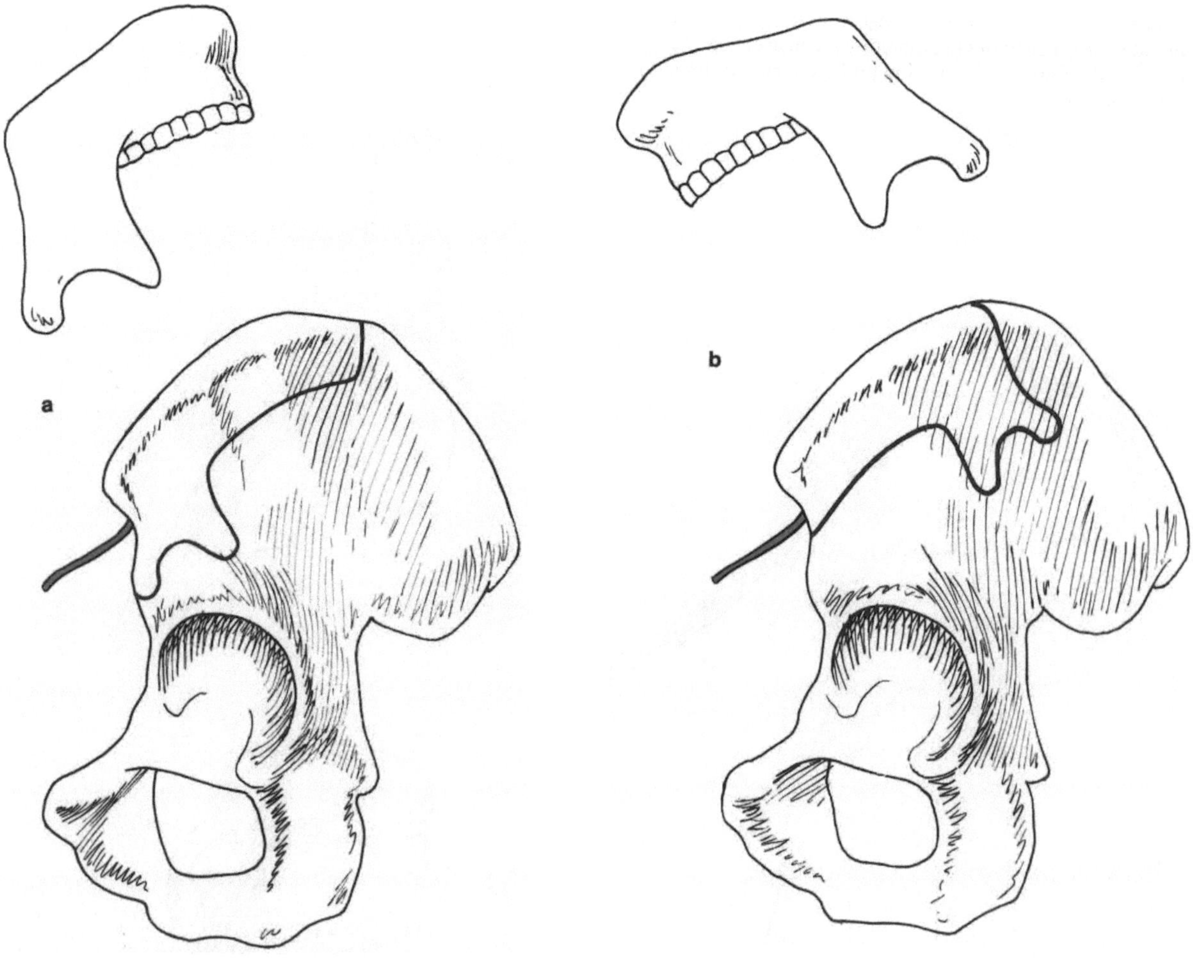

Fig. 16-7. a, b Two possible positions in which a lateral mandibular reconstruction may be taken from the ilium. As the pedicle will be located at the angle in (**a**) or at the mental prominence in (**b**), the site of the recipient vessels in the neck may determine which is the better position for the mandible

Fig. 16-8 a–c. For intra-oral coverage, the skin flap may be brought over (b) or under (c), the bony reconstruction. The portion of the flap which is buried under the chin or lip is de-epithelialized

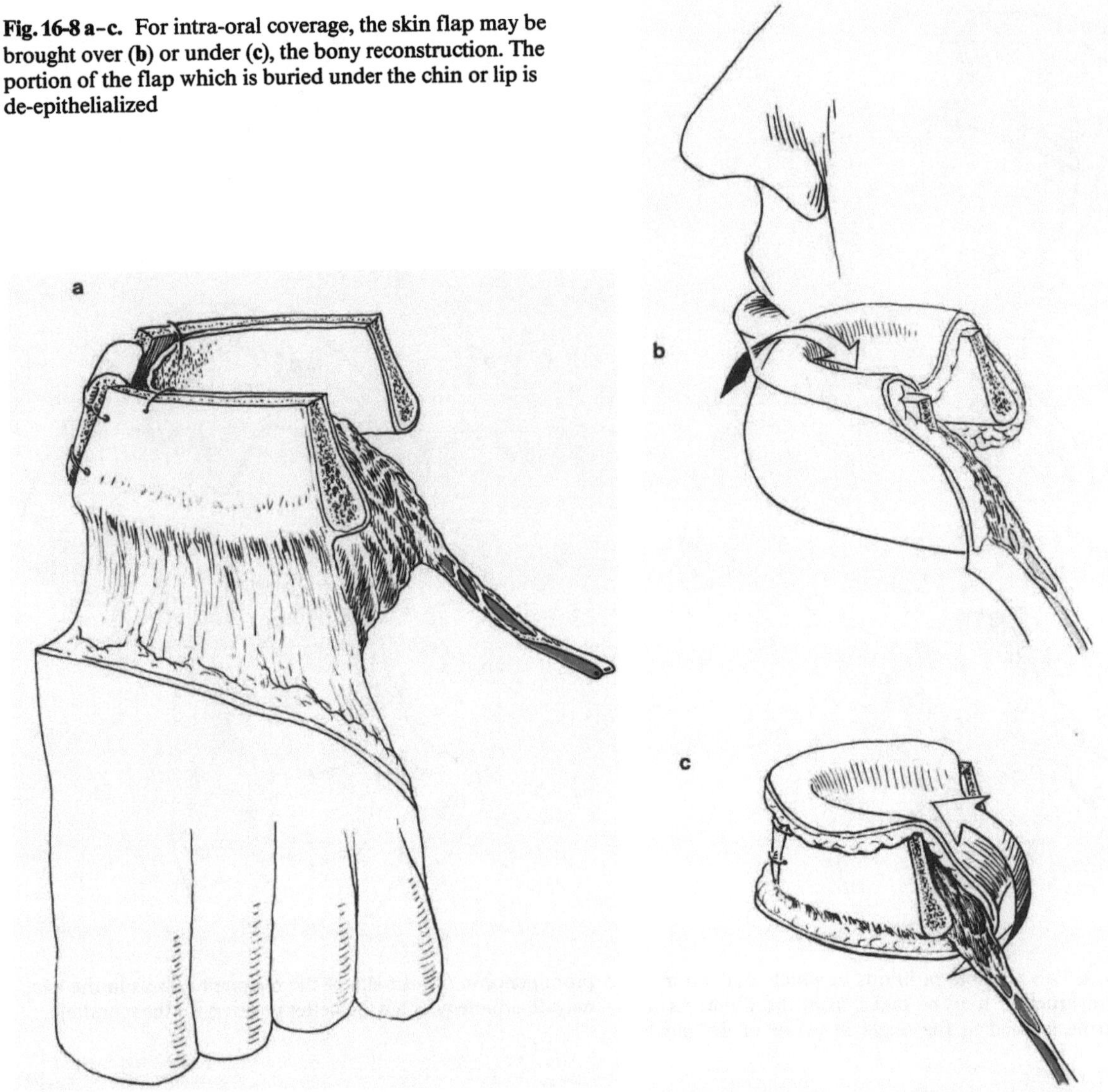

D. The Soft Tissue Reconstruction

Since the iliac crest is transferred upside down with the crest forming the inferior margin of the mandible, the skin flap will hang below the crest. This is an ideal location for coverage of the chin, cheek and submental area. Unfortunately, because of its bulk, when the flap is used for chin and submental coverage, it tends to hang under the mandible as a blob, and provides poor submental definition. This situation can be improved by secondary defatting. It is possible for a flap, particularly one which was cut with an extension inferior to the crest, to be brought up over the mandible into the mouth for intra-oral reconstruction. With this technique, a large flap may be used for combined intra-oral and external skin coverage. The flap does not need to be divided where it passes under the cheek and chin tissues, but merely de-epithelialized.

For intra-oral soft tissue coverage alone, the flap may be brought into the oral cavity over the top or under the bottom of the reconstruction (Fig. 16-8). Bringing it into the mouth under the bottom and medial to the bone may be difficult because of the bulk of the flap, unless at least a partial tongue resection was done with the tumour excision. In the latter situation, the bulk of the flap provides a replacement for the missing tongue. On occasion, suturing the intra-oral flap after bone fixation is particularly awkward. If this difficulty is anticipated, the wires should be inserted for bone fixation but left quite loose, and the skin flap sutured into the mouth before tightening the wires.

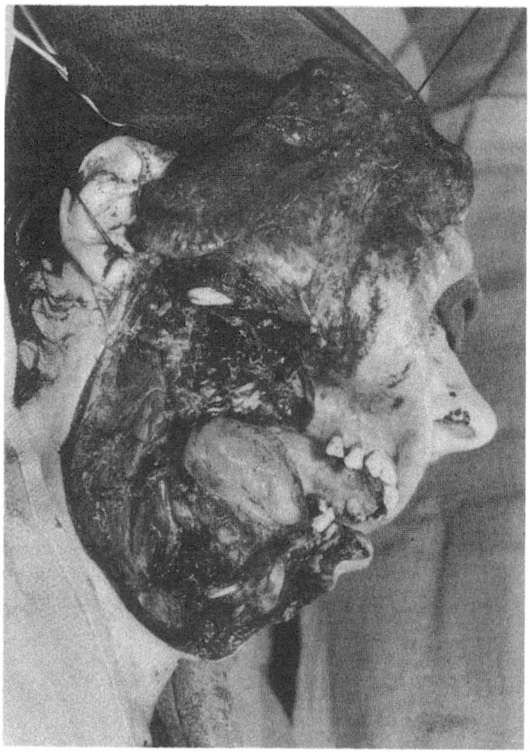

a

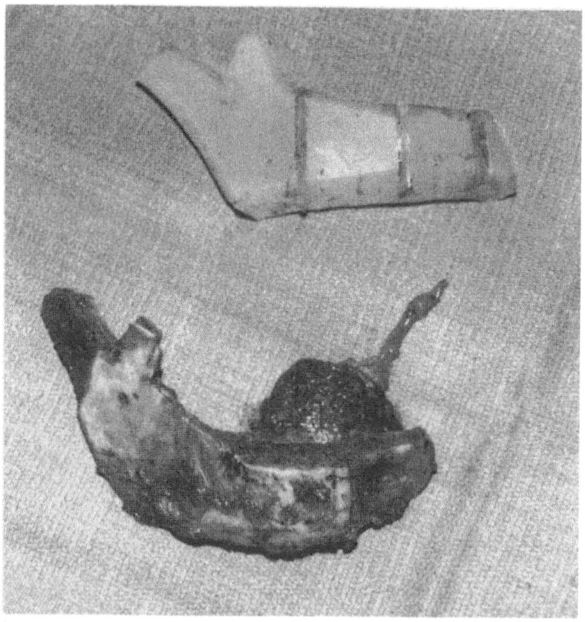

b

Fig. 16-9. **a** Defect following resection of left hemimandible for odontogenic sarcoma. Soft tissue excision is minimal. **b** Silastic model of the desired hemi-mandible was copied on the iliac crest. **c, d** One year following iliac crest reconstruction

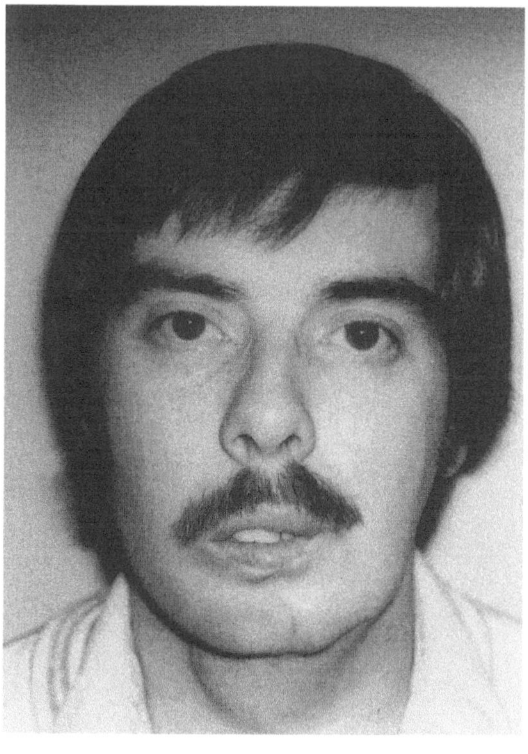

c

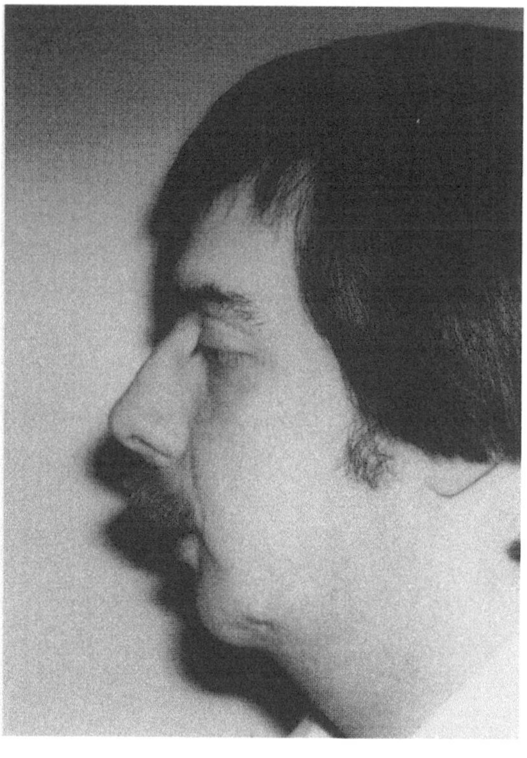

d

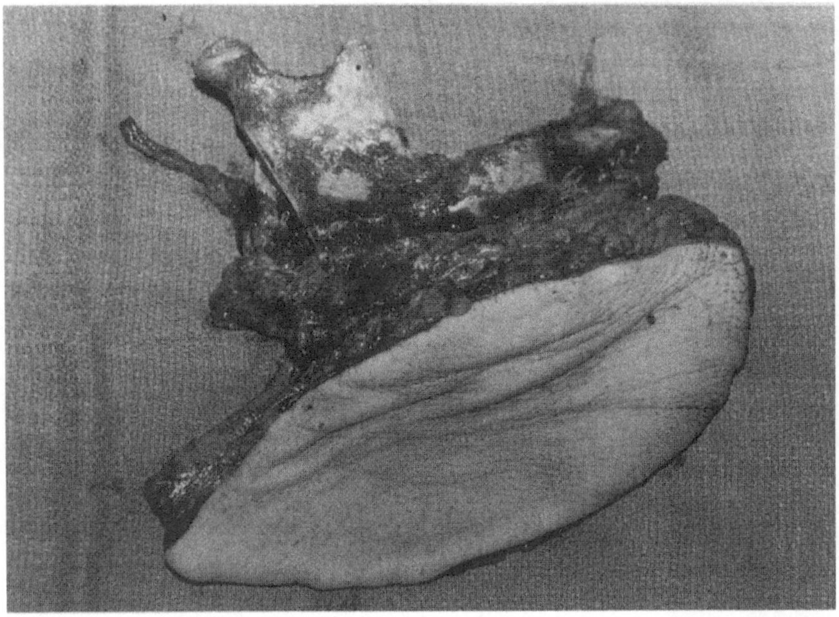

Fig. 16-10. Hemimandibular reconstruction of the left mandible with attached osteocutaneous transfer

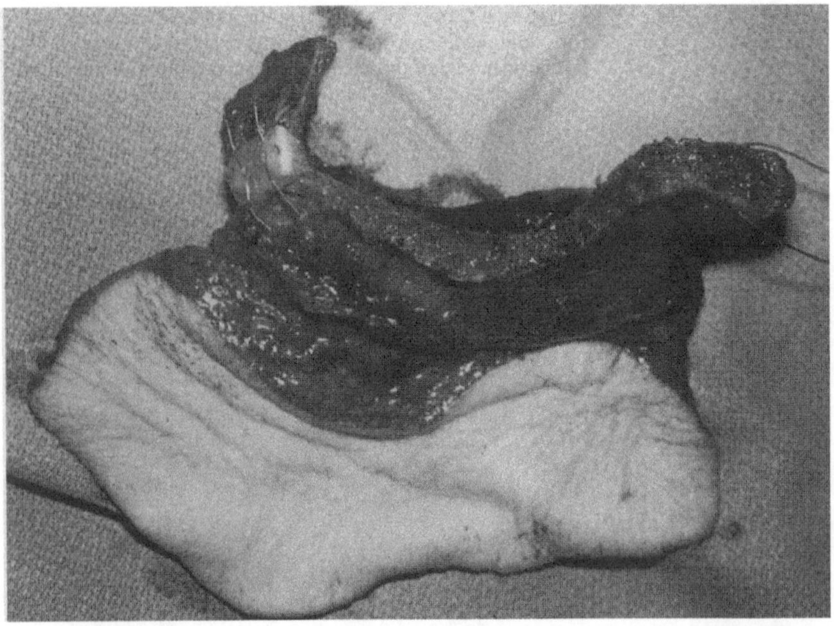

Fig. 16-11. Reconstruction of the left hemimandible mental prominence with bone block and portion of right body with attached cutaneous transfer

Mandibular Reconstruction with the Metatarsal

The vascularized metatarsal transfer provides an excellent bony reconstruction of the mandible. Taking the dorsal foot skin with the transfer provides a thin flexible flap which makes a good intra-oral lining. The large areas of well-vascularized cancellous bone at the head and base of the metatarsal result in rapid reliable bone union with the mandible. By removing a wedge of bone in the mid shaft, the surgeon can shape the metatarsal to a 'v' which simulates the shape of the anterior mandibular arch.

We have used this transfer 27 times as an osteocutaneous transfer, with complete survival 25 times. In the surviving grafts, solid bone union occurred at both ends of the graft in all cases except one. In this case of osteoradionecrosis of the mandible, nonunion occurred at one end because the mandibular resection was inadequate.

Operative Planning

Plan the reconstruction so that, when the metatarsal is in place, the vascular pedicle and its branches to the skin will lie on the labial side of the metatarsal reconstruction. If the pedicle lies on the lingual side with the pedicle and branches to the skin flap lying between the tongue and the metatarsal shaft, postoperative swelling of the tongue will compress the pedicle and its branches against the unyielding metatarsal shaft, and may result in loss of the transfer. In order that this labial position of the pedicle on the second metatarsal be accomplished, the donor foot should be from the side opposite to the neck recipient vessels.

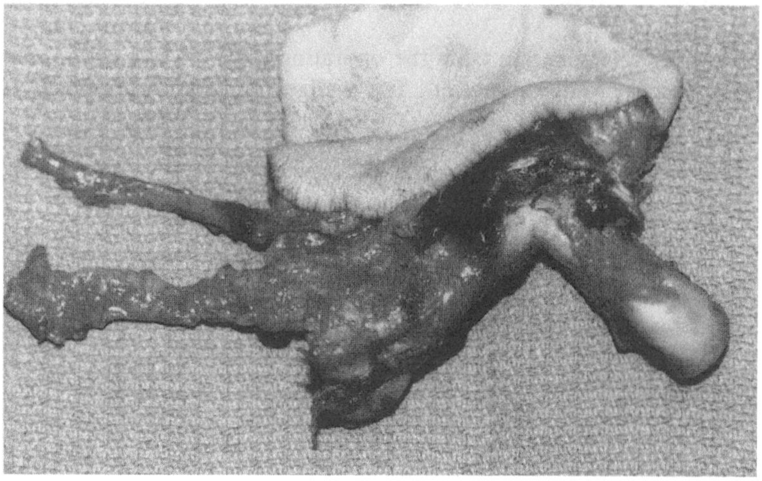

Fig. 16-12. Metatarsal osteocutaneous transfer with 75 degree wedge osteotomy. Saphenous vein and dorsalis pedis pedicle are seen to the left.

Surgical Technique

A. Preparation of the Face

The preparation is the same as that described for the iliac crest (p. 109).

B. Reconstruction of the Central Mandible

The technique of removing the metatarsal is described in chapter 11.

1. Evaluate the defect and determine the optimum size and shape of the metatarsal. If the reconstruction is being done immediately following a tumor resection, examine and measure the resected mandible. For an anterior reconstruction, measure the mental angle and length of bone on each side. Calculate the size of bone wedge which should be removed from the metatarsal to create the mental angle. The size of the angle of the removed wedge of bone determines the amount of angulation created in the metatarsal shaft. The degree of angulation determines the prominence of the chin and the width of the bony reconstruction (Fig. 16-13 a, b).

2. Use a table separate from the operating table to do a precise wedge resection. The wedge of bone may be removed from either the plantar or lateral surface of the metatarsal. Expose the required area of metatarsal shaft, elevate the periosteum and protect the interosseous muscle. An oscillating saw with a fine blade will produce a precise osteotomy. A green stick fracture is not possible as the bone is brittle. Place a single interosseous wire across the osteotomy to provide stable fixation.

3. Hold the angled metatarsal in the mandibular defect, and align ends with the lower margin of the mandible. Determine the optimum position of the mental prominence, which can be rotated caudal or cephalad like a bucket handle.

4. Use a butt joint between the metatarsal and the remaining mandible. It adds unnecessary complexity to try to create step joints between the mandible and graft. Holding the mandibular reconstruction in the face in the precise position that is desired, remove each end of the metatarsal with a saw to obtain surfaces parallel to the cut surfaces of the mandible to which it will be attached. The adjacent surfaces of the butt joints must be parallel in order that the reconstruction sit properly after interosseous wire fixation (Fig. 16-13 c). Two non-parallel interosseous wire loops at each butt joint provide firm fixation (Fig. 16-13 d). Intermaxillary fixation is undesirable.

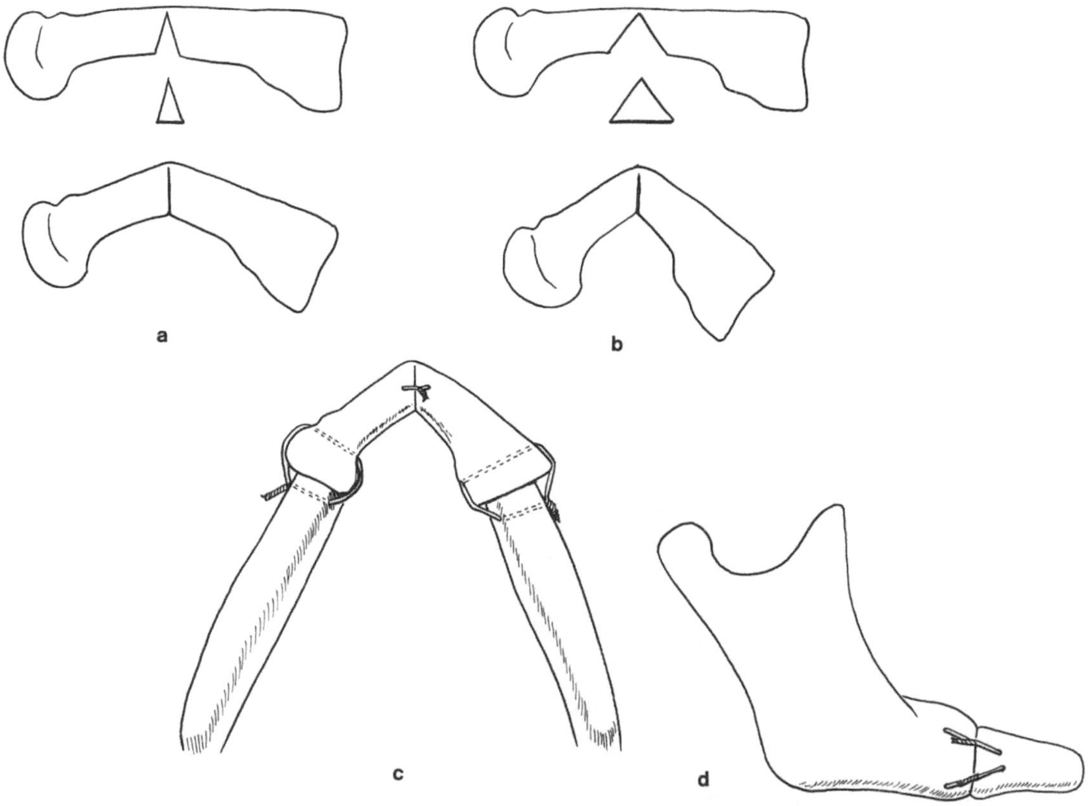

Fig. 16-13. a, b For anterior arch reconstruction with the metatarsal, a wedge of bone is removed from the mid shaft to provide a mental angle. The angle of the wedge determines the degree of angulation of the metatarsal. **c, d** Fixation of the wedge osteotomy is accomplished with a single interosseous wire loop, and fixation between the metatarsal and mandible is with two asymmetrical interosseous wire loops

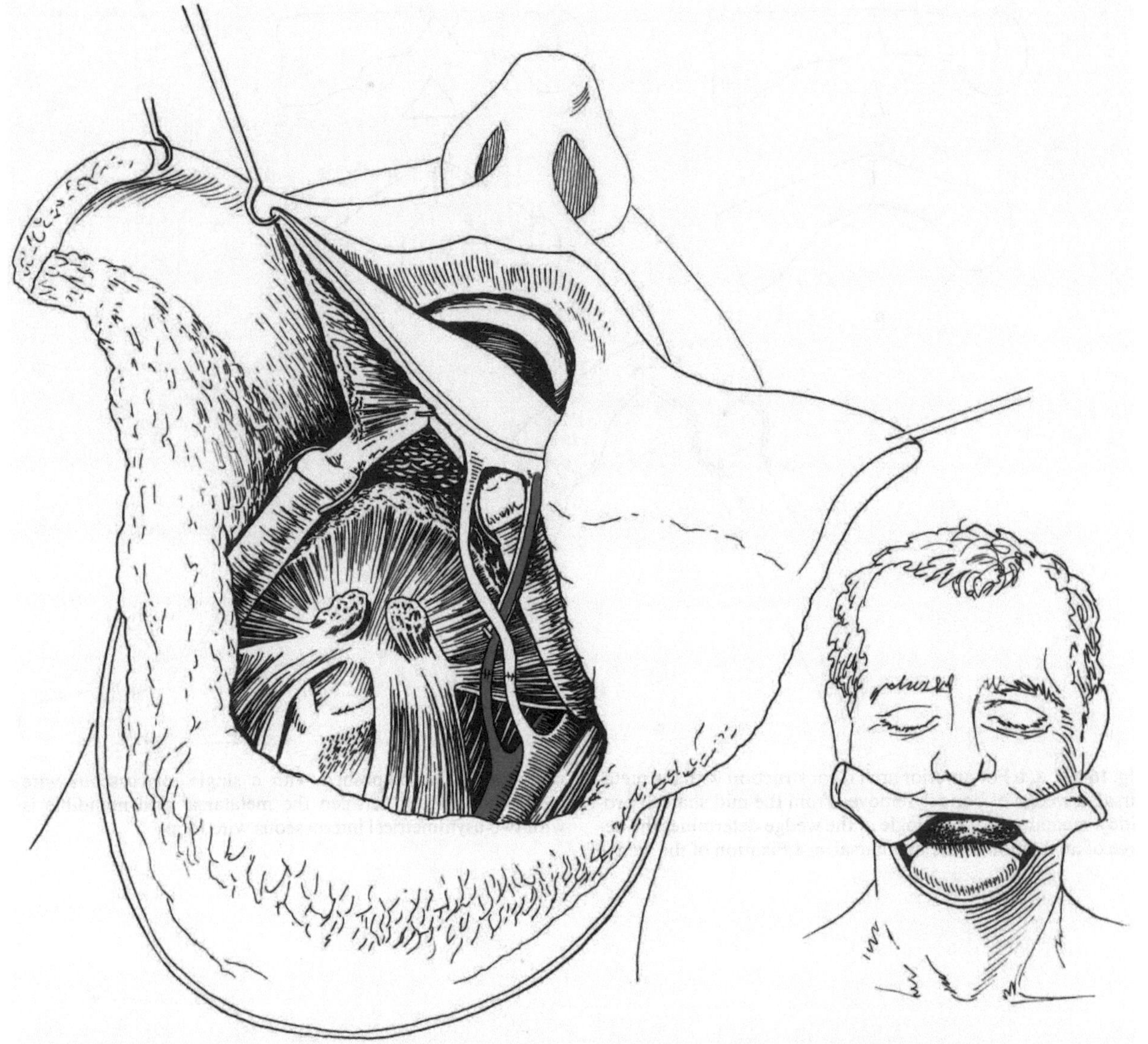

Fig. 16-14. Inferior view of the reconstruction with the skin flap lifted by a hook to reveal the osteotomized metatarsal. Anastomosis of the dorsalis pedis artery and the saphenous vein to the superior thyroid artery and vein

5. The usual vascular anastomoses are end to end to the facial or superior thyroid artery and vein. Be sure that there is adequate slackness in the pedicle to allow postoperative movement of the patient's head. Following the vascular anastomoses, bleeding will be observed from the drill holes in the bone fixation, and the skin flap will slowly become pink.

6. Replace the cheek flaps, evaluate the position of the chin reconstruction, trim the intra-oral flap and suture it to the floor of the mouth and buccal and labial mucosa. A two-layer suture repair over the mandible provides a reliable closure.

7. Close the neck skin flaps with suction drains secured so that they neither lie on nor can move onto and obstruct the pedicle.

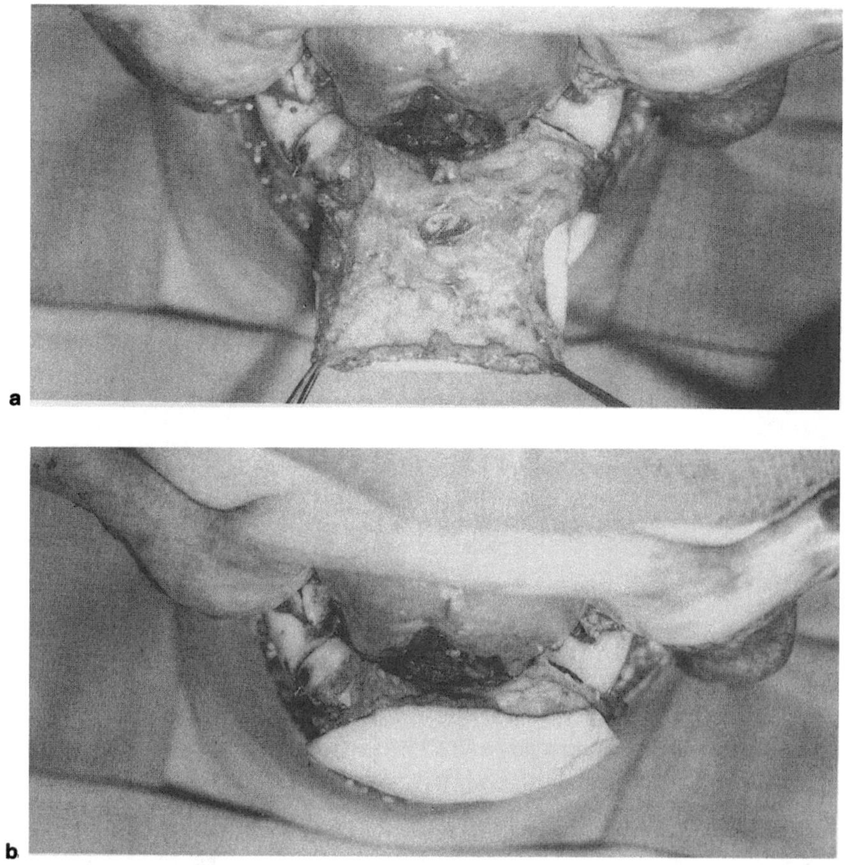

Fig. 16-15. **a** Superior view of the osteotomized metatarsal wired to the mandible, with the skin flap retracted. **b** The skin flap is now lying on the superior surface of the mandibular reconstruction to provide soft tissue coverage for the floor of the mouth

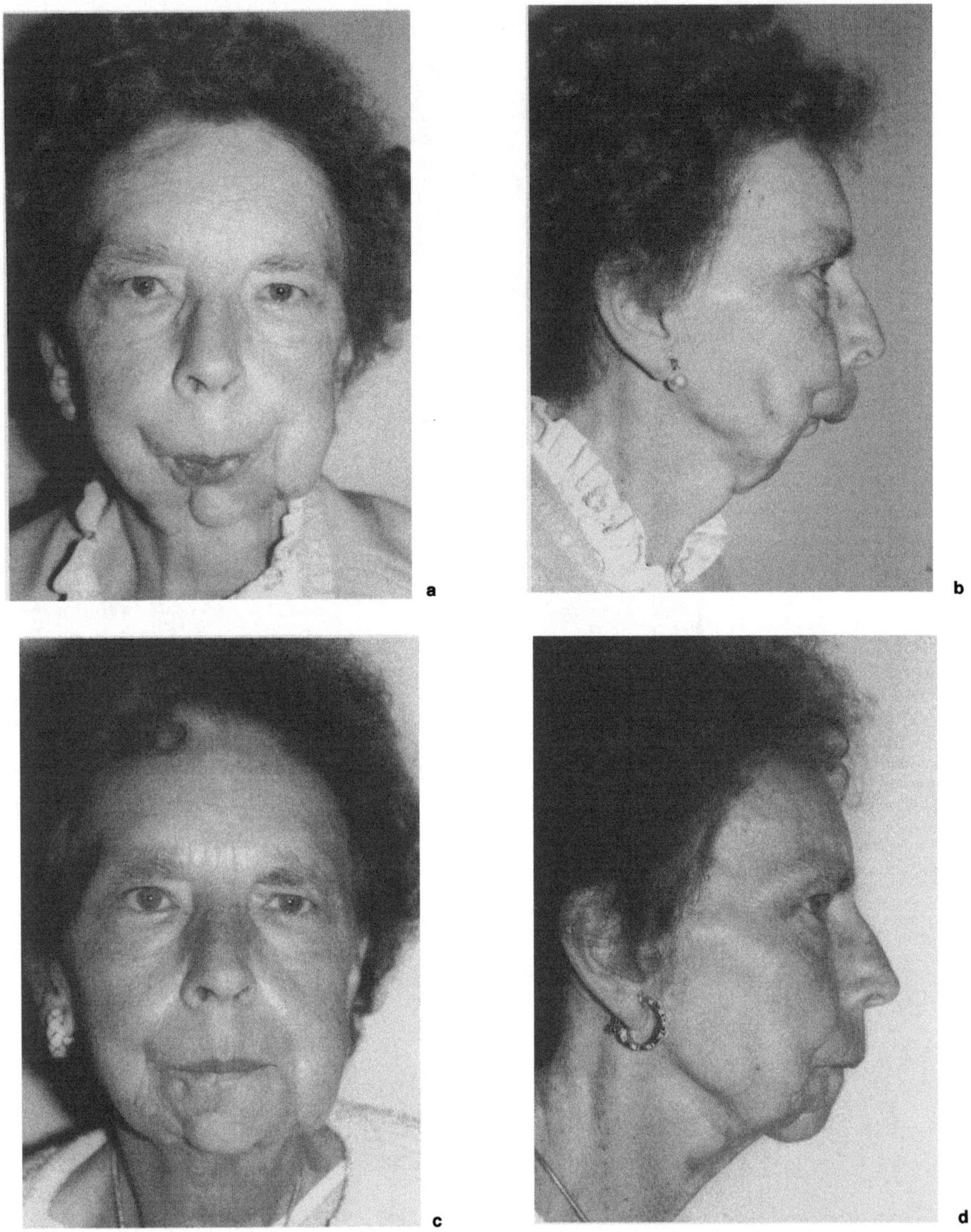

Fig. 16-16. a, b Appearance of patient who has had resection of the mandible from mid-body to mid-body, including the floor of the mouth. **c, d** Appearance following reconstruction with the metatarsal osteocutaneous transfer. **e** Appearance following additional onlay bone graft to anterior mandible

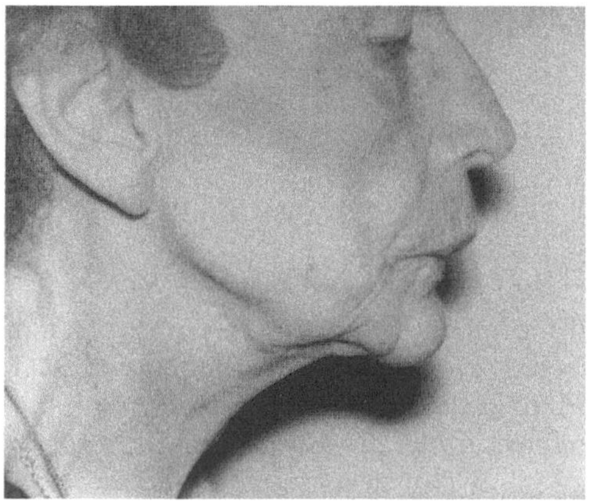

Fig. 16-16 e

References

1. MacLeod AM, Robinson DW (1982) Reconstruction of defects involving the mandible and floor of the mouth by free osteocutaneous flaps derived from the foot. Br J Plast Surg 35: 239
2. Manchester WM (1965) Immediate reconstruction of the mandible and temporal mandibular joint. Br J Plast Surg 18: 291
3. Manchester WM (1972) Some technical improvements in the reconstruction of the mandible and temporomandibular joint. Plast Reconstr Surg 50: 249
4. Rosen IB, Bell MSG, Barren PT, Zuker RM, Manktelow RT (1979) Use of microvascular flaps, including free osteocutaneous flaps in reconstruction after composite resection for radiation recurrent oral cancer. Am J Surg 138: 544
5. Taylor GI, Townsend P, Corlett R (1979) Superiority of the deep circumflex iliac vessels as the supply for free groin flaps: experimental work. Plast Reconstr Surg 64: 595
6. Taylor GI, Townsend P, Corlett R (1979) Superiority of the deep circumflex iliac vessels as the supply for free groin flaps: clinical work. Plast Reconstr Surg 64: 745
7. Taylor GI (1982) Reconstruction of the mandible with free composite iliac bone grafts. Ann Plast Surg 9: 361

Chapter 17. Facial Paralysis Reconstruction

Each patient with facial paralysis requires a unique plan of treatment based upon the individual's particular deformities and concerns. Innumerable procedures have been used for facial reconstruction. For mouth reconstruction, these include static and dynamic slings, muscle transfers and transplantations, nerve repairs, grafts and transfers, neurectomies and myectomies and various soft tissue procedures. Most of these procedures have a useful place in the correction of the deformities of facial paralysis. However, for smile reconstruction, vascularized muscle transplantation is gradually becoming the procedure of choice.

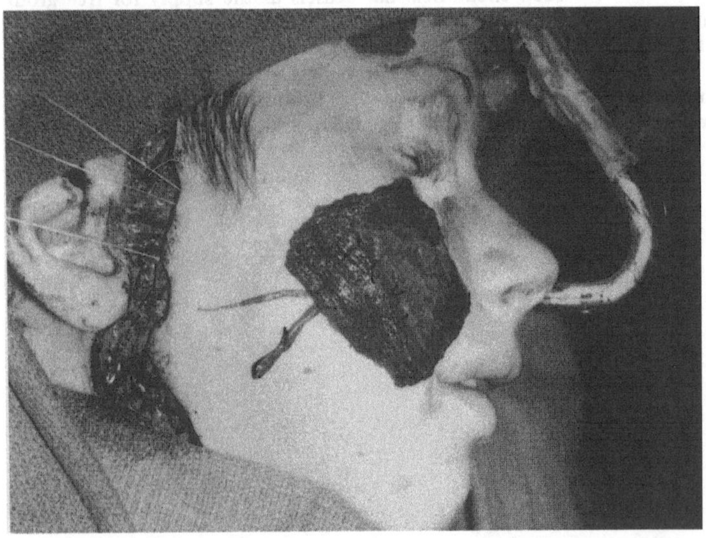

Fig. 17-1. Segment of gracilis muscle prepared for transplantation for smile reconstruction

Thompson transplanted the extensor digitorum brevis and palmaris longus muscles to the face. For their survival, he depended on the ingrowth of vessels from the surrounding tissues. Neurotization of the transplanted muscle took place through direct contact of the transplant with innervated facial musculature on the normal side, or by suture of the transplanted muscle's nerve to a branch of the normal facial nerve. The concept was ingenious. However, few surgeons were able to obtain a useful amount of movement from muscles transplanted with this technique because of inadequate muscle survival and/or insufficient reinnervation. With the advent of microvascular surgery, it became possible to transplant all or part of a muscle to the face and be sure of its survival. Since this procedure was described by Harii, it has been used by many surgeons [4, 5, 6, 10]. With its physiological basis, this surgical method carries great promise for improving facial paralysis reconstruction.

There are 18 separate muscles of facial expression which operate in combination with each other as a finely tuned system which provides not only facial tone and voluntary movement, but also involuntary facial expression. The surgeon's ability to transfer one or two contracting units does not allow for much sophistication in simulating the co-ordinated contractions of the multiple muscles of facial expression. However, the movement which many patients miss most is elevation of the corner of the mouth to produce a smile. Muscle transplantation can provide this active motion as well as a balanced symmetrical appearance to the mouth at rest. In my experience, this technique reconstructs the smile better than any other procedure.

If the facial nerve is used to reinnervate the transferred muscle, the smile can be spontaneous and not dependent upon conscious movements of the patient, such as clenching the teeth or moving the tongue, as it is in masseter muscle and hypoglossal nerve transfers. With vascularized muscle transplantation, because of the flexibility of the procedure, the surgeon can more accurately match the shape of the smile on the normal side of the face.

Preoperative Planning

Microneurovascular transfer with survival of muscle is not a difficult procedure. However, using this operation to create an adequate smile is a challenging task. The solution lies in choosing the correct amount of muscle, and selecting the optimum insertion, origin and tension for the muscle, and providing adequate reinnervation.

Muscle Selection

As the most successful applications of muscle transplantation have been smile reconstruction, this chapter will discuss only this procedure. Surgeons have used all or parts of the gracilis, latissimus dorsi, serratus anterior, pectoralis minor and extensor digitorum brevis. However, the specific muscle which is used may not be as important as the amount of muscle used and its placement. The muscle selected should produce no functional deficit following its removal, and should be at a site distant from the face so that simultaneous preparation of the face and the muscle can be done. If the surgeon wishes to provide an additional function, such as the replacement of the orbicularis occuli, it is desirable to have a muscle which can be divided into two separately functioning neuromuscular units, one for the mouth and one for the eye. The pectoralis minor, serratus anterior and gracilis have this anatomic capability. However, the reconstruction of orbicularis occuli function with vascularized muscle transplantation has not been very gratifying up to this time.

The most common objective of microvascular muscle transplantation is to elevate the corner of the mouth to create a smile. This requires a short muscle with a functional length of 4-7 cm, a contractile capability of 1-1.5 cm, and sufficient strength to overcome the forces of gravity and tissue resistance. The selected muscle must have a constant vessel and nerve anatomy to allow reliable microvascular transfer. The best way to obtain a piece of muscle of sufficient size and functional capability is to cut the piece from a larger muscle such as the gracilis, latissimus dorsi or serratus anterior (Fig. 17-1). The amount of functioning muscle which is transferred must vary with the individual requirements of each reconstruction. The patient with a powerful smile on the normal side and heavy facial tissues will require a larger piece of muscle than a patient who smiles weakly. When a cross-facial nerve graft is used, a larger piece of muscle should be transferred, as the graft does not have the same innervation capabilities as a direct nerve repair.

Muscle Innervation

Muscle neurotization may be achieved by using the facial nerve on the side of the paralysis, or the facial nerve on the normal side, or other motor nerves in the vicinity, such as the hypoglossal or the motor branches of the trigeminal. All three sources have been used with some success. Neurotization with the facial nerve is the preferred route as it is the only source of nerve impulses which are normally produced at the time of facial expression. Probably the only means of obtaining involuntary facial movements and spontaneous expression is to use the facial nerve.

In the patient who has a long standing facial paralysis as a result of peripheral facial nerve injury, the stumps of the facial nerve would appear to be the preferred source of innervation. However, this apparent solution is not as adequate as it might seem. The more distally in the face that these stumps are located, the more certain the surgeon can be that the branch is a buccal branch of the nerve. Nevertheless, a buccal branch may carry axons to many individual muscles, including the orbicularis oris and zygomaticus major, which have different and conflicting actions. Or, if the nerve branch carries orbicularis oris function as its primary activity, the muscle transplantation will receive a nerve impulse only when the patient tries to pucker the lips. Furthermore, if a proximal nerve stump is used, there is a two-thirds chance that it will have primarily orbicularis oris or orbicularis oculi function [3]. It is apparent that appropriate selective neurotization may be difficult, using facial nerve stumps.

If there are no suitable nerve stumps available on the paralyzed side, the preferred source of neurotization is the opposite facial nerve. This situation will prevail in the patient who has an intracranial nerve lesion following trauma, acoustic neuroma resection, Bell's palsy, or proximal nerve stumps on the paralyzed side. Nerve excitation is provided by a long nerve graft placed across the face from the normal to the paralyzed side. This cross-facial nerve graft is done 9–12 months prior to the muscle transplantation.

The cross-facial nerve graft was originally described by Anderl and Smith as a means of transmitting nerve impulses from the normal side of the face to the paralyzed side [1, 2]. The procedure involves dividing some of the branches of the facial nerve on the normal side and attaching the proximal ends to a nerve graft. The graft is placed across the face in a subcutaneous tunnel to the paralyzed side. On the paralyzed side, the comparable branches of the facial nerve are divided and their distal ends attached to the nerve graft.

The cross-facial nerve graft concept is appealing. There is good logic in tapping the normal nerve for appropriate neural impulses for the paralyzed side. Although other nerves have been used for facial reanimation, the seventh is the only nerve which can transmit neural impulses to provide spontaneous facial animation. However, for many surgeons, the results of this procedure have been disappointing. Although some patients do develop muscle contraction on the paralyzed side, the amount of movement has often been inadequate to satisfy the patient and surgeon. This may be the result of factors such as the long period of facial muscle denervation atrophy, the inadequacy of a long graft to provide a potent reinnervation, and the mixture of messages being collected by a nerve graft attached to many branches of the facial nerve.

A possible solution to the problem of denervation atrophy of facial muscles is to do a vascularized muscle transplantation after the cross-facial nerve graft has reinnervated [6]. If 6–12 months are allowed to elapse before the muscle transplantation is done, regenerating nerve axons will have reached the distal end of the graft and be available for immediate reinnervation of the transplanted muscle. Anticipating sone atrophy of the transplanted muscle, the surgeon can transplant a large piece of muscle.

The procedure of cross-facial nerve grafting is possible without harm to the normal facial nerve because there is a profuse supply of peripheral facial nerve branches with overlapping functions. Approximately 50% of the branches at the level of the medial border of the parotid can be divided and donated for innervation of nerve grafts without any apparent functional loss on the normal side.

After reinnervation of the graft, the patient will usually notice a buzzing sensation when the distal end of the graft is tapped. It is interesting that this Tinel-like sign localizes to the musculature of the previously divided facial nerve branches. When tapping the distal end of the nerve graft produces a buzzing sensation, nerve regeneration has taken place adequately for muscle transplantation to be done.

Patients who have a bilateral facial paralysis have no 7th nerve source for muscle neurotization. In these patients, we have used both the hypoglossal and the motor branches of the trigeminal nerve. When the hypoglossal nerve is used, it is identified deep in the neck and split longitudinally. This is usually a one fascicle nerve, and the splitting of the single fascicle cannot be carried through a very long length. However, two patients who have had this done bilaterally have not had any apparent loss of tongue function and have developed useful muscle contraction on both sides of the face. To obviate the technically difficult dissection and splitting of the hypoglossal nerve, we have used the motor branch of the masseter. This nerve is easily identified on the deep surface of the masseter where it comes under the zygomatic arch and enters the deep surface of the masseter. The disadvantage of using either of these nerves is the inappropriateness of the nerve impulses for movements of facial expression. However, with retraining, these patients develop the ability to consciously create a smile. In our hands, these muscle transplantations provide a stronger and more natural smile than temporalis and masseter transfers.

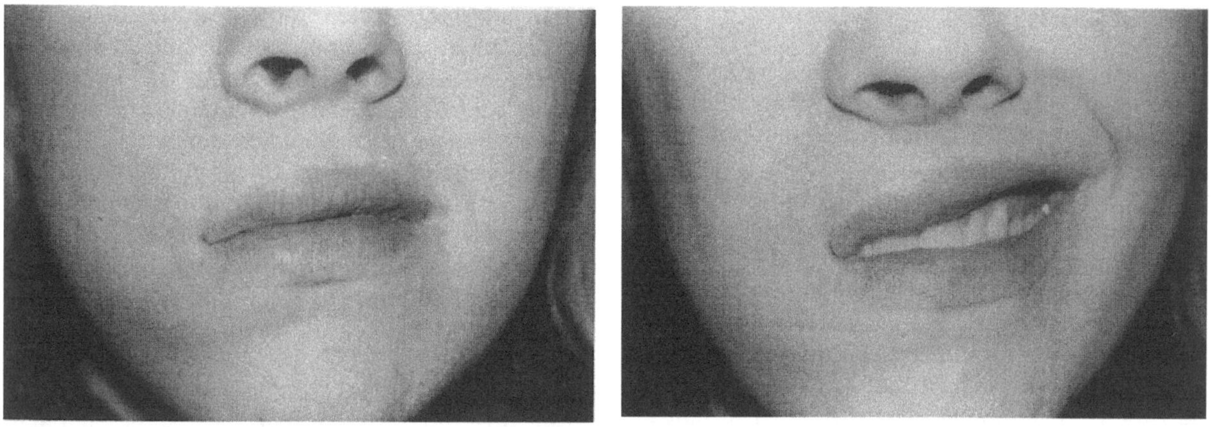

a b

Fig. 17-2. **a** 21 year old woman with uni-lateral facial paralysis secondary to Bell's palsy. She regained slight tone on her right side but was unable to smile. **b** She has a powerful smile on the left side. With a maximum smile, she forms a pointed commissure which moves 18 mm at an angle of 50° from the horizontal. There is a well-defined nasolabial fold which curves around the commissure

Muscle Placement

The correct position for the transplanted muscle is determined by a smile analysis of the non-paralyzed side of the face (Fig. 17-2a, b). Smile analysis involves an assessment of the shape of the mouth, location of skin creases, and measurement of the direction and amount of movement of the commissure.

Creases and Indentations
Smiling creates creases and indentations around the oral commissure and in the nasolabial region. The presence, location and extent of these creases vary from patient to patient.

Shape
The shape of the commissure may be pointed, round or square, depending to some extent on the force of the smile. Reconstructing a pointed shape for the commissure is relatively easy, whereas a square one is difficult as it requires a simultaneous downward and upward force to be exerted on the commissure.

Movement vector
The direction of movement of the commissure, which varies between 30-80 degrees from the horizontal, can be measured with a goniometer on the patient and on the projected photographs. With a maximum smile, the amount of movement of the commissure varies from 1-2 cm.

Following the evaluation of these components of a smile, the surgeon has a better idea of what he or she is trying to create with the muscle transplantation. The reconstruction on the paralyzed side should attempt to produce a smile which replicates the normal side. However, it must be remembered that the non-paralyzed side is not always normal in the patient with unilateral facial palsy. Frequently, there is an exaggerated depressor anguli oris which results in exposure of the lower canine when a large smile or laugh is produced. The extent of movement of the unopposed commissure is usually greater than normal as the entire mouth moves away from the paralyzed side.

Attaching the muscle to the mouth is a critical part of the procedure. The specific insertions are chosen intraoperatively by traction on the commissure and lip tissues, and observation of the shape of and creases about the commissure. The muscle is usually inserted into the fibres of the orbicularis oris above and below the commissure. It is the accuracy of the placement of these sutures which determines the shape of the smile. The direction of movement of the commissure is determined by the angle of muscle pull, which is determined by the origin of the muscle. This angle, which was determined by the smile analysis, will usually place the muscle's origin on the body and arch of the zygoma. The amount of movement of the commissure is determined by the cross-sectional area, length of the transferred muscle and degree of reinnervation. As the placement of the muscle origin determines the functioning muscle length, it also affects the amount of commissure excursion.

Recipient Vessels

The facial artery and vein are the preferred recipient vessels. The facial artery is usually 1 mm or larger in diameter. It can be identified by palpation where it passes over the body of the mandible and traced towards the corner of the mouth. The facial vein is usually found posterior to the artery and is slightly larger in size.

The superficial temporal artery and vein are the second choice for recipient vessels. They are a little further from the location of the muscle's vascular pedicle. However, we have had a few cases in which the superficial temporal vein was either absent or too small to use for a microvascular repair.

Technique of Cross-Facial Nerve Grafting Prior to Muscle Transplantation

Facial Nerve Preparation

1. Drape the entire face free from behind both ears and from forehead to submental region. Anaesthesia should be done without muscle paralysis.

2. Use a preauricular facelift-type incision. Visualization for the microneurovascular repairs requires the preauricular incision of exposure to be extended beneath the body of the mandible for about ¼ of its length (Fig. 17-3 a).

3. Elevate the skin flap at a plane superficial to the parotid fascia. Have the assistant place traction on the cheek skin towards the midline while you elevate the flap, allowing good visualization at the deepest part of the dissection. The assistant should observe the mouth and eye for facial nerve stimulation during the dissection.

4. At the medial margin of the parotid, carry the dissection slightly deeper and identify all branches of the facial nerve to the mouth and eye. These branches are 0.3 to 1.0 mm in diameter and require a nerve stimulator for confirmation (Fig. 17-3 b).

5. Draw a sterile sketch of the operative field, indicating each dissected branch of the facial nerve. Use a nerve stimulator which has both frequency and voltage control and a small curved electrode which allows elevation and separate stimulation of each branch of the facial nerve. Identify the exact facial movement function produced by the stimulation of each branch. This identification should be a detailed one which includes all movements such as a pucker, elevation of the upper lip, elevation of the commissure, lower lip depression, etc (Fig. 17-3 c, d).

6. Place a preauricular incision on the paralyzed opposite side and an incision at the base of each alar margin. Create a subcutaneous tunnel across the face from the dissected branches to the opposite preauricular area. The tunnel should be high in the cheek on the paralyzed side so that the nerve is not in the way of the muscle transplantation.

Sural Nerve Graft Preparation

The nerve graft may be taken simultaneously with the preparation of the face. With the patient lying supine and tilted towards the paralyzed side, both operative sites are well exposed.

1. Prep the leg free, with a tourniquet on the thigh.

2. Place an incision directly over the nerve at the ankle. It lies 2–4 cm anterior to the Achilles tendon on the lateral side of the ankle.

3. Identify the nerve and trace it proximally. Remove it through multiple small transverse incisions or a longitudinal incision directly over the nerve (Fig. 17-4 a).

A longitudinal incision with direct exposure of the nerve appears to be less traumatic than the avulsion technique and provides visualization of the branches of the nerve. However, this technique does leave a long visible incision on the posterior aspect of the calf.

If removing it through multiple transverse incisions, divide the nerve distally and withdraw it proximally to minimize the tearing of side branches from the nerve.

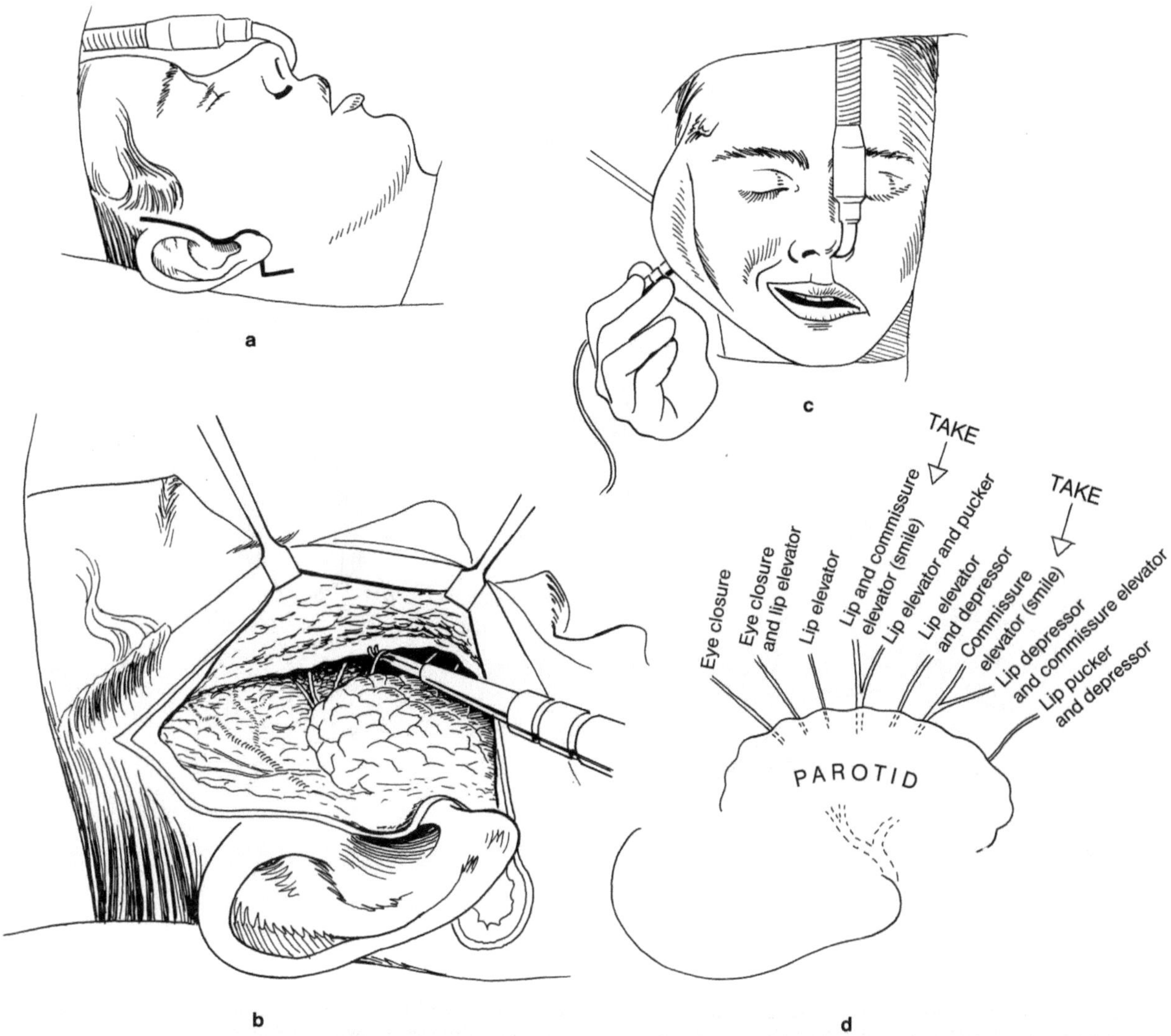

Fig. 17-3. **a** Incision for exposure of facial nerve. **b, c** A nerve stimulator is used to identify the function of each branch of the facial nerve. **d** An intraoperative record of the function of each branch of the facial nerve. For reinnervation of the nerve graft, facial nerve branches are selected which, when stimulated, produce a smile. Branches which produce lip elevation as well as lip pucker (pursing) should not be used

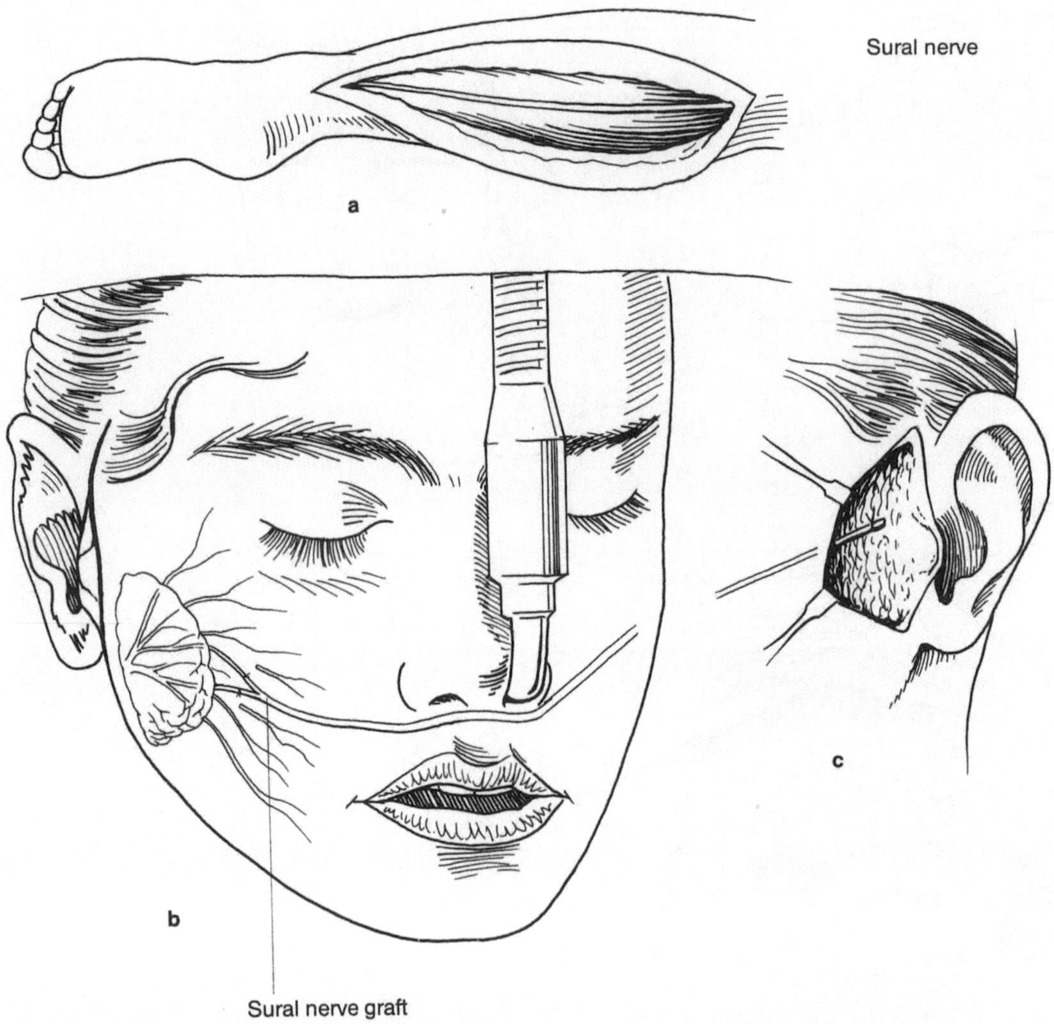

Fig. 17-4. **a** Direct exposure of sural nerve in the calf. **b** The completed cross-facial nerve graft sutured to the proximal ends of the facial nerve branches. **c** The free end of the sural nerve is 'banked' in front of the tragus for easy identification at the time of muscle transplantation

Insertion of Cross-Facial Sural Nerve Graft

1. Use a tendon tunneller or suitable instrument to draw the nerve graft through the subcutaneous tunnel with its proximal end on the paralyzed side. This position ensures that there is little chance of wasted fascicles through torn side branches of the sural nerve.

2. Select all of the dissected branches which produce a normal smile and no other movements.. Divide one half of the branches and suture their proximal ends to the nerve graft, using a meticulous fascicular repair with 11-0 nylon (Fig. 17-4b). It is difficult to obtain sufficient fascicles to cover the whole cross-sectional area of the sural nerve. A small nerve graft may be better than a large one as a higher proportion of its axons will likely be reinnervated.

Suture the opposite end of the graft with a large silk suture in the preauricular area so that it can be found easily at the time of the muscle transplantation (Fig. 17-4c).

3. Insert drains, close the incision and apply a gentle pressure dressing to the face and cheeks.

Postoperative care is relatively simple and the patient can be discharged as soon as the leg is comfortable with ambulation. Paresthesias in the foot may be bothersome for about one month and then they will disappear.

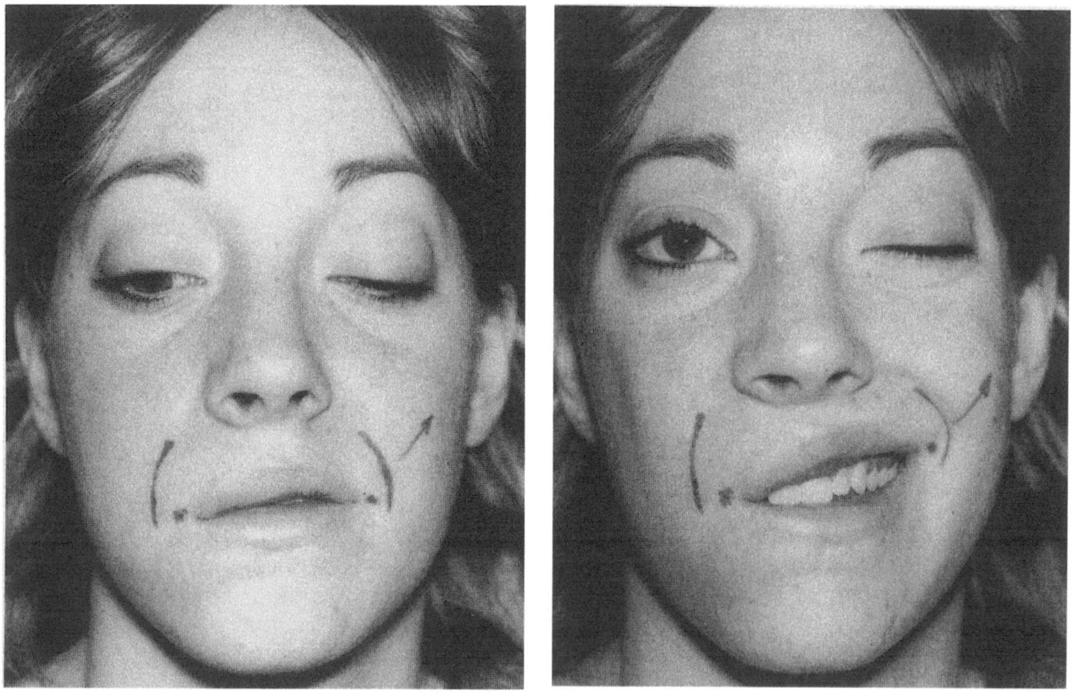

Fig. 17-5 a, b. Preoperative markings (same patient as 17-2 a, b) **a** The nasolabial fold has been marked on the patient's normal right side and the desired fold line marked on the paralyzed side. An indentation just lateral to the commissure is marked with a dot.

b The desired angle of commissure movement is marked by an arrow.

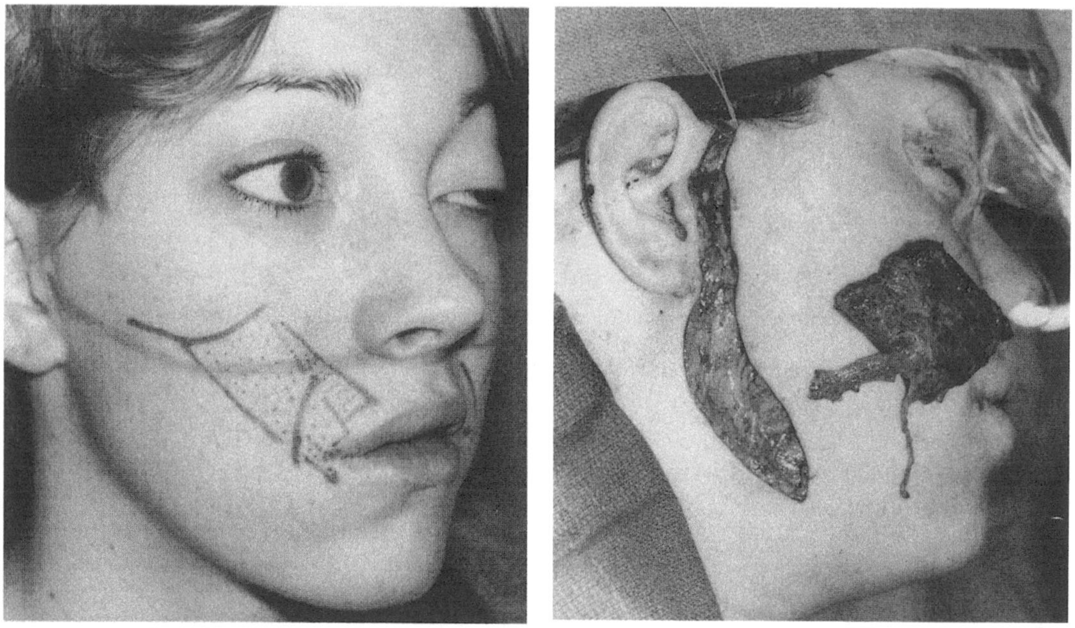

Fig. 17-5. c From these markings, the desired location and likely insertions of the muscle have been marked on the face. The location of the previously inserted cross-facial nerve graft is marked by a line passing across the cheek from the base of the nose to the ear.

d A piece of the gracilis, cut to the desired size, is placed on the face in the location outlined by the sketch. The vascular pedicle leads towards the angle of the jaw and the motor nerve leads inferiorly

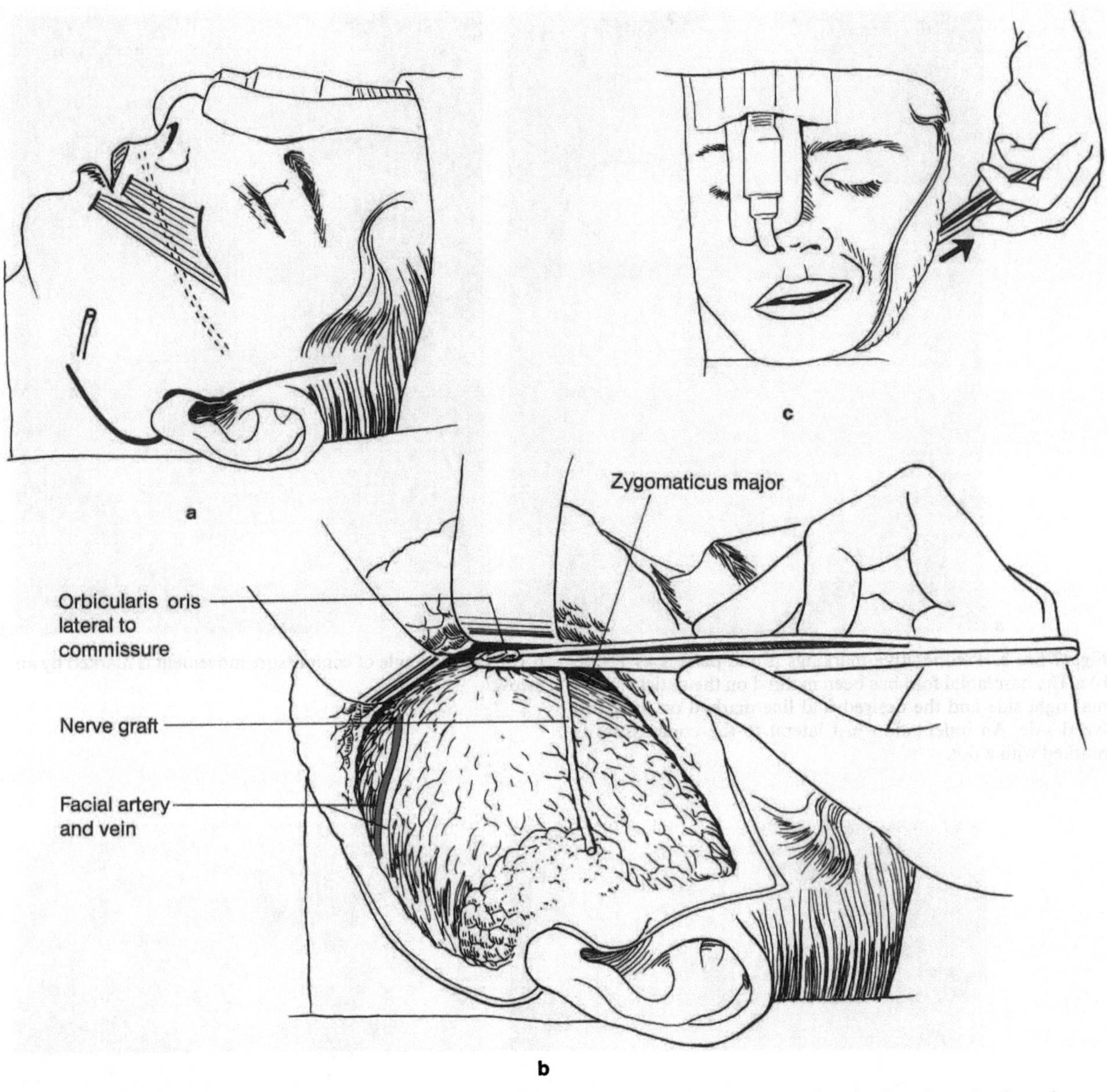

Fig. 17-6. **a** The desired location of the transplanted muscle is outlined on the patient's face. The cross-facial nerve graft passes through this area. The facial artery and preauricular incision are outlined. **b, c** Traction is placed on the deep tissues at the commissure at different locations until traction points are found which produce a smile shape to the mouth

Technique of Facial Paralysis Reconstruction with Muscle Transplantation

A. Preparation of the Face

1. Prior to administering the anaesthetic, observe the patient smiling and mark on the normal side of the face the creases which are created in the commissure, nasolabial fold and the direction of movement of commissure (Fig. 17-5 a–d). Place the same marks on the paralyzed side (Fig. 17-5 a, b). Outline on the face the desired location of the muscle transfer (Fig. 17-5 c). Identify the location of the end of the nerve which will be used for muscle reinnervation. Both the cross-facial nerve graft and facial nerve stumps have a Tinel's sign which can be elicited by percussion over the end of the nerve. Mark the nerve, the facial artery and the preauricular incision (Fig. 17-6 a).

2. Through the preauricular incision, elevate the facial flap superficially to the parotid fascia, with identification and preservation of the cross-facial nerve graft or facial nerve stumps. Carry the dissection medially until the desired site of the muscle's origin and insertion is exposed. Identify and prepare the facial artery and vein for anastomoses. Examine the nerve under magnification. A specimen may be sent to the neuropathologist for quick section evaluation. This examination allows identification of the fascicles which have the greatest concentration of regenerating axons.

3. Identify the optimum point of insertion of the zygomaticus musculature. These muscle fibres intermingle with the oribularis oris and insert directly into the skin and mucosa of the lip. Using forceps, apply traction at different points on the orbicularis oris and observe the effect on the face (Fig. 17-6b, c). Select this point or other points through which traction produces the most naturally shaped smile, which mimics that on the normal side. Try different areas until the optimum location is found. Usually the dominant point of traction is located at or immediately below the commissure. In addition, elevation needs to be applied to the lateral half of the upper lip. Photos of the patient attempting to smile should be available in the operating room for comparison. Insert two or three double-armed sutures into the sites of traction, and observe the appearance of the smile produced by traction on the sutures (Fig. 17-7a, b).

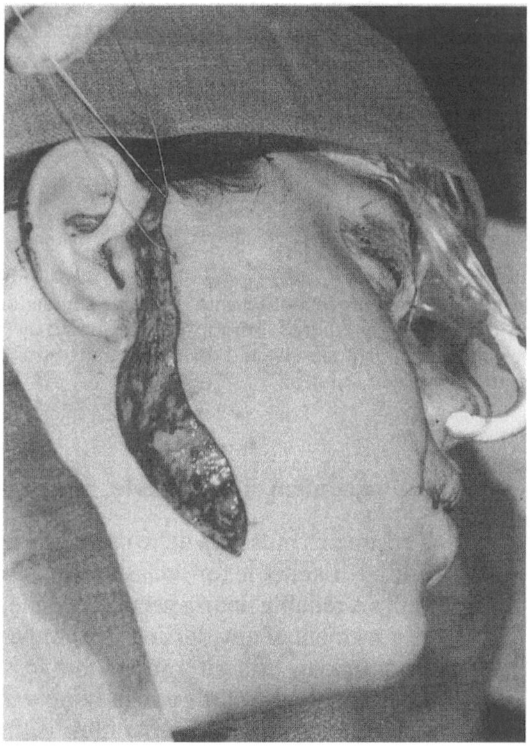
a

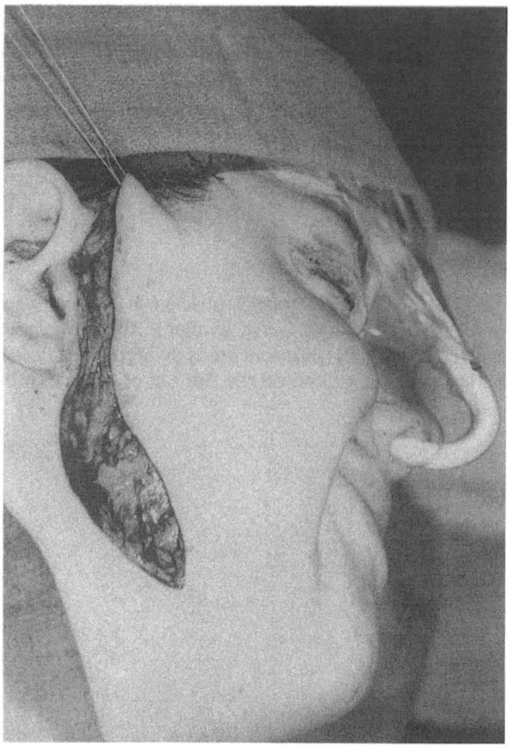
b

Fig. 17-7. **a** The adequacy of the position selected for the muscle's insertion is given a final assessment by placing the sutures which will hold the muscle into the desired locations about the commissure and lips. The suture ends are left long. **b** Traction is applied to the sutures in the direction of the desired commissure movement and the shape of the smile is observed. If the desired shape is not produced, sutures are repositioned until an adequate smile is produced which simulates that on the patient's other side

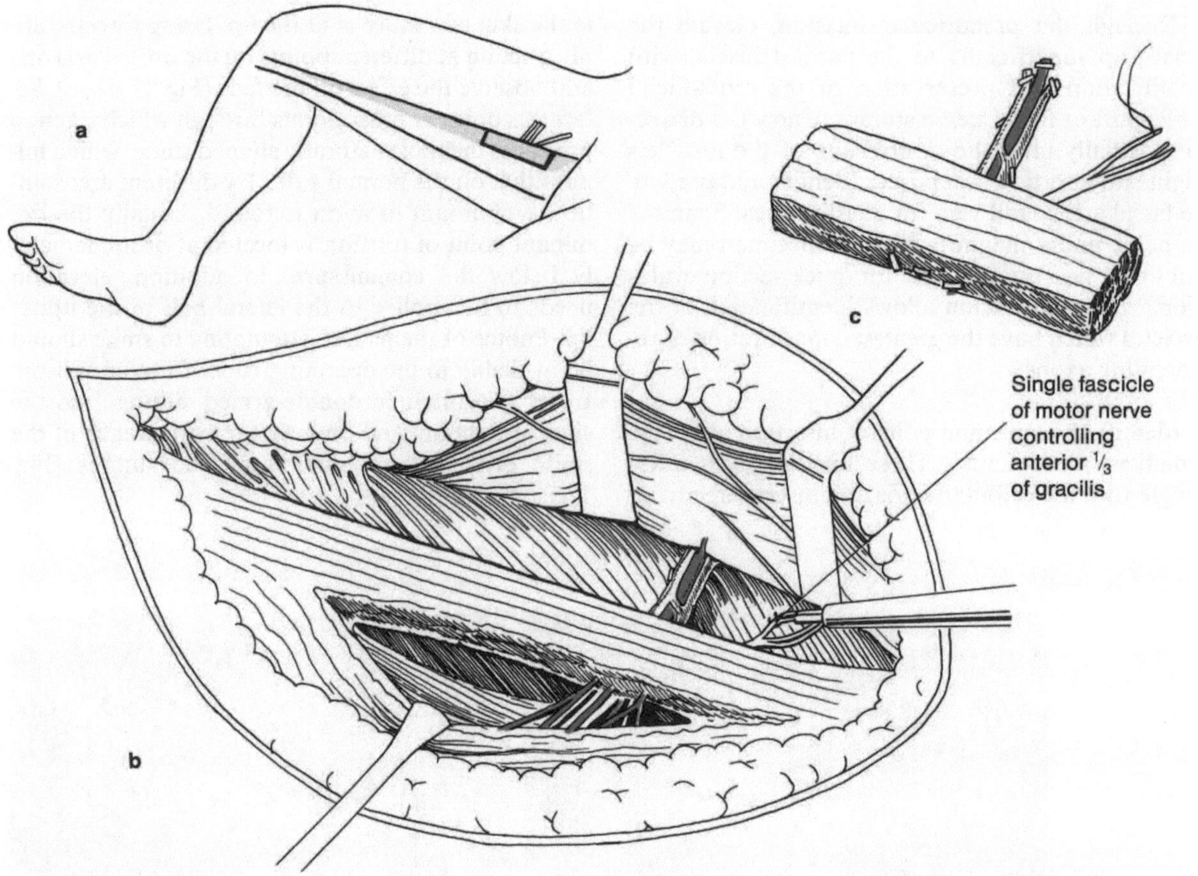

Fig. 17-8. **a** Portion of gracilis muscle which is transferred. **b** If there is limited facial nerve available for reinnervating the transfer, the gracilis motor nerve is divided longitudinally and the fascicles which control the portion of muscle to be transferred are identified with the nerve stimulator. The amount of muscle required for transfer is separated by splitting the muscle longitudinally and dividing it transversely. **c** The separated muscle segment

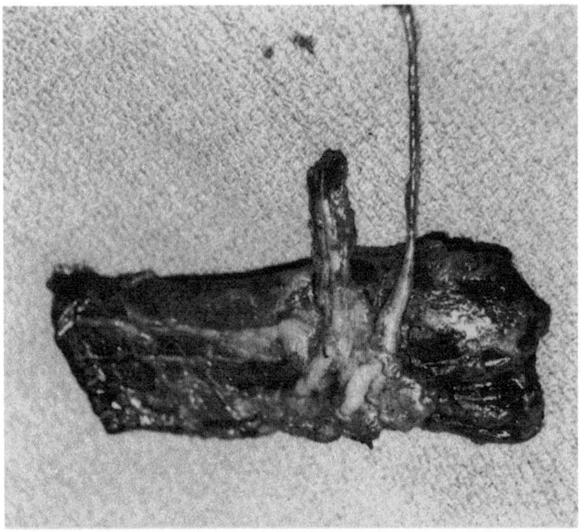

Fig. 17-9. A 9 cm long segment of the anterior third of the gracilis muscle motor nerve is to the upper right. Muscle appears shorter than 9 cm because of contraction

B. Preparation of the Muscle

The gracilis muscle will be used. The anatomy of this muscle is suitable for facial paralysis reconstruction. It has a reliable neurovascular pedicle, can be cut into a segment of any desired size, and can be removed from the leg without a functional loss or significant scar. The thigh is far enough removed from the face that a simultaneous preparation of the muscle and face is feasible. Either leg may be used as the muscle may be turned end for end without affecting its function.

See chapter 6 for a description of the general preparation of the gracilis muscle.

The amount of gracilis muscle to be taken depends upon the functional requirements and reinnervation potential within the face. Usually a short length of the anterior 25–50% of the gracilis is used (Fig. 17-1 a, 8 a).

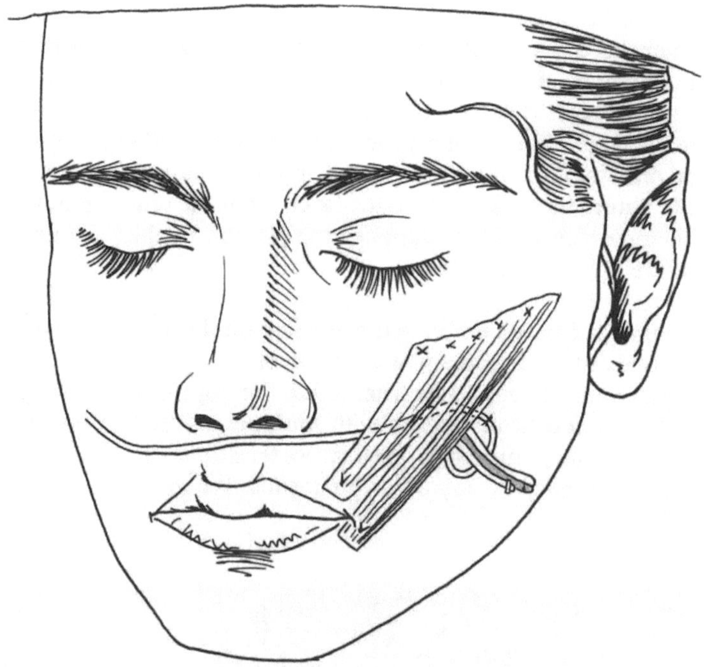

Fig. 17-10. Completed muscle transplantation

1. If there are only one or two good nerve fascicles available on the face for muscle innervation, it may be helpful to have a muscle which has only one or two fascicles. Divide the muscle's motor nerve longitudinally into separate fascicles at the approximate point where it will be sutured. Stimulate each fascicle and identify the portion of muscle which is under the control of that fascicle (Fig. 17-8 b). Usually one fascicle will control the anterior margin of the muscle, which constitutes 25-50% of the muscle width. This is the portion of the muscle usually used for transplantation. Usually, the rest of the nerve controls the posterior portion of the muscle.

2. Note the point of attachment of the neurovascular pedicle to the muscle. Be sure that it is entering the portion of the muscle which you are transferring. Usually, the pedicle enters the deep aspect of the anterior margin, but occasionally enters the deep surface of the central part of the muscle. Determine the length and width of the piece of muscle to be transferred and mark this on the muscle, centred on the neurovascular pedicle. At present, there are no guidelines except experience to indicate what is the appropriate cross-sectional area of muscle to be transferred. However, a 9 cm long strip of the anterior third of the gracilis is the average size removed and, after trimming and suturing of the ends, a 6 cm length of functioning muscle is transferred.

3. Separate the muscle longitudinally and transversely, cauterizing the vessels which pass across the area of division. Leave this piece of muscle attached by its pedicle while the facial dissection is completed, and observe the color of the muscle to assess its perfusion (Fig. 17-8 b, c, 9).

C. Muscle Transplantation

1. Place the muscle in the face, stretched to its final length, and review the location of the vessels and nerve before suturing it. Attach the muscle "insertion" into the commissure. If the muscle is thick at the insertion, it may be tapered by removing muscle fibres from the centre of the end to be inserted so that it does not produce a lump at the commissure. Take a generous bite of muscle fibres with each mattress suture and secure the insertion to the commissure. Tack the other end of the muscle to the zygoma prior to doing the vascular repairs.

2. Do microvascular anastomoses between the muscle and the recipient vessels as end to end repairs. The repairs must be technically perfect as the muscle cannot be monitored to identify an anastomosis thrombosis.

3. Do a fascicular nerve repair with 11-0 nylon between the cross-facial nerve graft and the muscle's motor nerve, and place the repair as close as possible to the muscle. If some fascicles of the graft have a greater concentration of regenerated axons than others, this situation will be identified in the quick section. Suture these fascicles to the fascicles of the gracilis motor nerve which supplies the portion of the muscle to be transplanted.

4. Fix the muscle's origin to the location on the arch and body of the zygoma which produces the desired angle of pull. It should be trimmed to the appropriate length and firmly tacked with multiple mattress sutures to the periosteum. The correct tension is difficult to identify by any objective means. We apply sufficient tension that the corner of the mouth is supported in the patient's normal rest position when awake. This may be a little more tension than appears to be present on the normal side during anaesthesia. However, tension adjustment is a very imprecise part of the operation and requires further studies. Apply non-compressive dressings and insert drains.

5. In the postoperative period, discourage mouth movements. A custom-made commissure retractor, fixed with a heavy suture to the scalp, is worn for 10 days postoperatively to prevent the muscle's being pulled from its insertion by smiling and laughing movements on the normal side of the face.

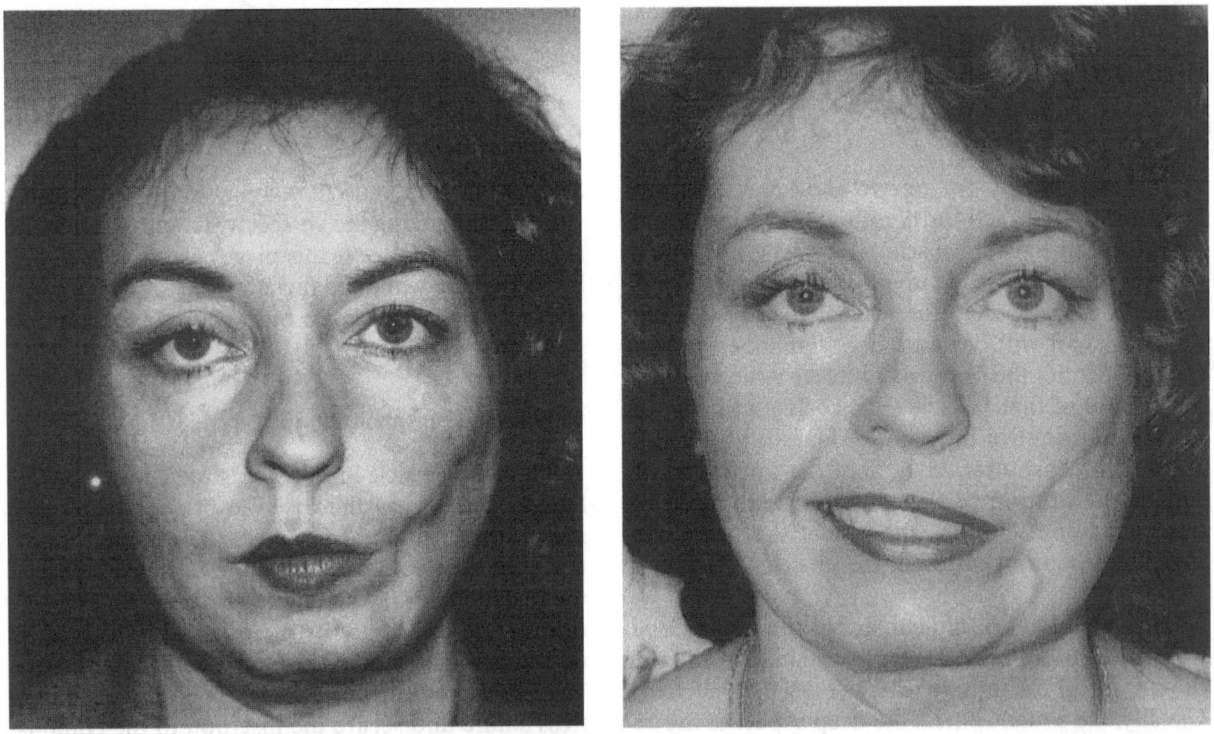

a b

Fig. 17-11. **a** A 33 year old woman with a partial facial paralysis following a fibrosarcoma excision of the left cheek nine years previously. At rest, her upper lip is deviated towards the normal side and there is a soft tissue defect of the left cheek.

b Three months following a gracilis muscle transplantation, which included vascularized subcutaneous fat. Reinnervation was achieved with a facial nerve stump from the left cheek. The patient is shown before reinnervation took place.

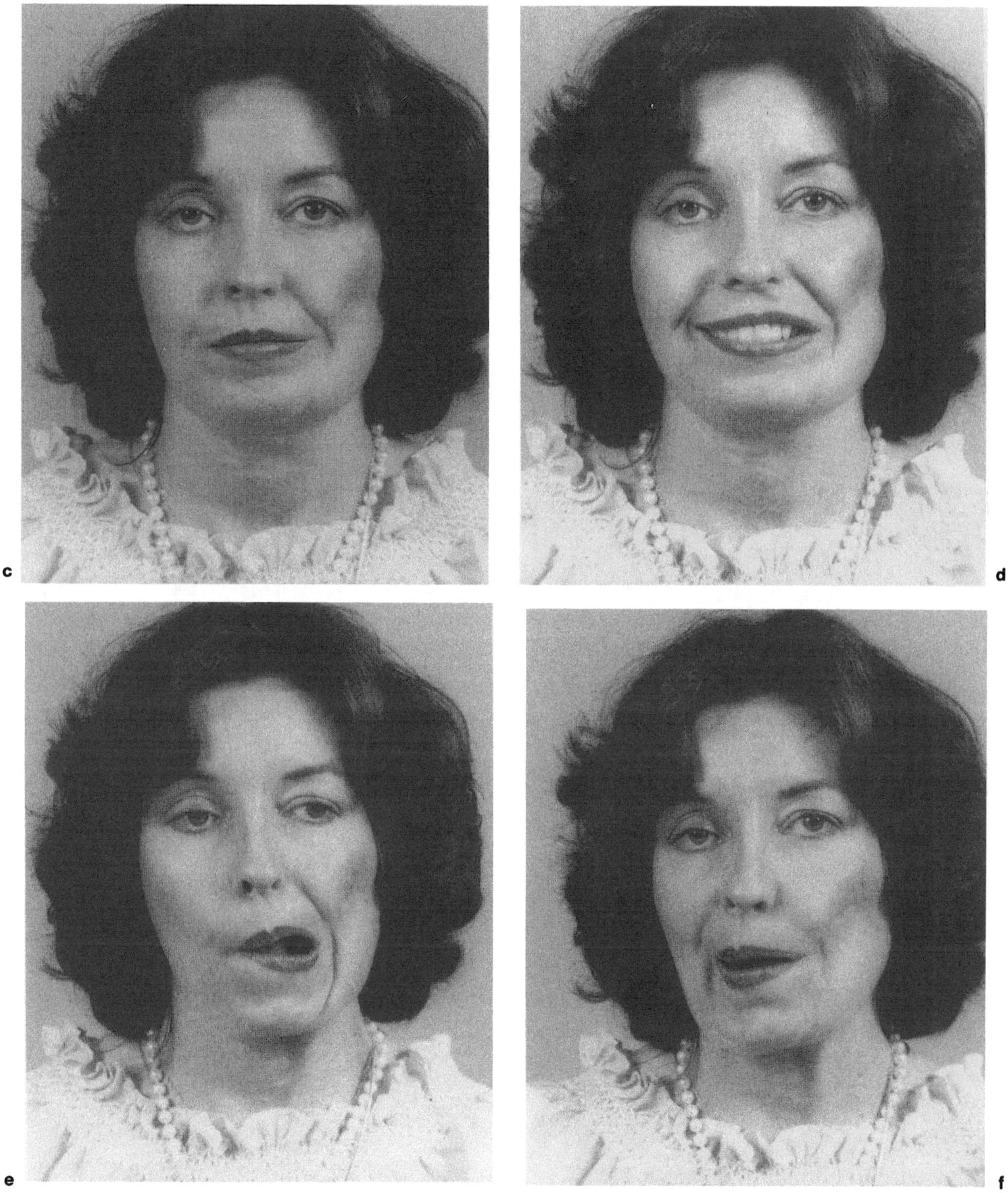

c One year postoperatively, the patient has a symmetrical appearance at rest. **d** The patient has a spontaneous and symmetrical smile. **e** Voluntary movement of the commissure towards the previously paralysed side, using transplanted muscle **f** Voluntary movement of the commissure towards the normal side, showing that the transplanted muscle can be stretched

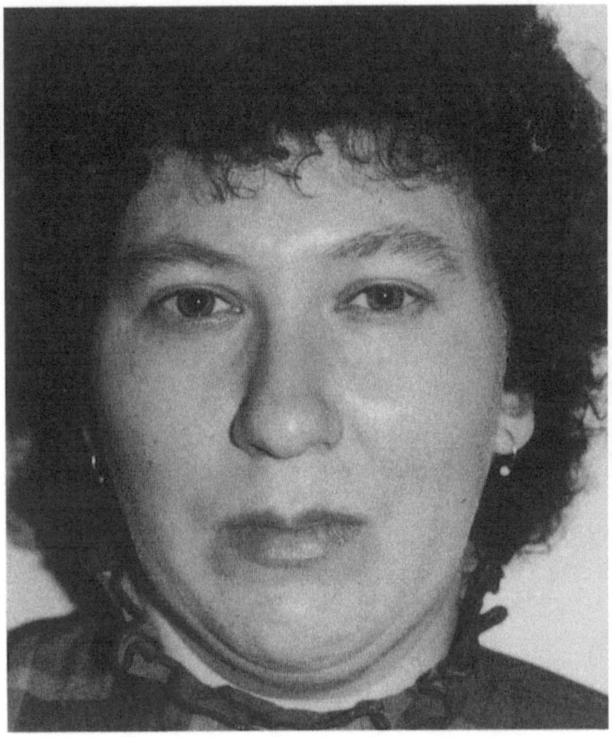

a

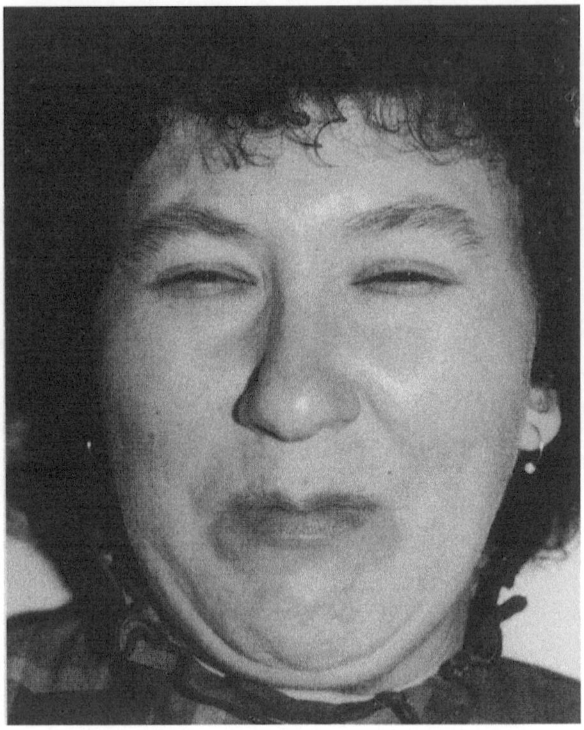

b

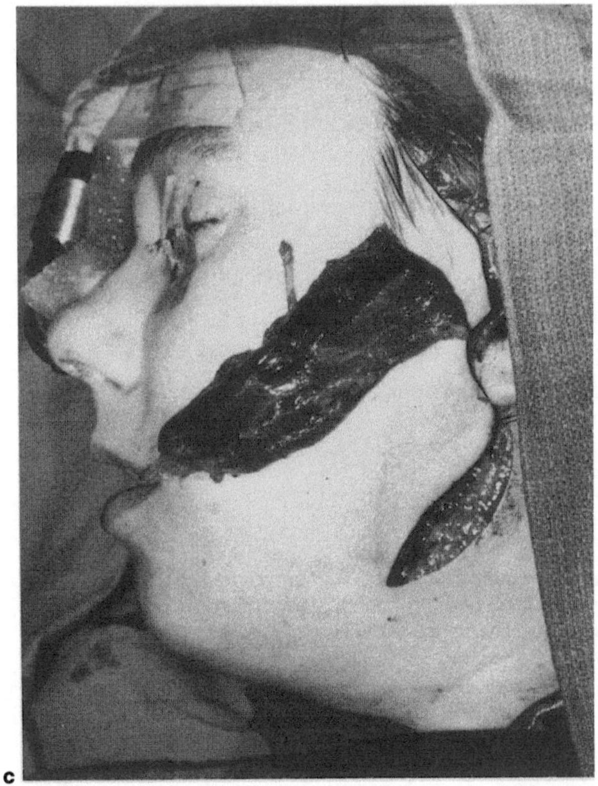

c

Fig. 17-12. **a** Following spontaneous recovery from a severe Guillame Barre syndrome, a 31 year old woman developed severe synkinesis. **b** On attempted smiling, all muscles of facial expression contract at once, producing a grimace. **c** A segmental gracilis muscle is seen lying on her left cheek prior to transplantation. The motor branch of the masseter was used for muscle innervation.

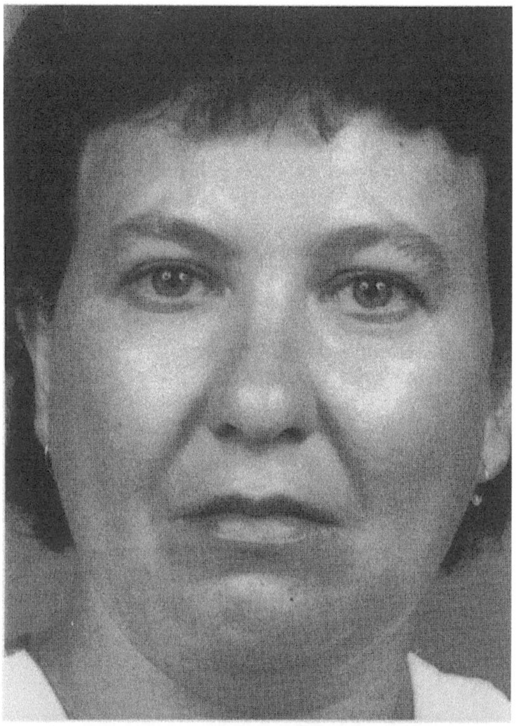

d

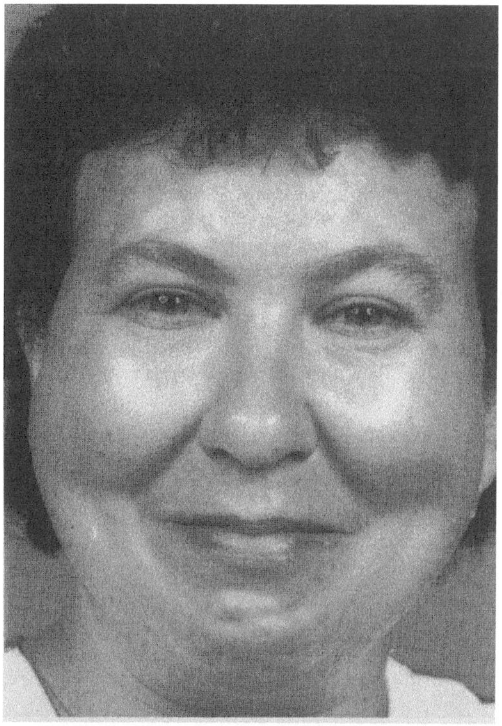

e

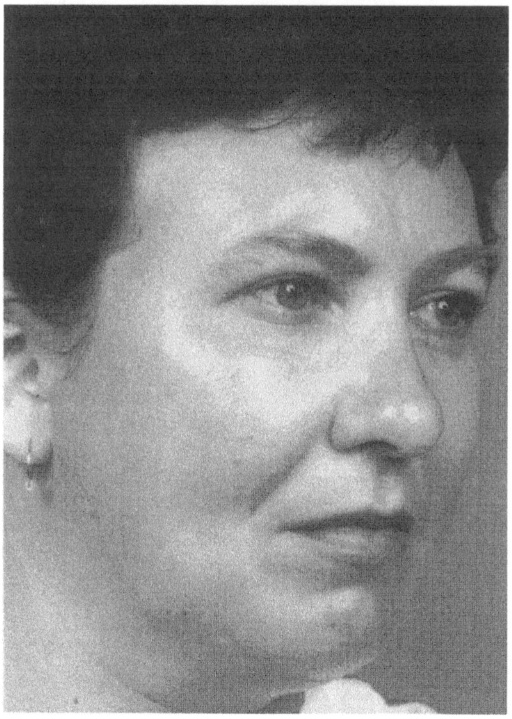

f

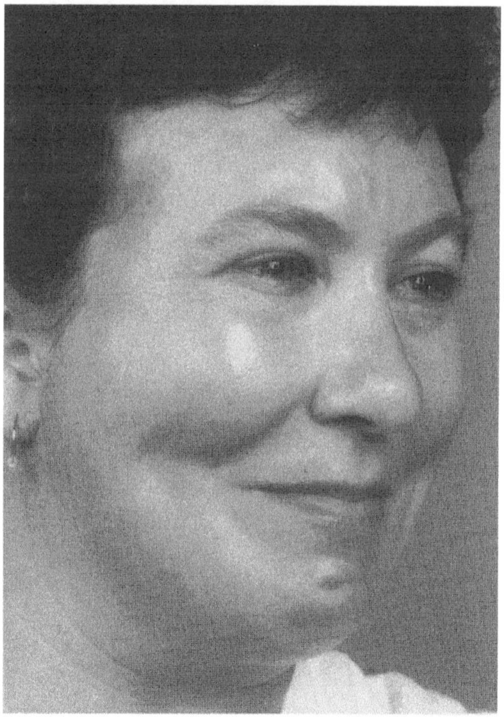

g

References

1. Anderl F (1973) Reconstruction of face through cross-face nerve transplantation in facial paralysis. Chirurgia Plastica 2: 17
2. Harii K, Ohmori K, Tori S (1976) Free gracilis muscle transplantation with microneurovascular anastomoses for the treatment of facial paralysis. Plast Reconstr Surg 57: 133
3. Kempe LG (1980) Topical organization of the distal portion of the facial nerve. J Neurosurg 52: 671
4. Manktelow RT, Zuker RM (1984) Muscle transplantation by fascicular territory. Plast Reconstr Surg 73: 751
5. Mayou BJ, Watson JS, Harrison DH (1981) Free microvascular and microneural transfer of the extensor digitorum brevis muscle for the treatment of unilateral facial paralysis. Br J Plast Surg 34: 362
6. O'Brien BM, Franklin JD, Morrison WA (1980) Cross-facial nerve grafts and microneurovascular free transfer for long established facial palsy. Br J Plast Surg 33: 202
7. Smith JW (1971) A new technique of facial animation. Transactions of the Fifth International Congress of Plastic and Reconstructive Surgery. Butterworths 83
8. Thompson N (1971) Autogenous free grafts and skeletal muscle. A preliminary experimental and clinical study. Plast Reconstr Surg 48: 11
9. Thompson N, Wynn Parry CB (1981) In: Freilinger G, Hole J and Carlsen M. Muscle Transplantation. New York, Springer Verlag
10. Tolhurst DE, Bos KE (1982) Free vascularized muscle grafts in facial paralysis. Plast Reconstr Surg 69: 760

Upper Extremity Reconstruction

The free tissue transfer has been accepted with great enthusiasm by surgeons doing upper extremity reconstruction. Not only is it useful for coverage problems and bone reconstruction, but it provides a unique reconstructive capability when functioning musculature has been lost and digits amputated. The toe and partial toe reconstruction have become the mainstay of thumb reconstruction. For patients who have lost the flexor muscle compartment, functioning muscle transplantation provides an excellent replacement of their missing musculature. A major advantage of a free tissue transfer for coverage is that it allows early hand mobilization and hand elevation.

Vascular Anastomoses in the Upper Extremity

Vascular anastomoses are more reliable in the upper extremity than the lower. Nevertheless, the surgeon must be particularly cautious that all the factors which affect peripheral perfusion are observed. These include maintenance of blood volume and pressure, and peripheral as well as core body temperature. The control of these factors, the prevention of spasm, and the importance of the zone of injury concept are described in detail in the introduction to Lower Extremity Reconstruction, page 185.

Arterial repairs may be either end to end, or end to side. In the proximal arm, a small branch such as the ulnar recurrent or anterior interosseous is available and provides an excellent vessel for end to end anastomosis. Both the radial and ulnar arteries are available within the forearm, and are particularly suited to end to side repairs. Within the palm, the ulnar artery is available and on the dorsum in the first web space, the radial artery is in a very accessible location.

In the forearm, superficial and deep veins are available for anastomoses. The superficial veins do not have the same tendency to develop spasm as the superficial veins of the leg. They are readily available and, if they have not been damaged by previous intravenous medication, are usually the veins of choice. If superficial veins are not available, venae comitantes may be used in the proximal forearm where they are a suitable size for flap transfers. Although the venae comitantes at the wrist and hand are often too small for reliable microanastomoses, there is a good supply of large dorsal veins in this area.

Chapter 18. Upper Extremity Coverage

The need for a free tissue transfer to cover a tissue defect is not as common in the upper extremity as it is in the lower. There are many other options available, including local flaps and distant pedicle flaps from the chest, abdomen and groin. Nevertheless, many complex injuries and reconstructions to the upper extremity require postoperative hand elevation, and early digit mobilization, and are not suited to two-stage dependent flap procedures. Since free tissue transfers are done in one stage, benefit from elevation and heal rapidly, they are particularly well suited to many complex hand injuries and reconstructions which require flap coverage. There are many free tissue transfers which are available, including skin only, muscle only, skin and muscle (myocutaneous), and fascial free tissue transfers.

A skin only transfer provides a flap with excellent appearance, durability and the potential of sensibility. The flaps most commonly used are the dorsal foot, forearm and the lateral arm flap. The disadvantages of the dorsal foot and forearm flaps are the undesirable appearance of each and the occasional functional problems in the foot. The lateral arm skin flap is an excellent, fairly thin flap, but it is limited to a width of about 6 cm if direct closure is to be obtained.

Muscle only flaps contour well to complex shapes and cavities. They take a skin graft well, and usually provide an acceptable cosmetic appearance. In addition, they provide a rich blood supply to the defect, which is often necessary to obtain tissue healing in a contaminated bed.

The myocutaneous flap has the biological and aesthetic advantages of both the skin and the muscle flaps, but often has the added disadvantage of too much bulk.

Fascial flaps appear to have a place, particularly for small tissue defects when minimal bulk is required. The temporalis fascia flap, covered with a small split thickness skin graft, can provide reliable and thin coverage for defects on the dorsum of the hand.

Any of the muscles previously described are suitable for coverage of the forearm. The size and shape of muscle required and size and length of pedicle will determine the most suitable muscle for transfer. The gracilis is a particularly suitable muscle as it can be prepared simultaneously with the forearm to minimize the total operative time. However, if a myocutaneous flap is desired, the latissimus dorsi or rectus abdominis is preferred because the skin flap is thinner and more reliable than the gracilis.

Technique of Forearm Coverage with a Latissimus Dorsi Myocutaneous Transfer

Preparation of the Forearm

1. Excise the margins of the defect until only undamaged healthy tissue remains (Fig. 18-1 a).

2. Expose the recipient vessels, identifying a suitable vein and artery. The proximal radial artery and a superficial vein are a good choice for this location of defect. If an end to end arterial repair is to be done, the artery should provide a vigorous spurt when divided. If an end to side arterial repair is planned, the artery should have a normal appearing wall with good pulsation.

3. Make a pattern of the defect with the location of the recipient vessels marked, and transfer this to the desired donor site.

Transplantation of the Flap to the Forearm

The technique of muscle elevation is described in chapter 7.

1. Place the muscle in the defect, tacking it loosely about the margins in its approximate final location.

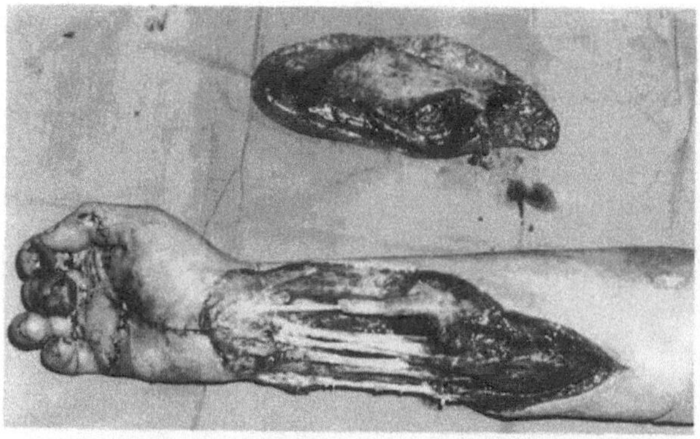
a

Fig. 18-1. a An injury to the right forearm in a 21 year old man resulted in loss of all soft tissues over the distal volar forearm, and exposure and injury to the flexor tendons and median nerve. A latissimus dorsi myocutaneous transfer is prepared for coverage.

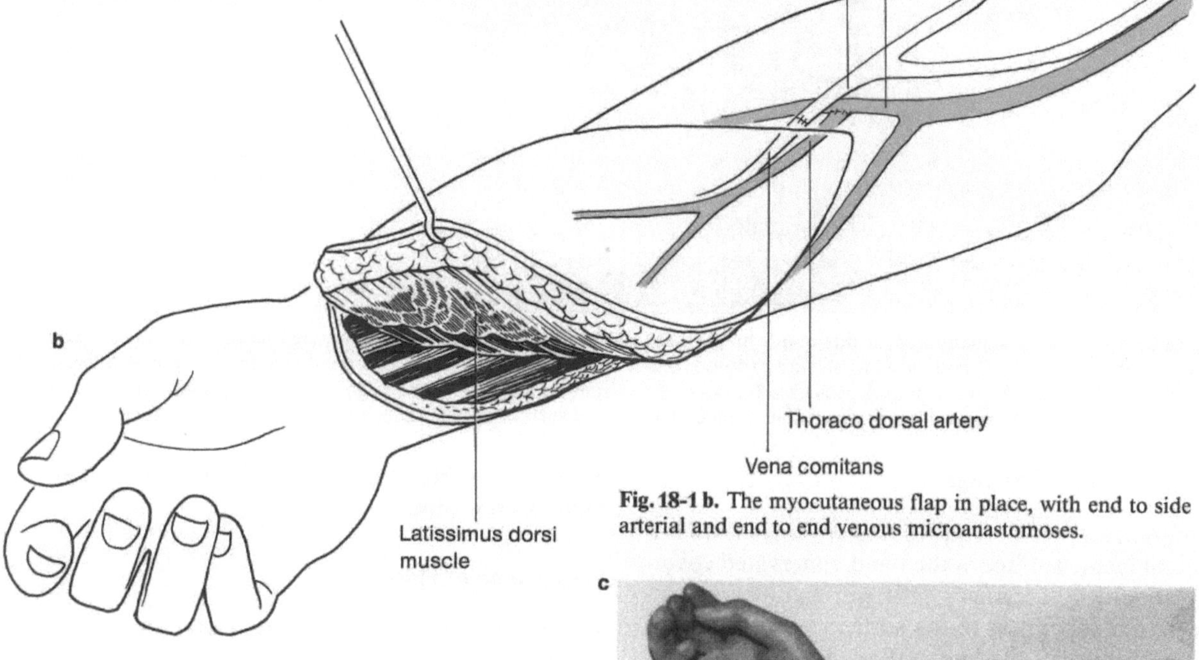

Fig. 18-1 b. The myocutaneous flap in place, with end to side arterial and end to end venous microanastomoses.

2. Take care that the pedicle is positioned in such a way that it passes from the muscle to the recipient vessels without kinking or obstruction. Select the point on the pedicle where the repair will be done. Do an end to end venous anastomosis and an end to end, or end to side arterial anastomosis (Fig. 18-1 b). Observe both skin and muscle to be sure that the entire transfer is perfusing well.

3. Insert a suction drain at the base of the flap and multiple small penrose drains about the periphery, paying special attention to the location of the pedicle so that the drains will not obstruct it.

4. After suturing the margins of the skin flap, reassess the color, capillary return, temperature and turgor of the flap to be sure that the pedicle is functioning normally.

5. Apply a posterior plaster slab to provide stabilization to the wrist and assist in supporting the arm for postoperative elevation. Leave a portion of the skin flap visible for postoperative evaluation.

c

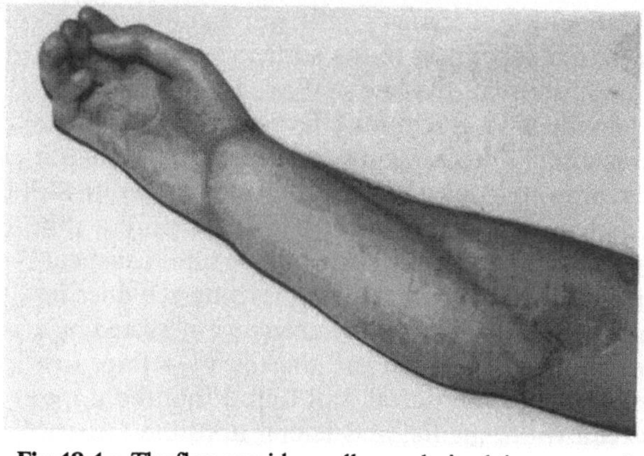

Fig. 18-1 c. The flap provides well-vascularized tissue cover for the devascularized tendons, preventing tendon rupture. A median nerve graft was routed through the latissimus muscle and provided useful sensation for his hand. As the subcutaneous fat over the latissimus dorsi is thicker than that normally on the forearm, these flaps tend to be bulky

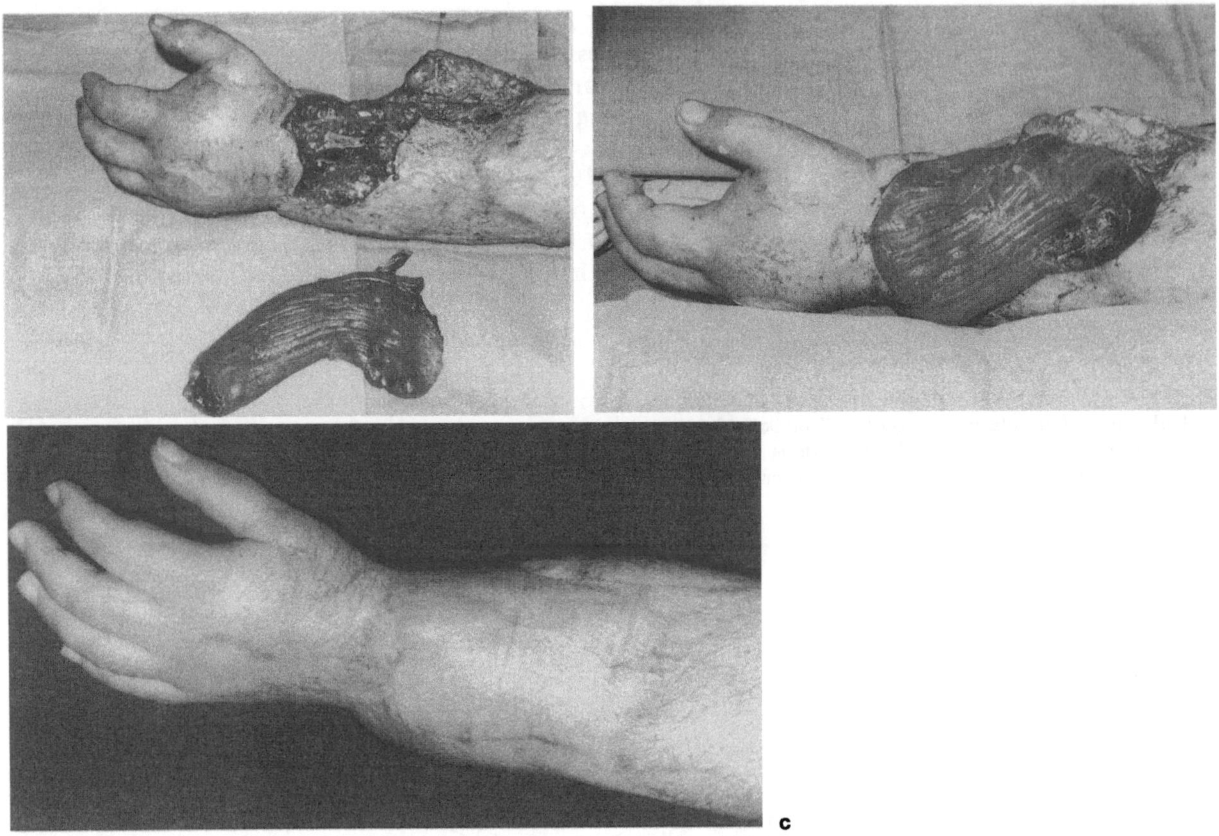

b

c

Fig. 18-2. a Following replantation of this man's hand, there was a tissue loss over the dorsal radial wrist, with exposed fixation plate and bone. b A gracilis muscle was used for coverage with a meshed split thickness skin graft on the surface. The flexible, well-vascularized muscle fills the irregular crevices in the defect without leaving dead spaces. c One year later, with muscle atrophy, there is an aesthetically satisfactory contour and surface appearance, and a durable skin surface

Innervated Skin Coverage

If the surface which requires flap coverage is an important tactile surface of the hand, innervated coverage should be supplied. This will significantly increase the usefulness of the surface and prevent ulceration through overuse and misuse. The physical requirements of a flap for a tactile surface are quite demanding. The flap skin should be durable, have at least protective sensation and be well attached to the underlying bony structures. If there is only a thin layer of intervening fat, there will be minimal shearing motion with gripping and pinching activities involving the flap. Flaps which can be innervated by a cutaneous nerve repair are the toe pulp flap, first web flap and the dorsal foot flap. From the upper extremity, the medial and lateral arm, the forearm and digital pulp flaps are available. Only the pulp flaps have all of the physical requirements of a tactile flap and they, unfortunately, are quite small. Our preference for a larger innervated flap is the dorsal foot flap.

Technique of Hand Coverage with an Innervated Dorsal Foot Flap

Preparation of Hand

1. Mark the area of unstable skin which requires innervated flap coverage (Fig. 18-3 a). Mark the expected location of the recipient vessels, in this case the radial artery and saphenous vein over the dorsum of the first web space. Identify the digital neuromas and digital nerves within the palm, as indicated by a Tinel's sign.

2. Make a pattern of the expected defect, marking the locations of the recipient vessels and nerves, and transfer this to dorsal foot skin.

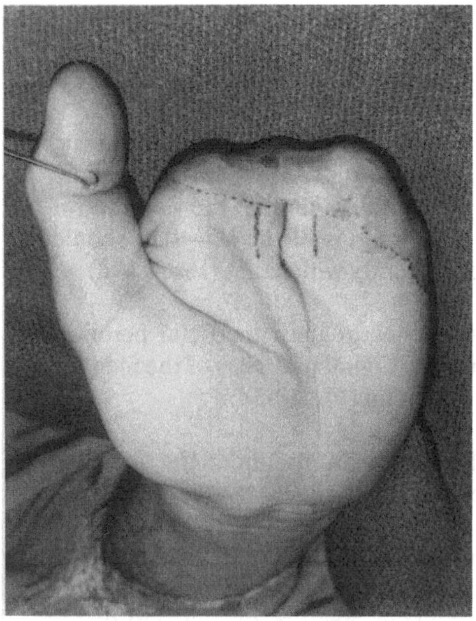

a

Fig. 18-3. **a** A farmer amputated 4 fingers in a corn picker, and degloved the distal palm. Skin grafts on the metacarpal heads were not durable and developed recurrent ulcerations. The area of unstable skin graft is marked distal to the dotted line and will be excised. **b** Dorsal foot flap is outlined from a pattern taken from the hand. The superficial peroneal nerve branches will be used for flap reinnervation. **c** The transferred flap is reinnervated by suturing the digital nerve branches in the palm to the superficial peroneal branches on the flap. **d** Flap revascularization is accomplished with end to side arterial and end to end venous microanastomoses. **e** The flap provided a durable innervated coverage for the metacarpal stump. The thinness of the flap allowed it to conform well to the end of the stump. With minimal subcutaneous fat, it developed very little shearing on use.

The farmer has used his hand for heavy physical work for eight years without any skin breakdown. Two point discrimination is 10 mm over the index metacarpal head - the surface which is used most for pinch functions. Light touch and protective sensibility are present over the rest of the flap

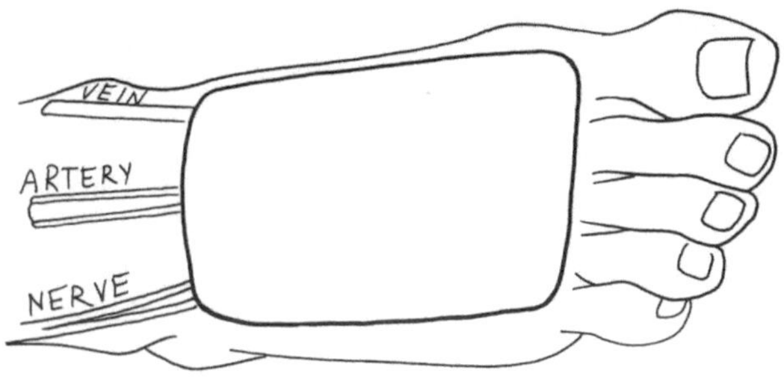

b

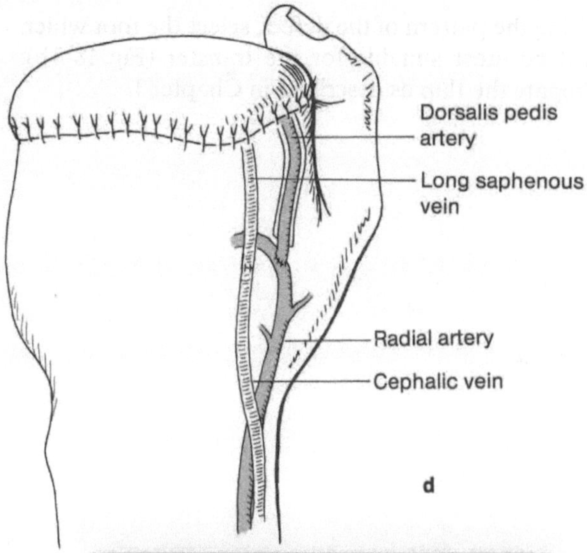

d

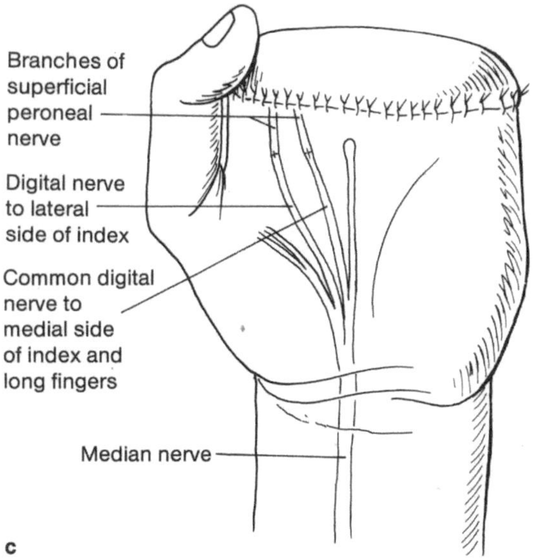

c

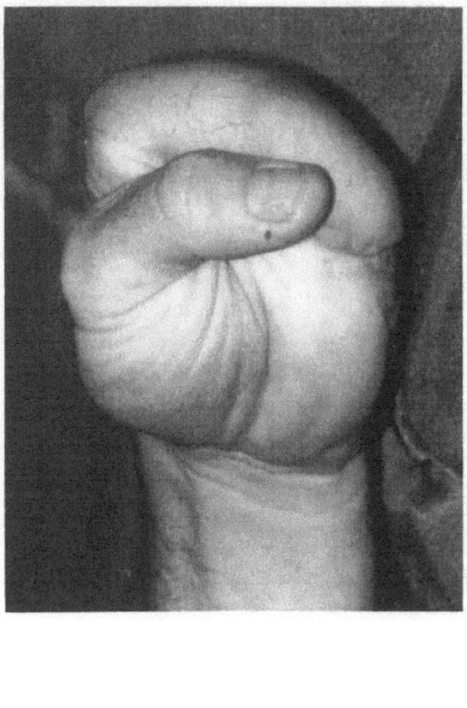

e

3. Excise the unstable skin over the amputation stumps.

4. Through a palmar incision, identify the digital nerve stumps to the long and index fingers. Using magnification, establish the point at which these nerves are undamaged and suitable for nerve repair.

5. Place an incision over the dorsum of the thumb index web space to provide exposure for the radial artery and branch of the saphenous vein. Identify and prepare the radial artery for end to side anastomosis, preferably distal to the extensor pollicis longus, and prepare the vein.

Preparation of Dorsal Foot Skin Flap

Using the pattern of the defect, select the foot which will be most suitable for the transfer (Fig. 18-3 b). Prepare the flap as described in Chapter 3.

Transplantation of Skin Flap to Hand

1. Loosely tack the skin flap in its expected location.

2. Do an end to end venous anastomosis and an end to side arterial anastomosis. Assess the color, capillary return, warmth and swelling of the flap following the repair. The margins of the skin flap should bleed when rubbed gently with gauze (Fig. 18-3 d).

3. Suture the branches of the superficial peroneal nerve to the common digital branches of the median, as identified in the palm (Fig. 18-3 c).

4. Insert small penrose drains under the skin flap margins before suturing in place.

5. The hand and wrist should be supported with an ulnar based plaster splint which provides stability to the wrist and prevents pressure on the flap or the anastomoses.

Chapter 19. Functioning Muscle Transplantation

Microneurovascular techniques allow the transplantation of a muscle from one location to another with maintenance of contractile capability. Reinnervation is produced by suturing an undamaged motor nerve in the recipient site to the transplanted muscle's motor nerve. This technique allows a major muscle deficit to be reconstructed using a functioning muscle transplantation.

The procedure was first reported by Tamai in 1970 when he successfully transplanted the dog rectus femoris using microneurovascular techniques. In 1973, surgeons at the Sixth Peoples Hospital in Shanghai transplanted a portion of the pectoralis major as a replacement for forearm flexor musculature in a patient who had Volkmann's ischemic contracture. The patient developed a good range of finger flexion and grip strength. Other authors have reported the application of other muscles for the replacement of skeletal musculature [8]. With subsequent experience, we have gradually refined the surgical technique and indications for the procedure [3-7].

For most muscle losses, tendon transfers, tenodeses or fusions will provide a useful functional reconstruction. In some patients, because of the nature or extent of the injury, there are no available muscles or tendons for transfer. In other situations, the available musculature is not adequate to provide the functional range and strength which the patient requires, and a muscle transplantation is indicated.

The most common application of muscle transplantation has been to replace the forearm flexor musculature. The procedure has also been used to replace extensor forearm musculature, elbow flexors, shoulder flexors and the anterior compartment musculature of the lower leg.

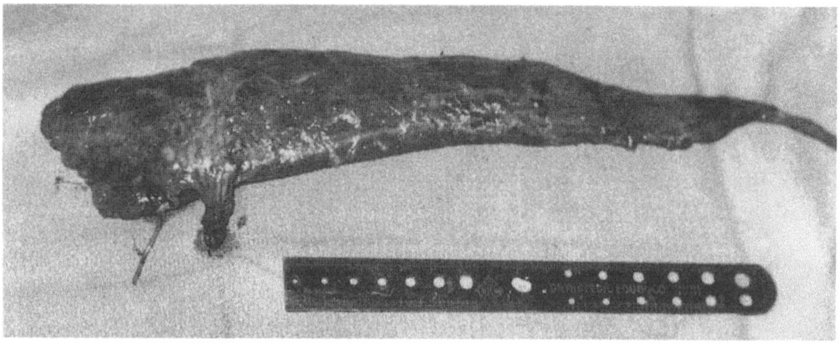

Fig. 19-1. A gracilis muscle prepared for microneurovascular transplantation beside a 15 cm rule

The usual causes of muscle loss in the upper extremity are direct trauma to the muscle compartments, usually through industrial accidents, Volkmann's ischemic contracture, and major electrical burns. Major proximal nerve injuries, such as brachial plexus injuries, present a problem in reconstruction as a motor nerve to reinnervate the muscle transplantation is usually not available.

Indications

Functioning muscle transplantation is indicated for those patients who have a major functional muscle loss for which alternate and simpler reconstructive techniques are not available.

Patient Selection

The candidate for forearm flexor muscle transplantation lacks finger flexion subsequent to a loss of the profundus and sublimus muscles. The hand must have mobile joints, good sensibility, and some intrin-

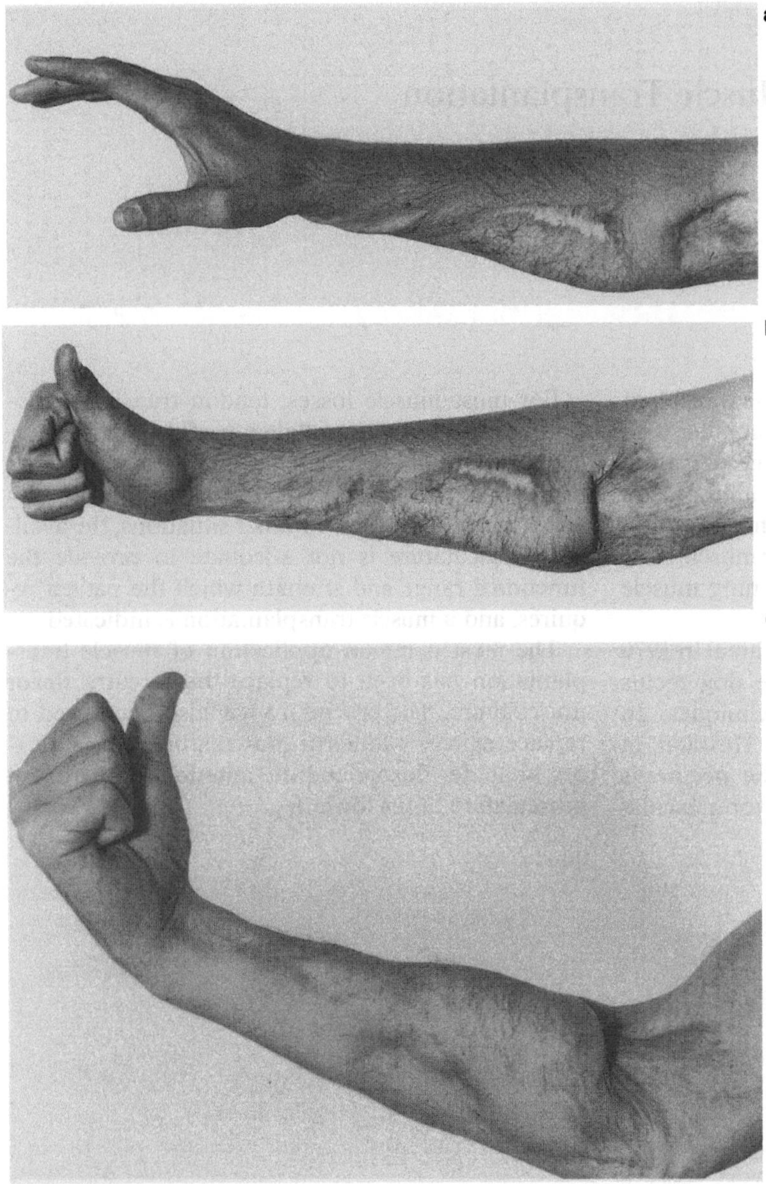

a

b

c

Fig. 19-2. a, b This patient lost all flexor forearm musculature, except for the flexor pollicis longus. A gracilis muscle transplantation provided a full range of flexion and allowed full extension. **c** The bulk of the contracting muscle can be seen in the proximal forearm. Grip strength was 42 lbs

sic function or the capability of reconstructing this function. A mechanism for finger and wrist extension must be present or an adequate reconstruction provided. There must be a good tissue bed for gliding of the distal portion of the muscle and tendon repairs, and good skin coverage in this area. A preliminary skin flap or transfer of the muscle as a myocutaneous flap may be necessary.

Following muscle transplantation, it takes one year for useful strength and range of motion to develop and two years to reach maximum strength. The complexities of this procedure and the long duration of time before a maximum functional result is obtained preclude its use when alternate adequate procedures such as tendon transfers are available. The extensor carpi radialis longus is a good transfer to provide long finger flexion and would be the usual first choice for this problem. However, in my experience, it does not provide the range of excursion or muscle strength which is provided by a gracilis for finger flexion. In an adult male, the gracilis can provide up to 40 pounds of grip strength and a full range of finger flexion in any position of the wrist. If the patient's particular work activities require a better function than can be provided by the ECRL transfer, then a muscle transplantation is indicated.

Preoperative Planning

If the patient satisfies the conditions in the previous section, the next step is to evaluate the technical feasibility of a muscle transplantation. This feasibility is determined by the gross and microneurovascular anatomy of the forearm. There must be an adequate recipient artery and vein, a normal undamaged motor nerve, a suitable muscle origin and insertion and adequate muscle coverage. The location of the vascular pedicle on most muscles will place the anastomoses in the proximal third of the forearm. The most common arteries for end to end anastomoses on the flexor surface in this area are the anterior interosseous and the ulnar recurrent. End to side repairs may be done with the ulnar, radial or brachial arteries. For a muscle transplantation to the extensor surface, the most common recipient vessel is the radial recurrent artery or the brachial artery. The extent of previous injury will usually determine the artery which is most suitable. The location and condition of forearm arteries are evaluated with a preoperative arteriogram. Either superficial or deep veins are used as recipient veins.

Recipient Nerve

The presence of an available undamaged motor nerve in the forearm is a critical requirement for muscle transplantation. All motor branches of the transplanted muscle must be sutured to appropriate nerves in the forearm or portions of the muscle may not become reinnervated. If there is any doubt about the availability of a motor nerve, an exploration of the arm should be done as a preliminary procedure, with identification of the nerve and nerve biopsy at the intended site of repair. If the nerve is suitable for reinnervating a muscle, it will be well packed with myelineated axons with minimal, if any, fibrosis. A motor nerve or branch which normally supplies finger long flexor musculature will provide the most appropriate neural messages. Suitable nerves include the anterior interosseous nerve, median nerve motor branches to the sublimus, and ulnar nerve motor branches to the flexor digitorum profundus.

Despite severe forearm trauma, the anterior interosseous nerve is often undamaged because of its deep location on the interosseous membrane and is readily distinguished from the other branches of the median nerve. In contrast, the finger flexor motor branches of the median and ulnar nerve may easily be confused with the wrist flexor branches. To find the anterior interosseous nerve, identify the median nerve proximally and follow it between the two heads of the pronator teres and under the sublimus muscle. Along this route are the motor branches to the pronator teres (1-4), the motor branch to the flexor carpi radialis (1), the branches to the flexor digitorum sublimus (2-7) and the branch to the palmaris longus. These branches may arise by common stems or as separate branches, and are usually given off in the order listed prior to the take off of the anterior interosseous nerve [2, 11]. A nerve of substantial size, the anterior interosseous nerve, is given off from the deep surface of the median nerve at a level 2-8 cm below the medial epicondyle. This nerve runs down the forearm, initially on the flexor digitorum profundus, and then between it and the flexor pollicis longus on the interosseous membrane. Often, despite severe trauma, small remnants of both of these muscles are still present. Stimulation of the nerve will produce muscle contraction and allow positive identification of the nerve.

If the flexor digitorum profundus motor branch of the ulnar nerve is used, follow the nerve into the forearm between the two heads of the flexor carpi ulnaris. The first branch of the nerve is an articular one to the elbow joint while subsequent branches are all motor. The first motor branches are to the flexor carpi ulnaris (1-4). The last branch is to the flexor digitorum profundus on its ulnar side and is usually solitary. However, sometimes one branch will supply both muscles. This last branch typically arises 3 cm below the medial epicondyle [10].

For transplantation to replace the finger extensor musculature, the appropriate branches of the posterior interosseous nerve (deep branch of the radial) are used. After this nerve emerges from the lower border of the supinator, it lies on the abductor pollicis longus and deep to the superficial group of muscles. The first group of branches goes to the extensor digitorum longus, extensor digiti minimi, and extensor carpi ulnaris. These branches may emerge by a common stem or in succession from the main nerve. They are the most appropriate branches for reinnervation of a muscle to be used to provide finger extension. The nerve then continues distally across the superficial surface of the abductor pollicus longus, giving off branches to the deep extensor muscles.

Insertion and Origin of Transplanted Muscle

The history of the injury will usually indicate the likely location of the flexor tendons. The position of the tendons will determine the length of muscle required. In some patients, there may be no flexor tendons within the forearm. This situation necessitates transfer of a muscle with a particularly long tendon which can reach into the palm, such as the gracilis. The usual site of tendon origin will be the fascia on the medial or lateral epicondyle for flexor or extensor muscle transplantation.

The distal half of the transferred muscle and tendon must lie under good skin coverage. This can be intact forearm skin or a skin flap, but not a split thickness skin graft. Good skin coverage will allow muscle and tendon gliding, and a tenolysis, should it be necessary at a later date.

Muscle Selection

The factors which determine the suitability of a specific muscle for transplantation are its anatomic configuration, neurovascular anatomy and functional capabilities. The size and shape of the muscle must fit the recipient area and provide a suitable origin and insertion.

After transplantation, the location of the muscle's neurovascular structures must match those in the recipient area. Reliable microvascular transfer requires that there be a single dominant vascular pedicle which supplies the muscle. Both artery and vein should have adequate length and diameter to allow a reliable repair. Although it is possible and sometimes desirable to use a muscle with multiple motor nerves, a single motor nerve makes the procedure simpler.

The muscle selected must provide strength of contraction and range of excursion adequate to replace the missing musculature. The strength of the muscle varies directly with the sum of the cross-sectional areas of the muscle fibres. A strap muscle which has long fibres will not be as strong as a pennate muscle of similar weight which has short muscle fibres with large aggregate cross-sectional area. The amount a muscle is capable of shortening is dependent upon the length of the individual muscle fibres. Muscle fibers can shorten at least 50% of their extended fibre length. Muscles with short fibres, such as pennate muscles, have a short excursion. In the rectus femoris, these fibres are approximately 6 cm long. With contraction, the entire muscle will shorten only about 3 cm. In a strap muscle with muscle fibres which extend its full length, muscle shortening is at least 50% of the muscle's entire length. In the case of the gracilis, with an average muscle fibre length of at least 25 cm, the entire muscle can shorten 10–15 cm (Fig. 19-3 a, b). It is helpful to transplant a muscle which has more excursion capability than is required in the arm, to allow some leeway in setting the muscle's tension after transplantation.

The function which is required in most extremity reconstructions will be provided best by a strap muscle with good bulk. Strap muscles which should be considered are the gracilis, latissimus dorsi, portions of the pectoralis major, one head of the gastrocnemius and the tensor fascia lata. The gracilis has a long muscle fibre length, a substantial cross-sectional area, good microneurovascular anatomy, a short tendon of origin and a long tendon for insertion. Its functional capability is adequate for forearm flexor musculature. As a musculocutaneous transfer, the bulky skin flap is not reliable over the distal portion of the muscle, which is the area that requires good skin coverage for tendon repairs.

The latissimus dorsi is a large powerful strap muscle with a reliable neurovascular pedicle. It carries a sometimes bulky but reliable skin flap over most of

a
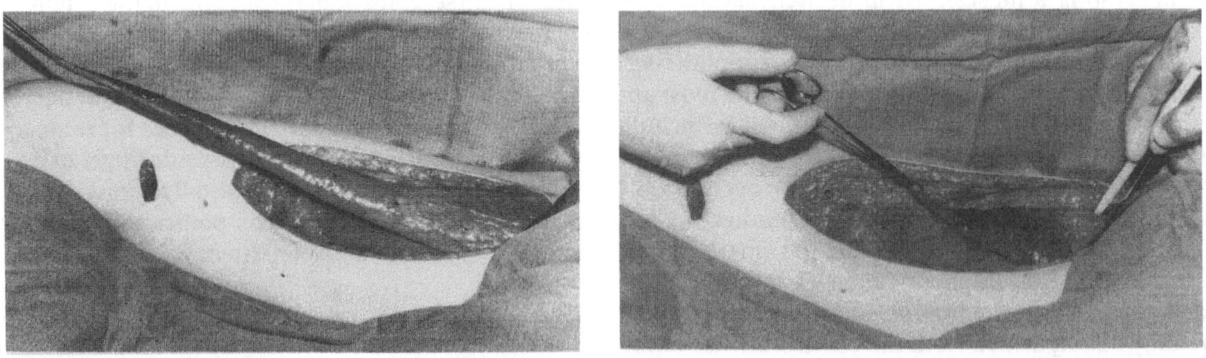
b

Fig. 19-3. a The gracilis muscle has been separated from its surrounding musculature and the insertion detached and held in the forceps. **b** With nerve stimulation of the intact motor nerve, the muscle shortens 15 cm

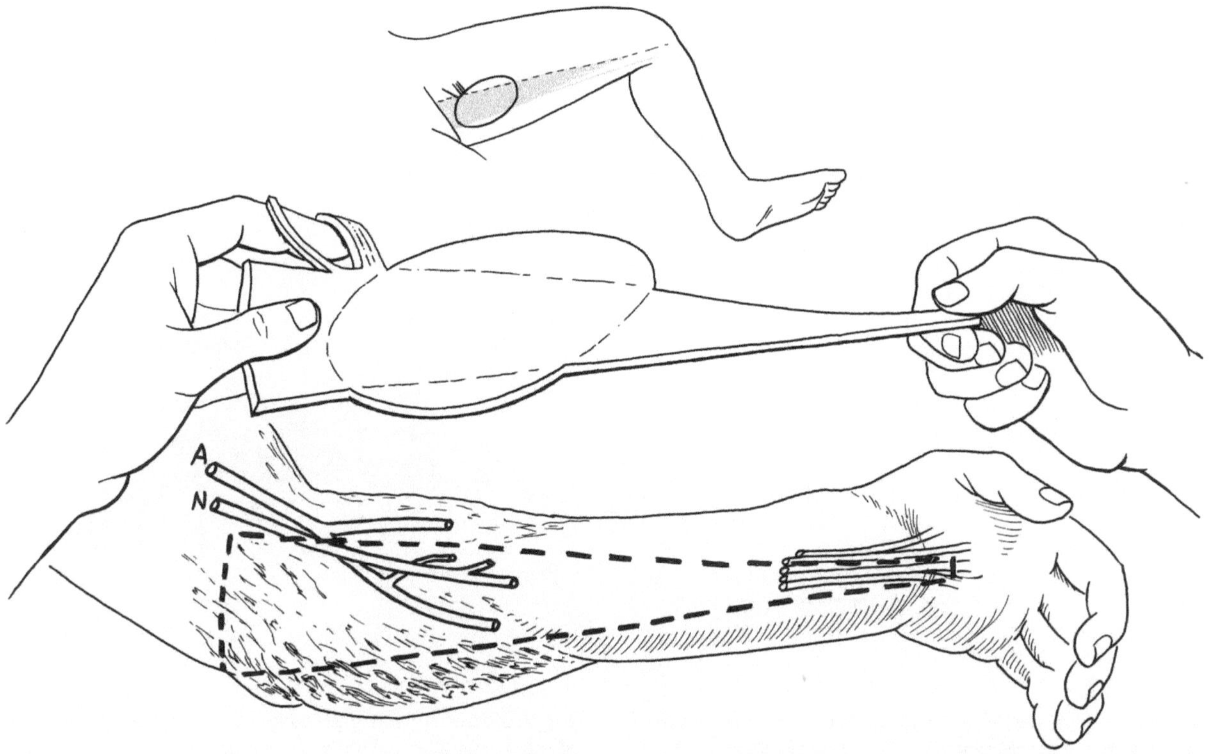

Fig. 19-4. Muscle selection is based upon the functional and anatomical requirements of the recipient site. This selection is facilitated by creating a pattern of the shape and size of the required muscle. The assessment of the location of arteries, nerves and tendons in this patient's forearm depended upon the angiogram and knowledge of the extent of his previous injury. The proximal forearm is covered by skin grafts and would benefit by flap coverage, as marked by the oval on the pattern. The pattern is then applied to potential muscle transfer sites and the one which best matches the pattern and provides adequate function is chosen. For this pattern, the gracilis provides an ideal match

the muscle. Disadvantages of this muscle are the shortness of the tendon of insertion, the broadness of the aponeurotic origin and the great length of the muscle belly.

The medial or lateral belly of gastrocnemius has a good tendon and good anatomic, functional and microvascular qualifications. It can also carry a reliable skin flap. However, the removal of this as a myocutaneous flap is a deforming procedure to the calf.

The tensor fascia lata, with its long fascial attachment for tendon insertion and reliable neurovascular pedicle, provides a good muscle for skeletal reconstruction.

The pectoralis major is a large powerful muscle with a reliable vascular pedicle but a complex innervation. Usually only a portion of the sternal head of the muscle is used. The fact that there are four to seven nerves to the sternal head may make reinnervation difficult [4]. As with the latissimus dorsi, its origin does not provide suitable tissue for suturing and the fan shaped muscle has short muscle fibres superiorly. The rectus abdominis fascia is taken in continuity with the pectoralis muscle's origin for insertion in the flexor tendons.

Some muscles, such as the gracilis, pectoralis major and latissimus dorsi, can be divided longitudinally into separately functioning neuromuscular units [4, 7]. The location of this division is determined by separating the motor nerve into fascicles and stimulating each separately. The portion of muscle which contracts when each fascicle is stimulated is identified and provides the anatomic basis of the muscle's division into two components (Fig. 19-7). This division allows the muscle to be used for two separate functions such as finger and thumb flexion. Only the distal portion of the muscle is separated into two parts. It may be difficult to find two nerves within the recipient area which have separate functional identities for reinnervation of the two separate neuromuscular components of the transplanted muscle.

Since the selection of the muscle will depend upon the status and location of the recipient structures in the forearm, it is helpful to draw these on the in-

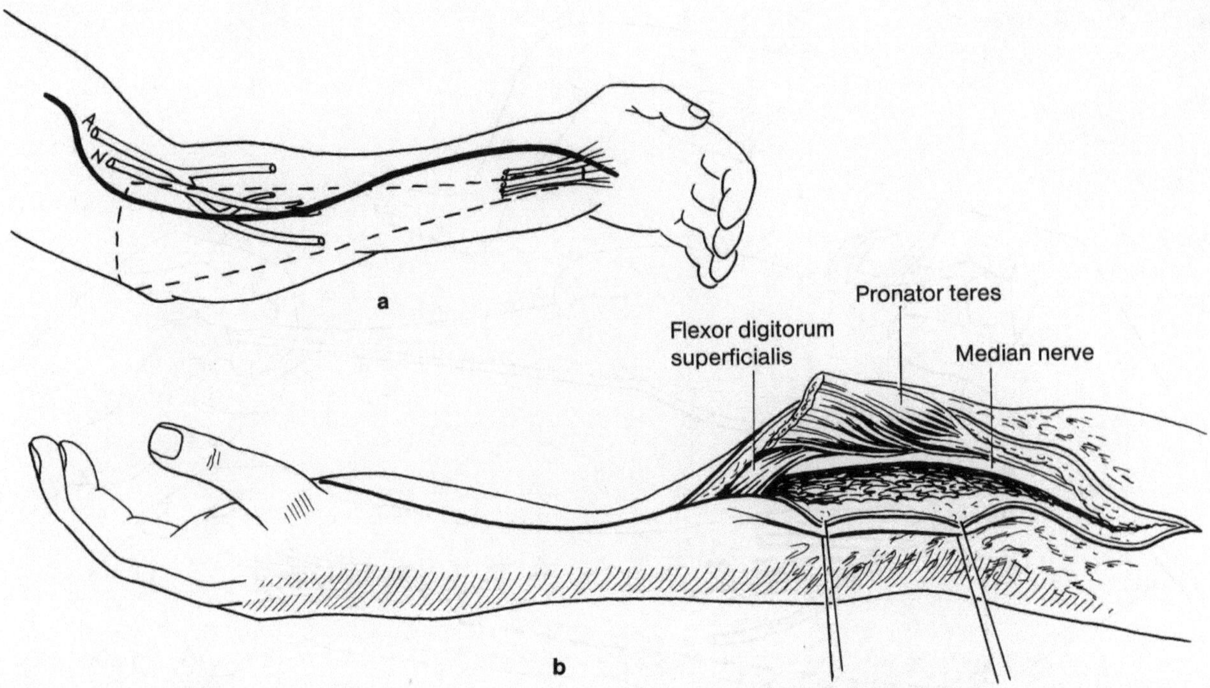

Fig. 19-5. **a** After outlining the location of the recipient structures, and the expected position of the transplanted muscle, an appropriate incision is planned. **b** Identification of neurovascular structures by starting proximally in normal tissue and tracing the structures distally

jured forearm along with the desired location of the transplanted muscle and skin flap (Fig. 19-4). In the forearm, the muscle must have sufficient length to go from the medial epicondyle to the flexor tendons. A pattern of muscle and skin flap shape with the desired location of its neurovascular pedicle can be taken off the forearm, and used to select and plan the most suitable muscle for transplantation (Fig. 19-5).

Technique of Muscle Transplantation for Finger Flexion

Preparation of the Forearm

1. Prep and drape the arm to above the elbow and apply a tourniquet loosely.

2. Mark on the skin all structures that will be used for the transfer, based on your preoperative clinical and radiological evaluations. These include possible recipient arteries, veins, the motor nerve, the origin which will be used for attaching the muscle and the expected location of the flexor tendons. The location of these structures is often a calculated guess. Draw the desired location of the muscle, usually from the medial epicondyle to the wrist. From this outline, it will be obvious where the best incision lines are to be placed for exposure of the structures and coverage of the muscle (Fig. 19-5 a). In the proximal forearm, it is common to skin graft the gracilis muscle rather than carry a bulky skin flap. In the distal half of the forearm, good skin coverage must be available to cover the tendon repairs and to allow distal muscle and tendon gliding.

3. Elevate the skin flaps and prepare the bed to receive the muscle. Identify and prepare each structure required in the transfer. If there are superficial veins available, prepare them for microanastomosis.

4. Identify an artery proximal to the level of injury. Usually this will be the brachial artery. Follow it distally to the site of desired anastomosis. If the artery is in an area of scar tissue, an end to side repair will be preferred as spasm is less likely.

5. Identify and follow the median nerve distally, identifying the branches to the superficial musculature, and the anterior interosseous nerve. Using magnification, ensure that the anterior interosseous is undamaged and therefore suitable for reinnervation of the muscle. Assess the nerve with a quick section at the point of intended nerve repair if there is any question about the quality of the nerve.

6. Identify and clean the common flexor origin over the medial epicondyle. Strong fascia is necessary for reliable fixation of the muscle.

7. Prepare the distal forearm flaps to accept the muscle, and identify the flexor tendons. Separate the tendons from scar tissue, exert traction on them and observe the range of finger excursion. If a few adhesions are present, it is worth removing them. However, if adhesions are extensive, a tenolysis should be reserved until muscle reinnervation has taken place and the muscle is able to contract and provide tendon gliding to prevent adhesions from reforming.

Preparation of the Muscle

See chapter 6 for the preparation of the gracilis muscle.

After the muscle is removed and placed in the arm, it is difficult to determine what is the tension at which the muscle will function best. Some authors have expressed concern that the muscle not be placed too tightly to affect the muscle perfusion. This is not a practical problem. The muscle should be placed in the forearm so that its excursion during finger flexion and extension is within the most powerful range of the length-tension curve of muscle contraction. The muscle will function within this range if the following technique is used. The technique employs pre- and post-transplantation muscle measurements to aid in setting the correct tension (Fig. 19-6 a).

1. After the gracilis has been separated from the surrounding muscles in the leg and is still attached to its origin and insertion, stretch it to its physiological maximum extended position by abducting the thigh and extending the knee.

2. With the muscle in this stretched position, place sutures on the surface of the muscle every 5 cm as markers. These markers will be used when the muscle has been transplanted to the forearm.

Prepare the motor nerve of the gracilis. If separately functioning neuromuscular groups are required for finger and thumb function, the following technique is used.

1. Divide the motor nerve longitudinally into its fascicles.

a

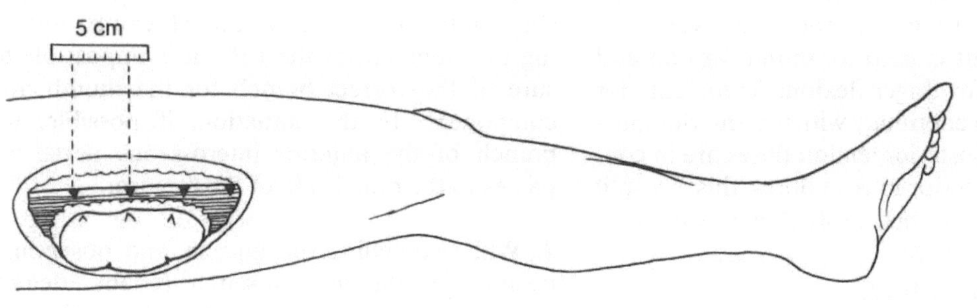

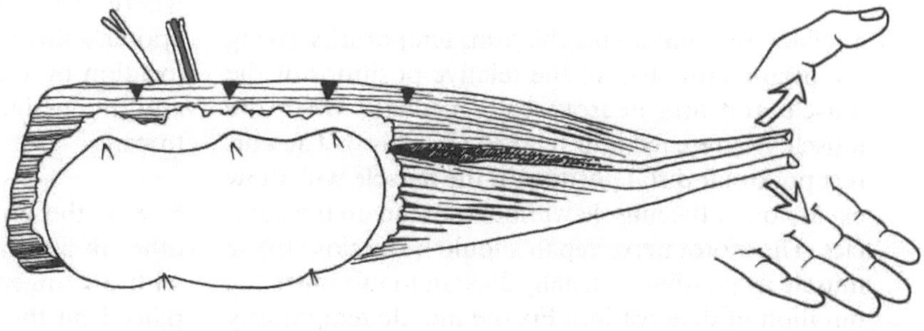

b

Fig. 19-6. a The gracilis is stretched to its physiological extended maximum by abducting the thigh and extending the knee. Suture markers are then applied every 5 cm on the surface of the muscle. **b** Distal muscle and tendon have been divided into two separate components for separate thumb and finger flexion

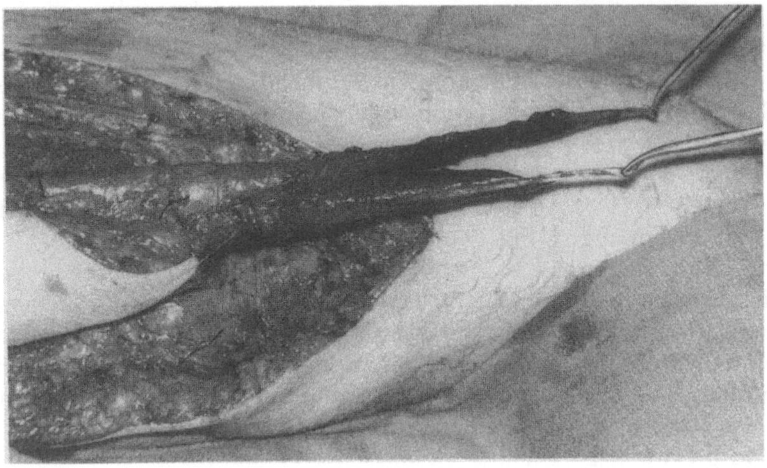

Fig. 19-7. The tendon and muscle of the gracilis have been split into two separate functioning units for separate thumb and finger flexion

2. Stimulate each fascicle separately with a nerve stimulator, using a micro probe. One fascicle usually controls the anterior 25–50% of the muscle and the other fascicles control the posterior portion of the muscle. The stimulator should have a variable frequency and voltage control which allow delivery of a stimulus which produces controlled muscle contraction. Identify and mark the portion of the muscle which is under the control of each fascicle by palpating the muscle during fascicular stimulation.

3. Split the distal portion of the muscle into anterior and posterior parts along the identified line of functional division, splitting the tendon as well. The smaller anterior part is used for thumb flexion and the posterior part for finger flexion. As the anterior tendon fibres are in continuity with the anterior muscle fibres and the posterior tendon fibres are in continuity with the posterior muscle fibres, this is a split which can be accomplished easily (Fig. 19-6b, 7).

Transplantation of the Muscle

1. Place the muscle on the arm, temporarily fixing the origin, and observe the relative positions of the muscle and arm neurovascular pedicles when the muscle is stretched and relaxed (Fig. 19-8). The correct proximal-distal position of the muscle will allow excursion of the muscle without traction on the pedicles. The motor nerve repair should be as close to the muscle as possible - usually 2–3 cm to minimize the duration of denervation. Fix the muscle temporarily in place with sutures to prevent accidental traction on the vessel and nerve repairs.

2. Do a venous, followed by an arterial, anastomosis. Technically perfect repairs are required.

3. The motor nerve of the gracilis contains considerable fatty connective tissue. Strip this back to expose the fascicles. Do a fascicular repair with 11-0 nylon between the branches of the anterior interosseous nerve and the gracilis motor nerve. If the distal end of the gracilis is split into one component for the thumb and one for the fingers, the appropriate gracilis motor fascicle controlling the thumb component should be sutured to the branch of the anterior interosseous which supplied the flexor pollicis longus (Fig. 19-9). Unless a nerve branch can be found going to a remnant of the FPL, it is impossible to be sure of the correct branch for the thumb muscle component. In this situation, if possible, use a branch of the anterior interosseous nerve which passes to the radial side of the forearm.

4. While stretching the muscle, and observing the position of the microvascular repairs, determine where the muscle's origin should go. Suture the aponeurotic origin of the gracilis to the appropriate location on the fascia of the common flexor origin and the medial epicondyle, with heavy mattress sutures.

5. Sew the profundus tendons side to side to each other in a position which produces a balanced grip with all fingers flexing in unison when traction is placed on the tendons as a group (Fig. 19-10a). At rest, the ulnar fingers should sit in slightly more flexion than the radial fingers.

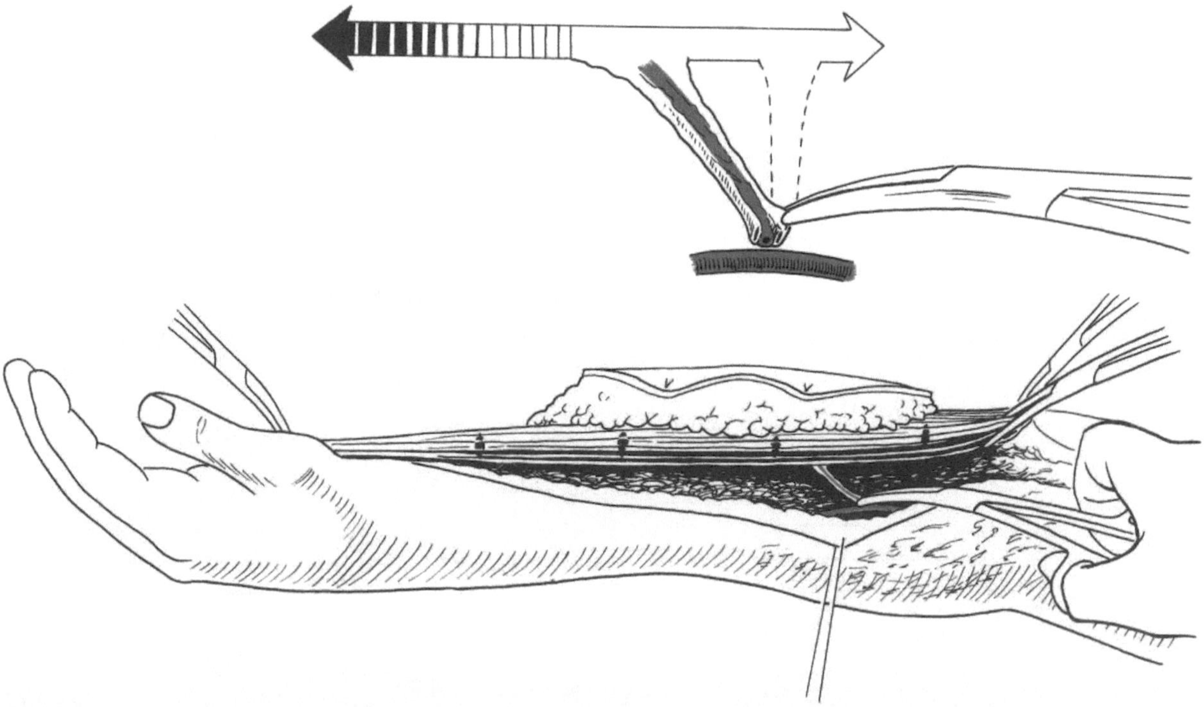

Fig. 19-8. Selecting a location for the neurovascular repairs so that they will not be under tension when muscle contraction and relaxation occur

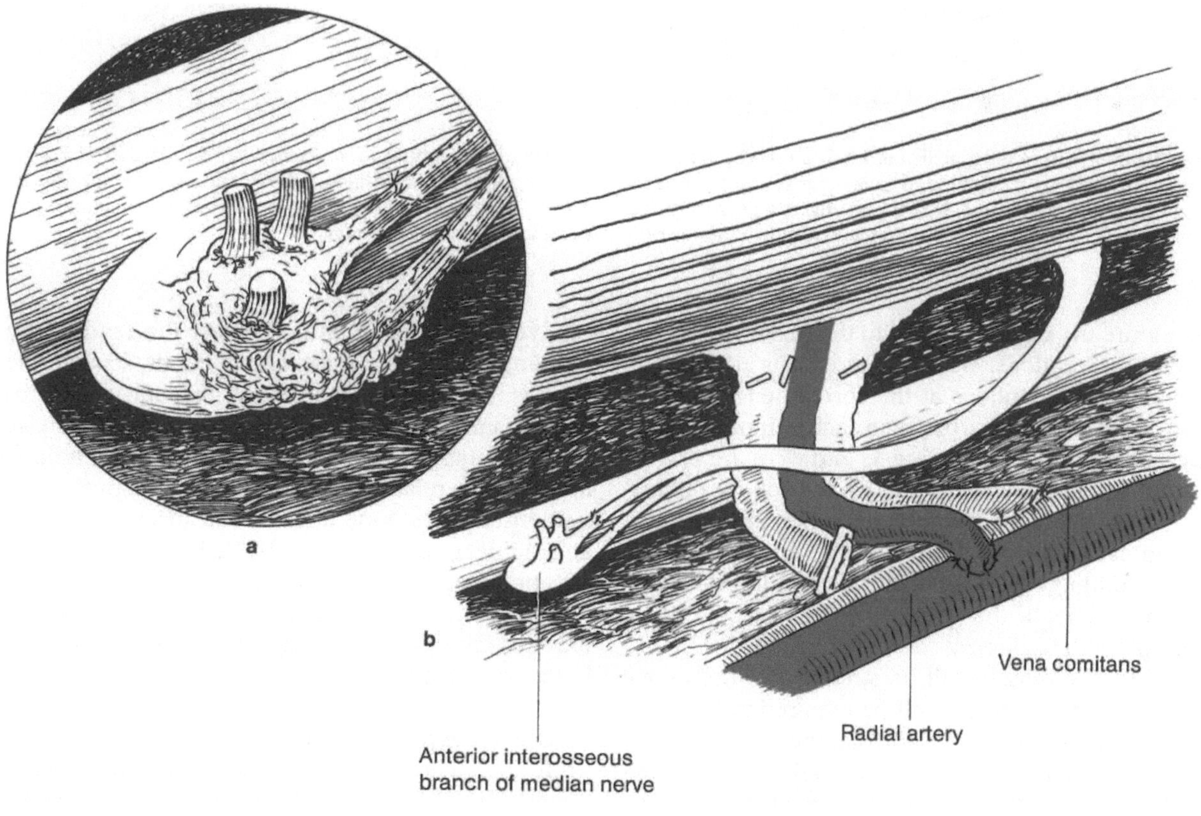

Fig. 19-9. **a** Fascicular motor nerve repair between the gracilis and the anterior interosseous. **b** End to side repairs to the radial artery and its vena comitans

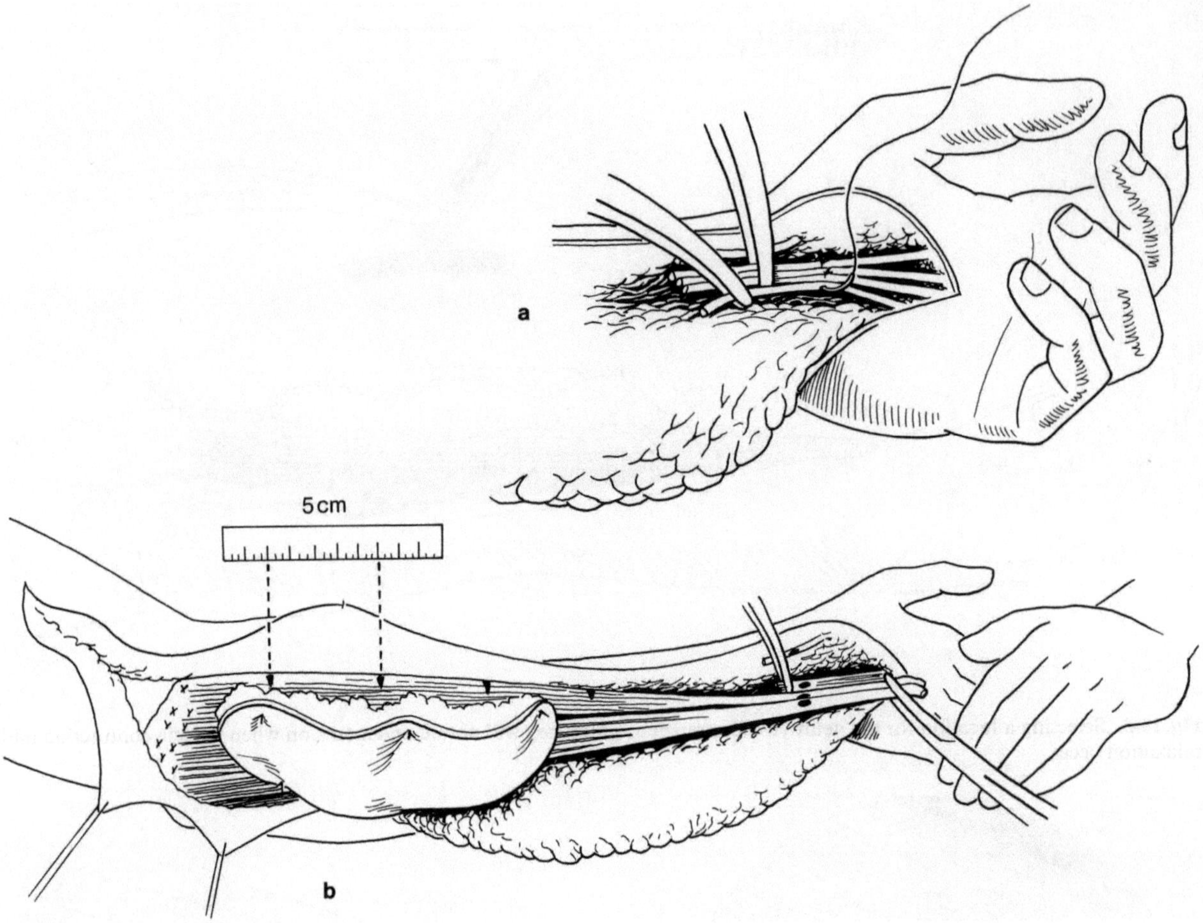

Fig. 19-10. a Before the gracilis tendon is attached, the flexor digitorum tendons are sutured to each other so that the fingers flex in a balanced position. **b** With the fingers and wrist in full passive extension, the gracilis is stretched distally until the previously placed sutures on its surface are 5 cm apart. Marks are placed opposite each other on the flexor digitorum profundus and on the gracilis tendon to locate the point at which the tendons should be sutured together

6. Suture the gracilis tendon to the flexor digitorum profundus tendons. When the gracilis is attached to the profundus tendons at the correct tension, there will be a 5 cm distance between each pair of the muscle's markings when the fingers and wrist are placed in full extension. Determine this tension by pulling the gracilis tendon distally until the distance between each pair of markers on the muscle is 5 cm. While holding the fingers and wrist in full extension, locate and mark the position of the flexor tendon stumps on the tendon of the stretched gracilis. In this position, the muscle will be stretched to the maximum length in which it will be required to function in the arm, which is the same maximum length as it was required to function in the leg. The flexor tendon stumps should be sutured to the gracilis muscle tendon in the marked positions (Fig. 19-10b). With the wrist and fingers in flexion, the tension is not excessive for tendon repair. Connect the tendons by weaving each of the profundus tendons through the gracilis, and the gracilis tendon through each profundus, into a smooth and solid tendon "knot". Use multiple mattress sutures for fixation. Slight adjustments of the relative tightness of the four profundus tendons can be done at this time to ensure a balanced finger position (Fig. 19-11 a, b). When the fingers and wrist are passively extended completely, the muscle markers will be 5 cm apart. As this extension requires considerable force, you may not be willing to test your tendon sutures to this extent.

7. The flexor pollicis longus can be inserted with the profundus tendons or attached to a separate slip of the gracilis. If inserted with the profundus tendons, it should be inserted with less tension. Traction on the gracilis tendon should produce finger flexion,

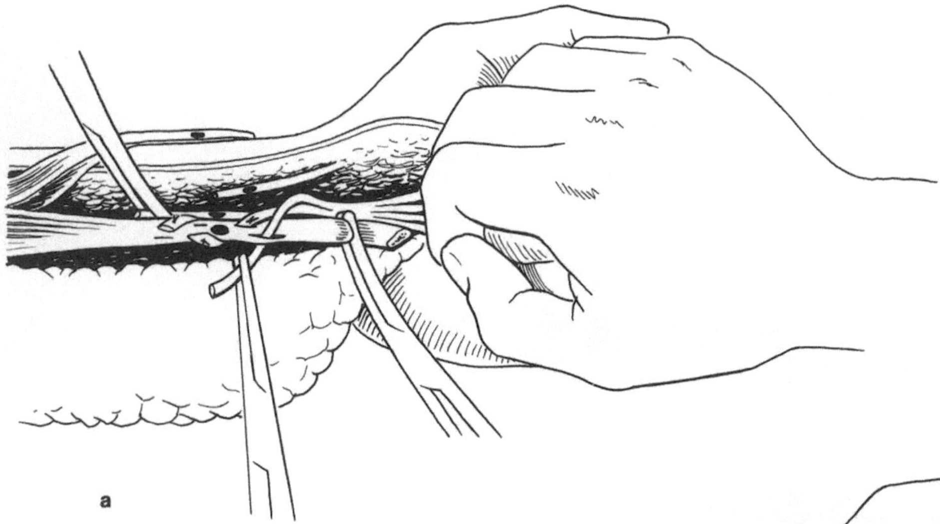

a

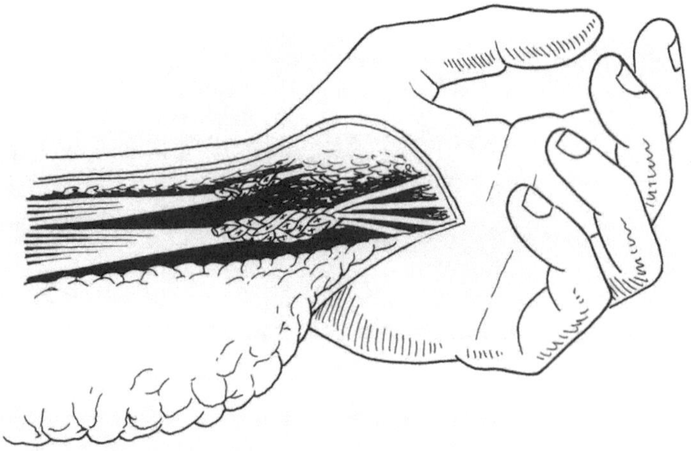

b

Fig. 19-11. a Each flexor digitorum profundus tendon is woven through the gracilis tendon so that the dots are opposite each other. **b** There is a separate portion of the gracilis tendon for the flexor pollicis longus

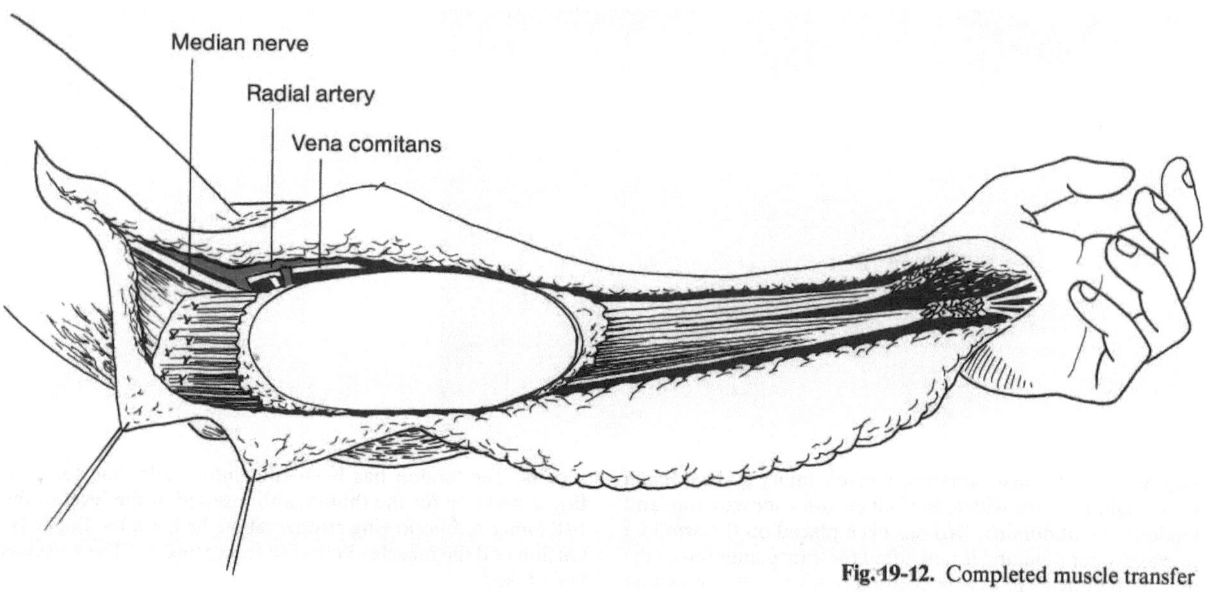

Fig. 19-12. Completed muscle transfer

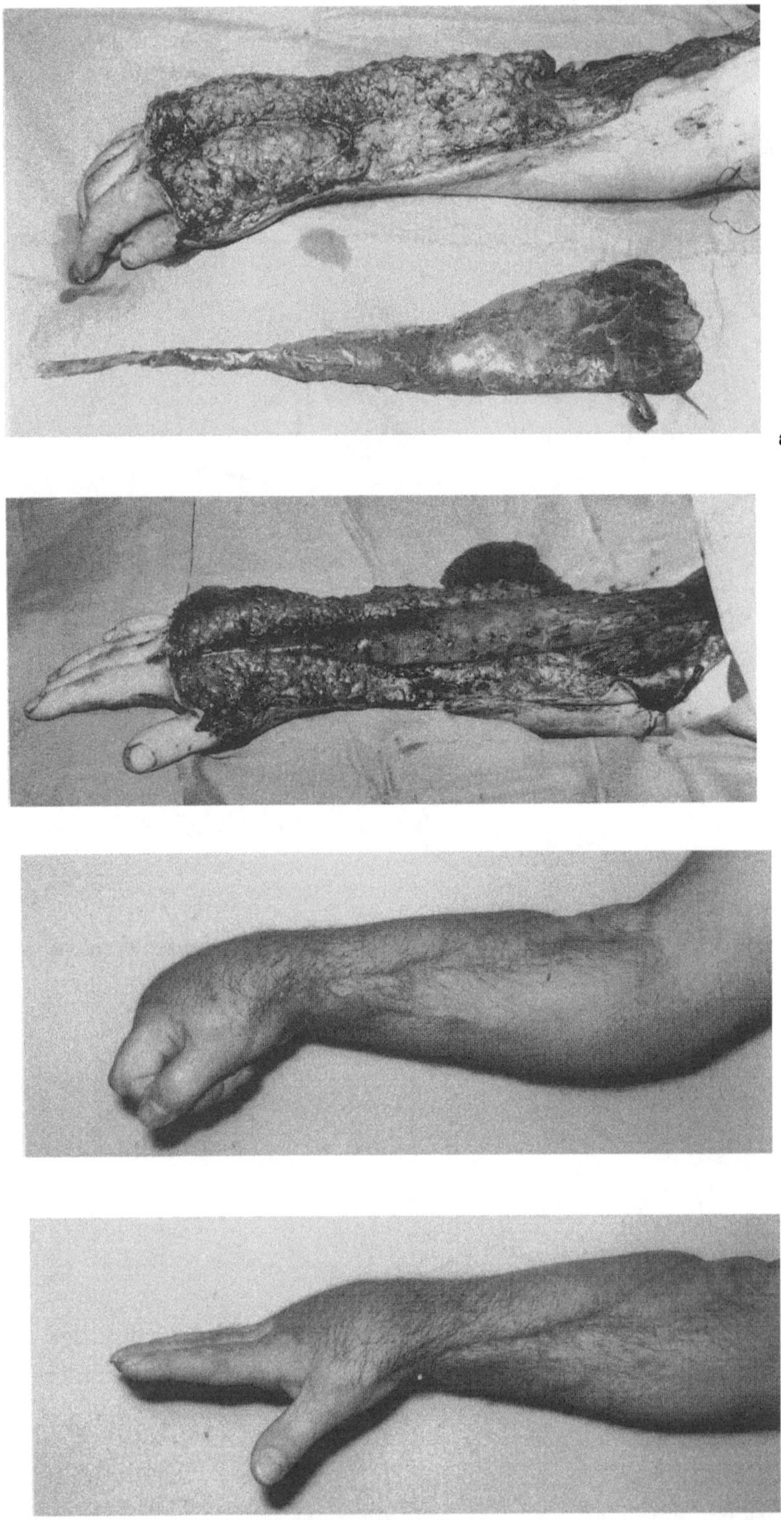

a

b

c

d

Fig. 19-13. **a** This man sustained a severe injury to the dorsum of his right forearm with loss of all extensor musculature and tendons. An abdominal flap has been placed on the arm in a previous operation and is now lifted for transplantation of the gracilis. **b** Gracilis muscle in position following neurovascular repairs. The tendon has been split into 5 tails, one for each finger and one for the thumb, and inserted at the level of the MP joints. **c, d** Following reinnervation, he has good finger extension and the muscle allows full finger flexion. The wrist has been fused

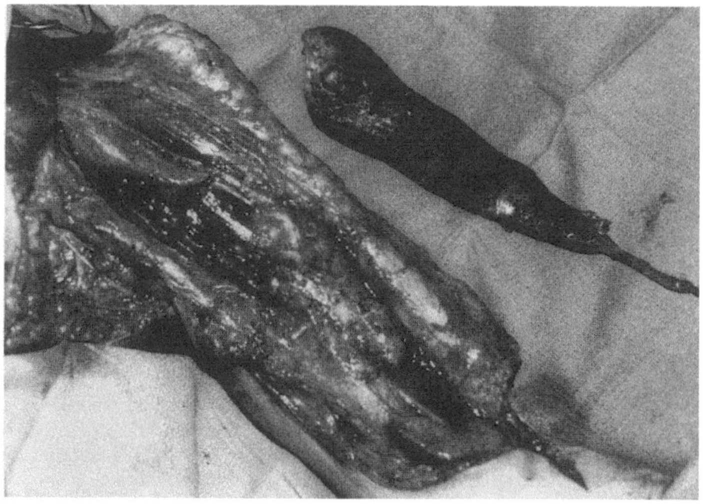

a

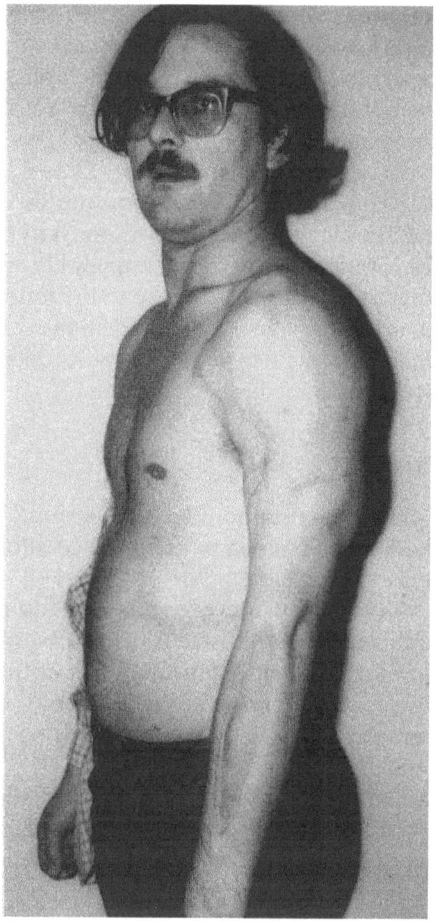

b

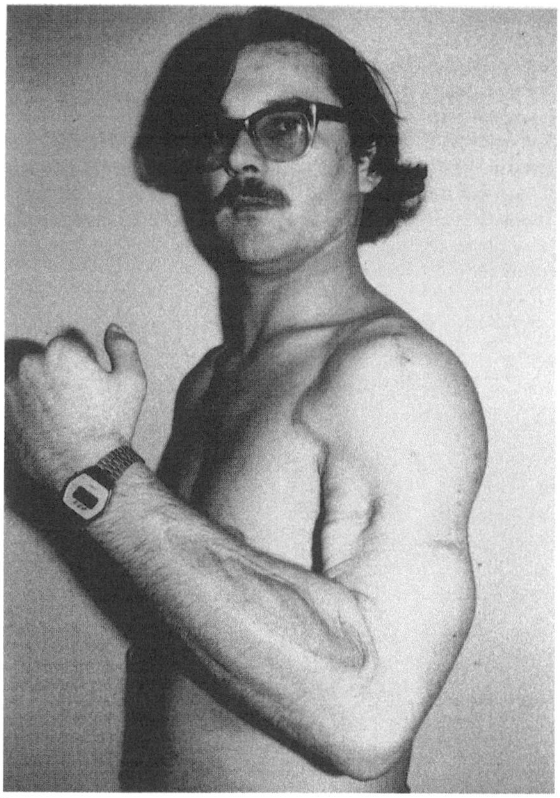

c

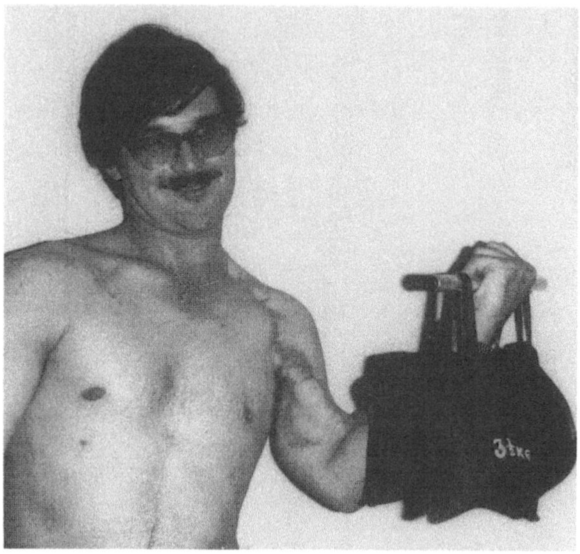

d

Fig. 19.14. **a** Patient received a severe crush injury to his upper arm and lost all biceps and brachialis musculature. Anterior compartment of the upper arm is prepared for transplantation. Gracilis is seen lying above the arm, prior to transfer. **b** Motor portion of the musculocutaneous nerve was used for reinnervation and the muscle was attached to the coricoid and biceps tendon. **c** Muscle provides full elbow flexion. **d** He can lift 7 kg from a fully extended position to full flexion

followed by thumb flexion. This should bring the thumb against the middle phalanx of the index for key pinch. If the flexor pollicis longus is too tight, the thumb will flex into the palm before the fingers come into flexion.

8. Replace the skin flap over the distal portion of the muscle with care. If forearm skin coverage over the proximal muscle is impossible, apply a split thickness skin graft directly to the muscle belly. The muscle will have been placed in the forearm so that the neurovascular pedicle is on its deep surface and is well protected.

Postoperative Care

Splint the wrist and fingers in flexion. After 3 weeks, tendon healing will be adequate to allow passive extension exercises.

Within a few weeks or longer, a full range of wrist and finger passive extension will be obtained. This develops the gliding mechanisms at the muscle tendon junction and distal muscle belly which will be necessary when active contraction occurs following reinnervation.

The first clinical signs of reinnervation occur 2–4 months postoperatively. As reinnervation progresses, the patient develops an increasing range of active muscle excursion. When a good excursion has developed, give the patient a program of resisted exercises. These exercises appear to improve the eventual strength of the muscle. The grip strength will continue to improve for 2 years following surgery.

References

1. Ikuta Y, Kubo T, Tsuge K (1976) Free muscle transplantation by microsurgical technique to treat severe Volkmann's contracture. Plast Reconstr Surg 58: 407
2. Linnell EA (1921) The distribution of nerves in the upper limb with reference to variabilities and their clinical significance. J Anat 55: 79
3. Manktelow RT, McKee NH (1978) Free muscle transplantation to provide active finger flexion. J Hand Surg 3: 416
4. Manktelow RT, McKee NH, Vettese T (1980) An anatomical study of the pectoralis major muscle as related to functioning free muscle transplantation. Plast Reconstr Surg 65: 610
5. Manktelow RT, Zuker RM, McKee NH (1984) Functioning free muscle transplantation. J Hand Surg 9 A: 32
6. Manktelow RT (1985) In New Trends in Peripheral Nerve Surgery. (ed) Terzis J. Functioning Muscle Transplantation to the Arm. W. B. Saunders, Co., Philadelphia
7. Manktelow RT, Zuker RM (1984) Muscle transplantation by fascicular territory. Plast Reconstr Surg 73: 751
8. O'Brien MBcC (1977) In Microvascular and Reconstructive Surgery. Churchill Livingstone, Edinburgh 290
9. Shanghai Sixth Peoples Hospital (1976) Free muscle transplantation by microsurgical neurovascular anastomoses. Chinese Med 2: 47
10. Sunderland S, Hughes SR (1946) Metrical and non metrical features of the muscular branches of the ulnar nerve. J Comp Neurol 85: 11
11. Sunderland S, Ray LJ (1946) Metrical and non metrical features of the muscular branches of the median nerve. J Comp Neurol 85: 191
12. Tamai S, Komatsu S, Sakamoto H et al. (1970) Free muscle transplants in dogs with microsurgical neurovascular anastomoses. Plast Reconstr Surg 46: 219

Chapter 20. Toe to Thumb Transfer

Surgical Options for Thumb Reconstruction

There are many techniques of thumb reconstruction. These include:

1. web space deepening
2. Gilles bone graft and cocked hat flap
3. distraction lengthening of the metacarpal
4. osteoplastic reconstruction
5. pollicization of a finger or portion of a finger
6. toe transfer (first toe or second toe)
7. microvascular wrap around flap

A modest increase in functional length can be obtained reliably with a web space deepening, and is particularly useful for amputations through the thumb IP joint or distal portion of the proximal phalanx.

The Gilles cocked hat flap and bone graft produces a moderate lengthening for patients who have amputations at the MP joint level and do not require a normal length of thumb [6]. The disadvantage is that the maximum lengthening obtained is 2 cm and the bone graft is prone to atrophy. Distraction lengthening of the metacarpal, as described by Matev, is a more reliable method of gaining stump length.

The osteoplastic reconstruction, a tubed pedicle with bone graft and neurovascular island transfer, has provided a useful thumb reconstruction for many patients [14]. The disadvantages of this procedure include the multiple procedures required, the lack of articulation, a neurovascular island flap which flip flops on the underlying bone graft and the perception, when the thumb is touched, that it is really the donor finger being touched. The lack of thumb nail and tubular appearance of the flap mark the thumb reconstruction as abnormal.

Pollicization provides a good thumb reconstruction which has precise sensibility and an excellent range of motion [2]. However, the pollicized digit may appear spindly and provide a relatively weak pinch. Because of the loss of a finger, there is loss of grip strength and torsion strength. Surprisingly, despite its long history of use, there is scant documentation of the functional results of this procedure in the medical literature.

The most recent thumb reconstructions employ microvascular techniques. Toe to hand transfer is a useful technique for replacing a missing thumb or finger. This technique provides a significant functional and cosmetic improvement to a hand which has lost a thumb [3, 5, 7]. Although first described by Nicoladoni as a two-stage pedicled transfer beginning with the hand attached to the foot, the present day procedure employs microsurgical free tissue transfer techniques.

Careful patient selection is critical in the decision about which type of thumb reconstruction is most appropriate. Following a traumatic loss of the thumb or digits, the patient should attempt to return to work, resume normal hand activities, and develop adaptations as possible. Surgeon and patient should then assess the degree of functional disability related to that particular individual's job and lifestyle, and select the procedure which fits the patient best. There is no one technique which provides the solution for all patients. An individual who has functioned without a thumb for some time will be in a better position to accept a reconstruction which appears less than normal, but may have difficulty incorporating a reconstruction into functional activities after having learned alternate coping mechanisms.

The present era of microsurgical toe transfer was ushered in by Buncke with his work in the Rhesus monkey, and by Cobbett who did a microsurgical transfer of the first toe in 1969. The first toe transfer quickly became popular in the west, while the second toe transfer became popular in the east. Surgeons were quick to recognize that the toe transfer provided a useful addition to the reconstructions previously available. In this technique, the tendons and nerves of the toe are attached to the appropriate tendons and nerves which had supplied the thumb. In its new location, the brain recognizes the transplant as a thumb, and the patient quickly integrates it into functional activities. Of all the techniques of thumb reconstruction, there are more well-documented assessments of toe transfer than any other procedure [4, 7, 13, 15].

The 'wrap around' procedure of Morrison is a useful alternative to toe transfer. It has the advantages of preserving some of the first toe and providing a reconstruction which is the correct thumb size. In this procedure, a first toe soft tissue microvascular fillet is wrapped around an iliac bone graft and placed on the thumb stump. Skin grafts and flaps to the first toe provide at least partial preservation of the first toe. This technique allows the surgeon to make the reconstructed thumb the same size as the thumb on the normal hand. The disadvantages of this procedure are the lack of an interphalangeal joint and the slight drumstick-like swelling of the distal joint. Atrophy and fracture of the bony graft may occur unless a portion of toe distal phalanx is transferred. Healing problems are common in the foot.

A compromise between toe transfer and wrap around, which carries articulation but allows reduction in size of the first toe, is the trimmed toe transfer designed by Fu Chan Wei from Taipai. In this procedure, the first toe is transferred and the medial side and tip are debulked. A piece of tissue is removed containing a strip of nail bed, skin, and bone sufficient to decrease the toe's size to that of a thumb.

First Toe versus Second Toe

The choice in toe transfer lies between the first and the second toe. There are cosmetic and functional advantages and disadvantages to each transfer. These pros and cons must be presented to the patient who can then make an informed selection.

Cosmesis, both in the hand and the foot, plays a major part in selecting the best toe for transfer. Either toe is usually removed at the MT joint level to prevent significant functional problems with the foot. When the first toe is removed at this joint, there is a significant cosmetic deformity. However, when the second toe is removed and the web space tightly closed with approximation of the first and third toes, there is minimal cosmetic foot deformity (Fig. 20-1,2).

Toe size, both diameter and length, relative to the missing thumb and to the remaining fingers, is a major cosmetic criterion in determining which toe will best replace the thumb. Buncke's experience with the first toe is that it will shrink in size [13]. This decrease in size has been recorded by Frickman, when assessing the Melbourne group's toe transfers, as a 5% reduction in circumference [4]. With large first toes, the 'wrap around' procedure of Morrison may be indicated.

The other factor which determines the selection of the toe is the functional requirement of the patient. A big toe can be expected to provide a broader, more stable surface area for pinch and grasp than the second toe and be more suitable for some types of manual labor. However, the second toe may provide a more precise fine pinch and manipulating capability. Our experience with pinch strength has been equally good with regard to the second and first toes, with a pinch strength as high as 80% of a normal hand.

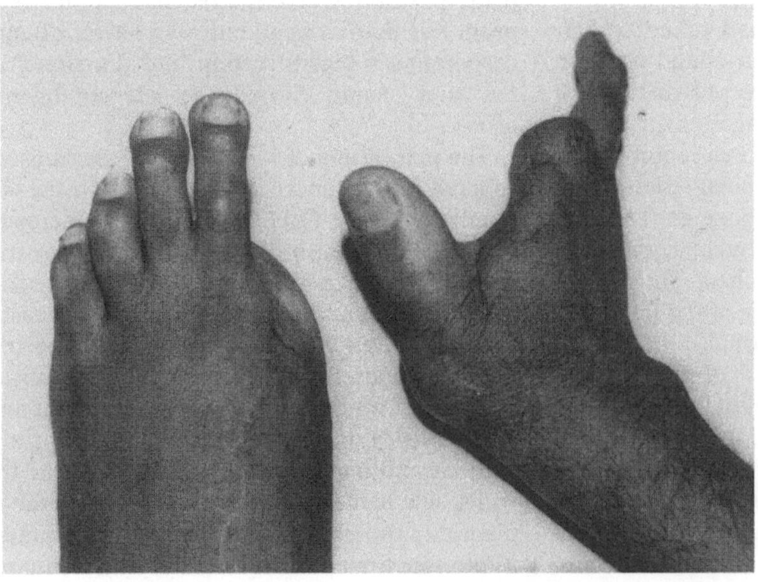

Fig. 20-1. The removal of the first toe at the MT joint is deforming. This patient requested a first toe transfer in order that he might have a broad surface against which he could pinch and grip with the remaining little finger

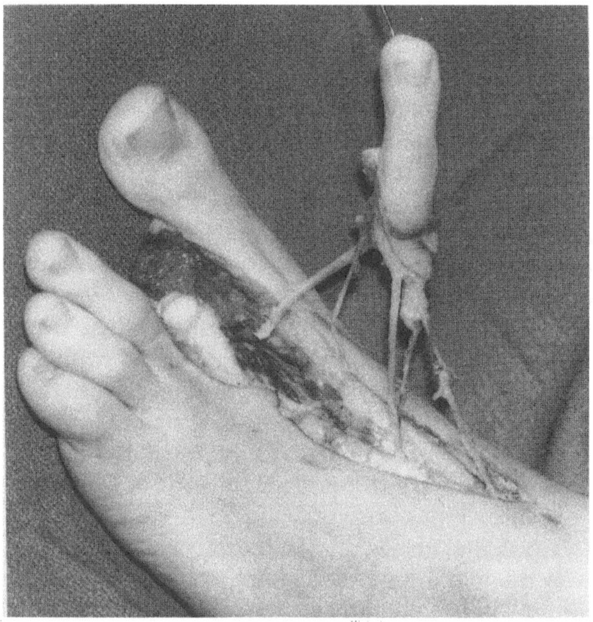

a

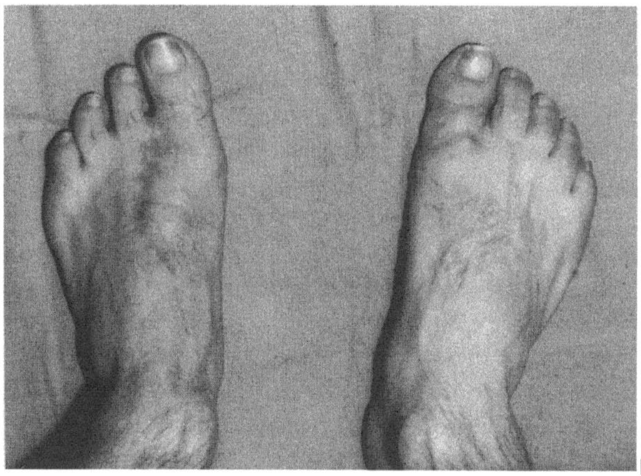

b

Fig. 20-2. a The second toe has been removed at the MT joint. b The toes must be counted to recognize that one is missing

However, pinch strength is related more to the integrity of the remaining thenar musculature and metacarpal than the particular toe added. The toe adds only an increase in length but not power to the ray.

Selection is also affected by the length of toe required. The second toe is usually not transferred with the metatarsal phalangeal joint, as the transfer of a three joint system without separate motors on each joint is susceptible to instability. However, the first toe, having a single interphalangeal joint, can be transferred with its metatarsal phalangeal joint with the expectation of stable motion and pinch. However, if the first metatarsal head is removed, foot function may be affected. The compromise is to remove the distal and dorsal half of the head as described by May. With this technique, the first toe can provide 1-2 cm more length than a second toe transfer.

Although gait analysis reveals changes when either toe is removed at the metatarsal phalangeal joint, there does not appear to be a significant alteration in walking or running capabilities. Although plantar discomfort is not uncommon with both toe transfers, it is almost always transitory.

Vascular Anatomy of Toe Transfers

(See Dorsal Foot, Chapter 3 for detailed discussion of vascular anatomy of the foot)

The arterial pedicle for a toe transfer can be designed on either the dorsal or plantar vasculature. The dorsal pedicle is the dorsalis pedis, the first dorsal metatarsal artery, and the digital arteries. The volar pedicle is the plantar metatarsal and digital arteries. As the dorsal pedicle is usually longer, easier to expose, and usually larger in diameter, it is the preferred pedicle. Even if the first dorsal metatarsal artery is smaller than the plantar metatarsal artery, the dorsal is preferred because of the relative ease of dissection and length of pedicle produced. However, a very small, absent or abnormal first dorsal metatarsal artery will prevent the use of the dorsal pedicle. Gilbert, in his anatomical dissections, found the dorsal metatarsal artery inadequate in 10% of patients. We have found it inadequate in 20% and Lister in 30% of toe transfers. In these situations, the plantar metatarsal artery is used for the arterial pedicle.

The selection of the more suitable pedicle may be aided by preoperative angiography of the foot. Both lateral and anterior posterior views are required. Peripheral vasodilation must be produced before contrast is injected. Warming the feet, posterior tibial and anterior tibial nerve block, or epidural blocks are used to produce vasodilation. Although the angiogram provides useful information about the location and anatomic pattern of vessels, it does not always indicate the calibre of the vessels unless there is good vasodilation. If only small vessels are seen on the angiogram, they may be their full size or the vessels may be in spasm. The final decision about the choice of pedicle is made at the time of the surgical exploration.

Preoperative Planning

Models of the toe to be transferred are very helpful to both surgeon and patient. The length of toe required and the optimum orientation of the toe become more apparent when the replica of the toe is placed on the hand. Seeing the model on the hand also aids in the patient's choice of which toe is to be used, and expectations of the cosmetic result are likely to be more appropriate. Models can be done simply and quickly in the office, using plasticine modelling clay or plaster cast models of the toes (Fig. 20-3). However, plaster cast models are rigid, and the length and shape cannot be modified easily while working with the patient.

After the selection of either the first or second toe, the technical steps in the procedure must be planned. They include the repair of each structure in the transfer: bones, joints, tendons, nerves, vessels and skin.

As the location of recipient vessels is fixed, they should be identified first and then the appropriate foot chosen so that the arterial and venous pedicles in the toe go directly to those in the hand. Usually, the preferred site for the arterial repair is the radial artery immediately distal to the extensor pollicis longus. The toe is selected so that the arterial pedicle will lie on the ulnar side of the thumb and go directly to the radial artery without having to cross over or under the extensor tendons. This route prevents pedicle obstruction by tendon compression. If the arterial pedicle is on the radial side of the thumb, the arterial repair is placed radial to the extensor pollicis longus in the snuff box, or in the radial wrist to obviate the need to cross tendons. On many feet, the first toe curves laterally. Since this curve will look best on the hand if it curves toward the fingers, the ipsilateral first toe is more aesthetically pleasing.

Unless there has been injury to the dorsum of the hand and wrist, a generous supply of veins is usually present and can be visualized with a venous tourniquet. The arterial supply is usually evident by palpation and Doppler. The adequacy of the ulnar artery in supplying the hand can be assessed with the Allen's test. However, the usual arterial repair is end to side so that the blood supply to the hand is not altered. A hand arteriogram is useful if the arterial anatomy appears to be inadequate or is within the zone of previous injury.

The digital nerves may be located by a Tinel's sign over the neuroma. If this is not present, the type of injury will usually indicate the location of the nerve ends. Avulsion injuries present a problem, as the digital branches to the thumb may be avulsed from the median nerve at the level of the carpal tunnel. For recipient nerves, it may be necessary to either use dorsal branches of the radial nerve or do a digital nerve transfer from one of the other fingers.

The extensor pollicis longus can usually be identified by palpation. The flexor pollicis longus may not be as easy to identify by palpation and its location may be unknown until surgical exploration.

The standard toe skin flaps are distally based triangles of skin on both the dorsal and the plantar aspect of the foot. Usually, toe removal is planned so

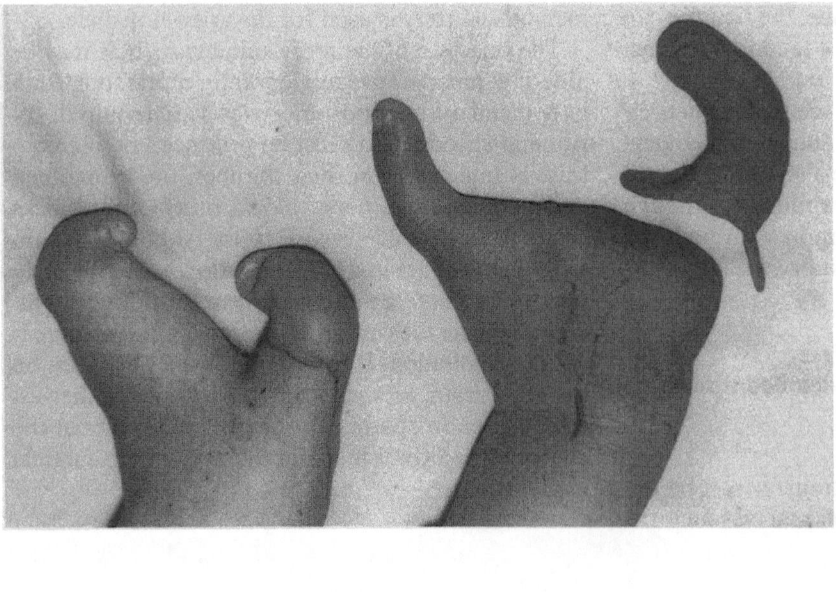

Fig. 20-3. Plasticine model of the large toe from a child born with a lobster claw foot deformity *(left)*. When placed on the hand *(right)*, the model assists in assessing cosmesis, provides the patient with realistic expectations, and assists in planning. The optimum toe length and position, and position of the skin flaps become readily apparent

that the foot can be closed directly. On occasion, a larger piece of skin will be taken with the toe as an attached dorsal foot skin flap to aid in the coverage of the hand. A split thickness skin graft is then applied to the dorsal aspect of the foot. First toe transplantation must be planned so that direct skin closure is possible on the plantar and medial aspects of the foot.

With distally based triangles of plantar and dorsal skin on the toe, the best incisions on the thumb stump will be longitudinal palmar and dorsal incisions which meet on the end of the stump. The location of these incisions depends upon the position in which the toe will be placed on the hand and the skin coverage available on the thumb stump. The use of plasticine models will aid in determining the best location for these incisions.

The incision on the sole of the foot should be kept as short as possible in order to minimize the area of scarring. As the flexor digitorum longus does not divide into separate tendons to the toes until it reaches the mid plantar area of the foot, the length of flexor tendon which may be taken with the second toe is limited.

Veins can be determined and outlined preoperatively by placing the foot in a dependent position or using a venous tourniquet. All veins should be marked. At the time of surgical dissection, the veins to be used will be determined by which veins are found to actually drain the dorsal skin flap.

Technique of Second Toe to Thumb Transfer

I. Preparation of the Second Toe

Transfers from the foot are more sensitive to cooling than any other tissue transfer. If the patient's core temperature is not maintained, the foot will become cold and the transfer vessels will go into spasm. The toe skin will be pale and it will be impossible to evaluate the adequacy of the vascular pedicle following the dissection of the toe.

In our first 25 toe to hand transfers, only one did not survive. That toe never pinked up after dissection, had borderline perfusion for 4 days after transfer, and then died. Perhaps the arterial pedicle had marginally inadequate vascular connections to the toe and should have been abandoned in favour of another artery, or perhaps the patient's vessel had a strong tendency to go into and remain in spasm. If the patient and the foot are not warm, it is impossible to evaluate the anatomic adequacy of the vascular network.

The toe dissection is done at the same time as the thumb stump is prepared. The 'thumb surgeon' identifies, and prepares, in order, the veins, dorsal nerves, extensor tendon, recipient artery, bone stump, flexor tendon and volar digital nerves. The distance from the site of bone fusion to the point of repair of each structure is identified and reported to the 'toe surgeon'. The 'toe surgeon' removes the desired length of each structure with a little to spare.

Surgical Technique

The toe is prepared under tourniquet control without exanguination of the limb.

1. Draw a long triangular flap based on the toe on both the dorsal and plantar surfaces. Each flap should be as wide as possible to still allow comfortable closure. Leave one half of the width of the web space skin on each side of the toe in order to allow web closure (Fig. 20-4a).

2. Make a curving skin incision on the dorsum of the foot, elevate the margins and identify the veins.

3. Identify proximal dorsal foot veins and trace them distally into the triangle of dorsal skin on the toe. Preserve all dorsal veins until you have decided which ones best drain the toe. Prepare branches of the superficial and deep peroneal nerves to the dorsum of the second toe.

4. The key to the preparation of the toe is the arterial pedicle.

a) Identify the dorsalis pedis and its venae comitantes over the mid tarsus by retracting the extensor hallucis brevis laterally. Identify the cutaneous branch of the deep peroneal nerve lying lateral to the artery.

b) Divide the extensor hallucis brevis and follow the dorsalis pedis artery distally. Identify the origin of the first dorsal metatarsal artery from the plantar communicating branch.

c) Follow the first dorsal metatarsal artery distally to the web space. Spread the toes and identify all of the digital arteries to the 1st and 2nd toes (Fig. 20-4b). Usually, the plantar digital vessels are largest but the dorsal may be dominant. As the metatarsal, communicating, and digital vessels have a variable pattern, it is necessary to identify the complete arterial pattern in the web space before dividing vessels. If the first dorsal metatarsal artery deviates towards the first toe before giving off the digital arteries, it may be inaccurately identified as the first

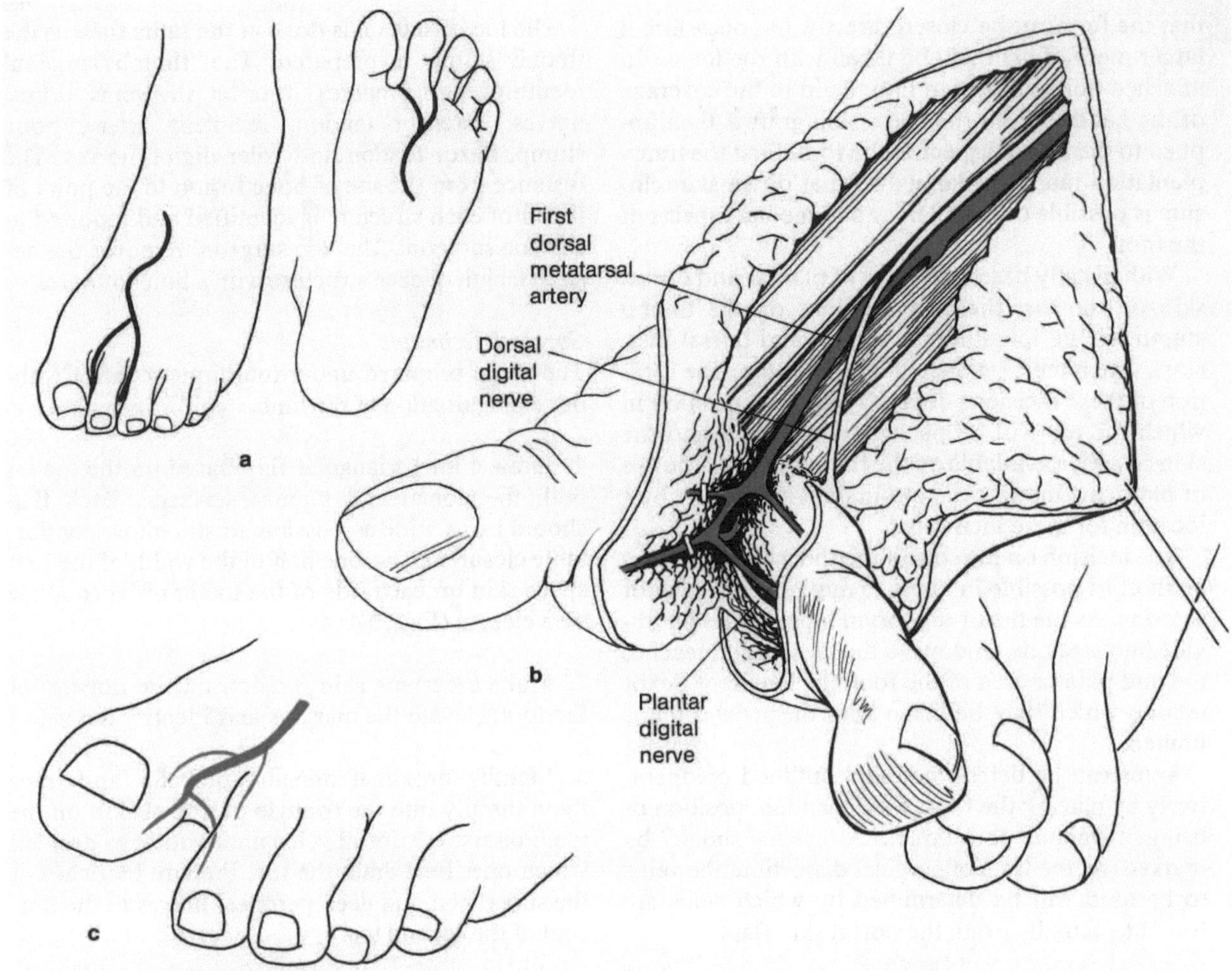

Fig. 20-4. **a** Distally based triangles of skin are outlined on the dorsal and plantar surface at the base of the second toe. **b** Dissection of the arterial pedicle. The dorsal and plantar digital arteries to both toes and the communicating branch to the plantar metatarsal artery are clearly identified before the arteries to the first toe are divided. The metatarsal artery is frequently tortuous and may deviate to one side or the other **(c)**, and be inadvertently divided if the entire vascular pattern is not identified

dorsal digital artery and mistakenly divided (Fig. 20-4c).

5. Through the dorsal exposure, identify the plantar digital nerves lying immediately deep to the digital arteries.

6. Incise the plantar triangle of skin. Elevate this flap, leaving most of the plantar fat on the foot. If the digital nerves are first identified and kept in view, dissection from the plantar surface through the thick plantar fat is easy. If the plantar triangle of skin is not defatted, there will be a thick wad of subcutaneous fat on the palmar side of the thumb reconstruction.

7. Incise the plantar skin proximally to provide exposure for the flexor tendon and digital nerves. Place this incision between the metatarsal heads to minimize the possibility of a tender scar. Divide the flexor digitorum longus and brevis and the digital nerves. As the flexor digitorum tendons have a common origin at the level of the proximal metatarsals, a useful tendon cannot be removed proximal to this site. The common digital nerve divides to form digital nerves to the sides of adjacent toes. The common digital nerve may be split surgically to the proximal metatarsal level to provide the length required on the hand. Split the nerve under magnification in order that the adjacent toe not be denervated. The nerves are always divided proximal to the metatarsal heads,

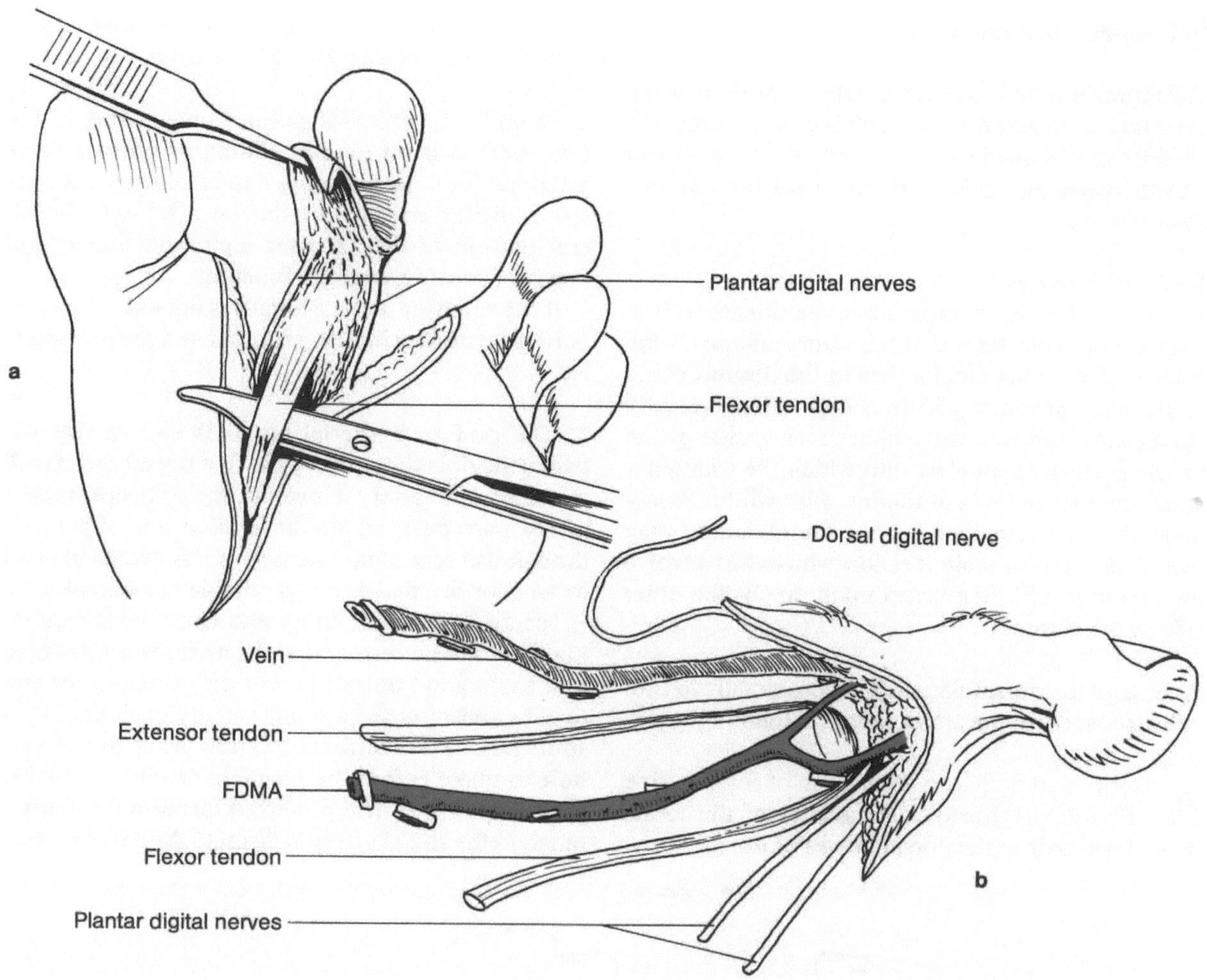

Fig. 20-5. a Plantar dissection to prepare the flexor tendon and complete the dissection of the digital nerves. **b** The second toe has been disarticulated at the MT joint. The FDMA supplies both dorsal and plantar digital arteries

so that neuroma formation is unlikely to cause symptoms.

8. Disarticulate the toe at the metatarsal phalangeal joint by dividing the volar plate and collateral ligaments, and divide the extensor digitorum longus tendon (Fig. 20-5b).

9. Place the disarticulated toe back into place, wrap the foot with gauze and release the tourniquet. The toe may take a few minutes to become pink. Do not transfer it if there is inadequate arterial input. The vasospasm should be recovered before transplantation in order that you can be assured that the vascular connections into the toe are adequate. If the toe does not become pink, the pedicle must be examined under magnification to see if there is an obstruction or injury to the pedicle.

10. If the plantar metatarsal artery is required, the dissection is difficult proximal to the metatarsal heads. The plantar metatarsal artery is best found by identifying the plantar digital artery at the web space, working proximally on the plantar surface of the foot while stretching the toes apart and retracting the soft tissues of the foot. Proximally, the plantar metatarsal artery hugs the metatarsal neck in a relatively inaccessible location. Good retraction with retractors on both sides of the pedicle and a headlight will aid in the dissection of the proximal pedicle.

11. Obtain good hemostasis and close the foot with interrupted everting sutures in the skin. If the first and third toes are difficult to approximate, place a deep suture in the subcutaneous tissues of the web.

II. Preparation of the Hand

The thumb stump is prepared at the same time as the toe, and the structures are identified in the same order as they will be identified on the toe: veins, dorsal nerves, extensor tendon, artery, flexor tendon and volar nerves.

Surgical Technique

1. Place a straight incision along the dorsum of the metacarpal, over the end of the stump and down the volar surface. This incision lies in the desired plane of flexion/extension of the thumb (Fig. 20-6a, b). Undermine and retract the skin on each side of the incision, creating a defect into which the triangular volar and dorsal flaps of the toe skin will fit. Sometimes the skin remaining on the thumb stump may dictate a more suitable incision which will involve the elevation of a flap based upon one or the other side of the stump.

2. Extend the dorsal skin incision proximally to provide exposure for the artery, vein and tendon repairs.

3. Identify and prepare a dorsal vein of suitable size. Identify and prepare distal branches of the radial nerve for repair to the dorsal nerves of the toe.

4. Clean the bone stump of fibrous tissue and determine the point of intended bone fusion.

5. Identify the extensor pollicis longus and ensure that there is good tendon gliding or go to a more proximal level. Repair only one extensor, as the extensor digitorum brevis on the toe attaches to the lateral portion of the extensor digitorum longus and does not provide separate function.

If the extensor pollicis longus is not available, prepare the extensor indicis proprius as a tendon transfer.

6. The preferred arterial repair is end to side between the dorsalis pedis or the first dorsal metatarsal and the radial artery. However, the princeps pollicis artery may be used for an end to end repair, although its volar ulnar location is less accessible and its smaller size makes a less reliable anastomosis.

Identify the radial artery and clear the surrounding tissues to be certain that the artery is undamaged and has a good pulsation. Vessels prepared for end to side anastomoses are not usually evaluated by a spurt test, as it is difficult to know what size of side hole to make before the recipient artery is available at the repair site. The preferred location for anastomosis to the radial artery is distal to the extensor pol-

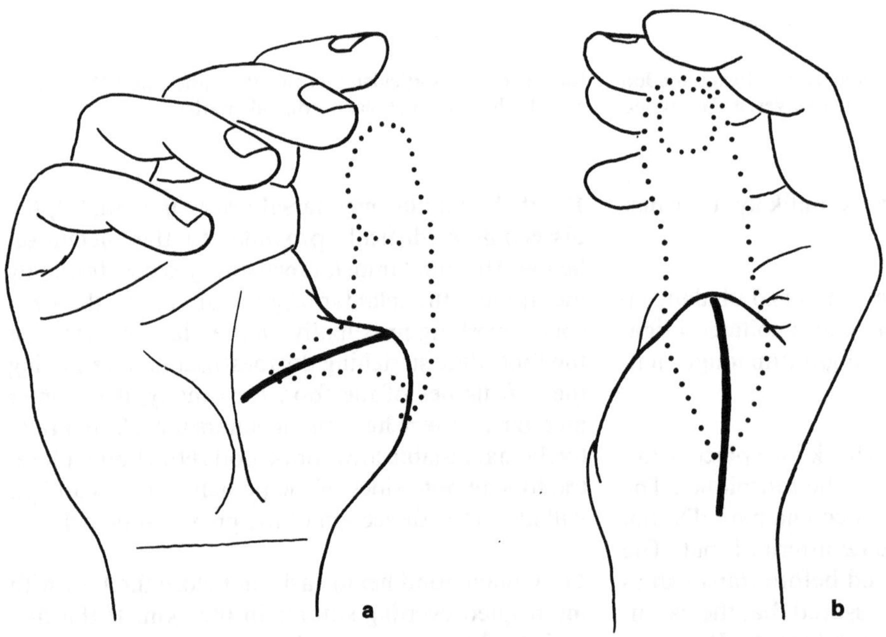

Fig. 20-6a, b. The volar and dorsal skin incision is commonly a straight line which lies along the axis of flexion and extension of the thumb. When the toe is correctly positioned, and the stump incisions spread apart, a volar and dorsal skin defect is produced which will accept the volar and dorsal triangles of toe skin. These flaps allow a relaxed skin closure over the pedicles

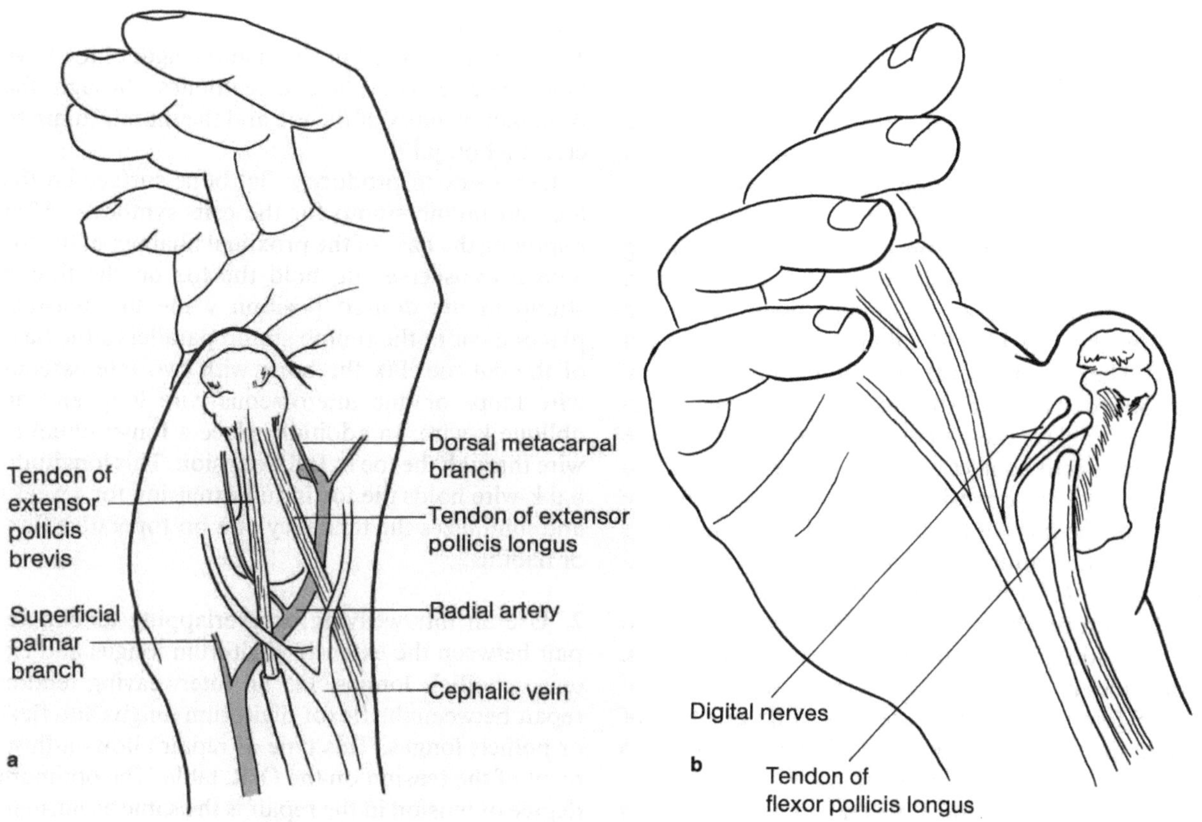

Fig. 20-7 a, b. The recipient structures on the base of the amputated thumb

licis longus before it passes into the first dorsal interosseous muscle (Fig. 20-7a).

7. Through the volar incisions, identify the digital nerves. If the amputation was an avulsion injury, carry the dissection into the carpal tunnel and identify the digital nerve stumps on the median nerve. If these stumps are not present, do a nerve transfer using either an ulnar digital nerve of the long or ring finger or the dorsal digital nerves of the radial nerve. The single ulnar digital nerve will be shared by both plantar nerves on the toe. Identify the flexor pollicis longus and ensure that there is good tendon gliding (Fig. 20-7b). As the second toe does not provide a long flexor tendon, it is occasionally necessary to prolong it with a flexor tendon graft if the end of the flexor pollicis terminates at the wrist.

If the flexor pollicis longus has been avulsed, prepare the sublimus from the long or ring finger as a tendon transfer.

III. Transplantation of the Second Toe

Fixation of the toe in the optimum position for function is a difficult part of the procedure. The objective is to place the new thumb in a position where it can come into good opposition to the fingers for pinch and grip functions and still have good extensor capability to allow the grasping of large objects. Taking into account abnormalities in the other fingers and the amount of remaining thumb tissue, each toe transfer must be individually positioned to fit each hand. The potential for thumb abduction-adduction, flexion-extension and opposition must be determined. Axial rotation is correct when the pulp of the toe comes into contact with that of the fingers when the thumb is in opposition. The angle between the plane of the pulp of the thumb and the plane of the palm of the hand is approximately 80° at rest and changes to 45° when in opposition (Fig. 20-8a, b).

Traction on the extensor pollicis longus, prior to bone fixation, will test the toe's extensor capabilities. Some toes lack 20–30° of active extension at each of the IP joints. It may be beneficial to fix this type of toe to the thumb in a position of hyperextension to compensate for the flexor habitus.

If possible, the toe transfer should provide a thumb length which is the same length as a normal thumb.

Surgical Technique

1. When the desired position and length of toe have been determined, place osteotomies through the proximal phalanx of the toe and the thumb stump to create a butt joint.

Use a saw to produce a flat bone surface on the toe and thumb stump for the osteosynthesis. After removing the base of the proximal phalanx of the toe with a transverse cut, hold the toe on the thumb stump in the desired position while the assistant places a cut in the thumb stump parallel to the base of the cut toe. Fix the bone with two interosseous wire loops or one interosseous wire loop and an oblique k-wire. In addition, place a longitudinal k-wire through the toe in full extension. This longitudinal k-wire holds the toe in full extension for 4 weeks and minimizes the tendency of a postoperative flexor habitus.

2. Use an interweaving or overlapping tendon repair between the extensor digitorum longus and extensor pollicis longus. Do an interweaving tendon repair between the flexor digitorum longus and flexor pollicis longus. This type of repair allows adjustment of the tension on the O. R. table. The optimum degree of tension in the repair is the same as normally present in the thumb's tendons. Tend to more extensor tightness than flexor to prevent a flexor habitus.

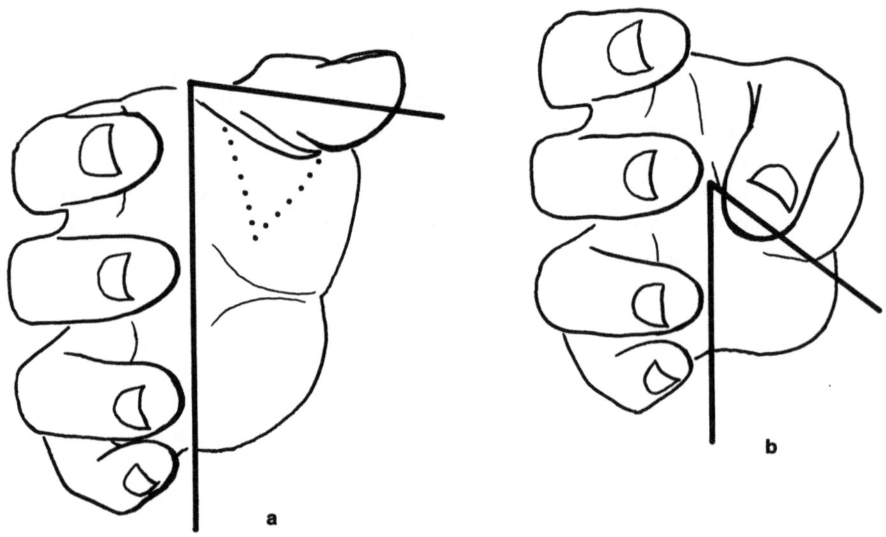

Fig. 20-8 a, b. The correct position of the thumb for pinch and grip functions. **a** In the neutral position, the plane of the touch surface of the thumb is slightly less than 90 degrees to the plane of the palmar surfaces of the fingers. **b** With opposition, the angle between the plane of the thumb and plane of the palm decreases to approximately 45 degrees as the touch surfaces of the fingers approach the position of opposition. The toe must be placed on the metacarpal carefully in order to obtain normal opposition

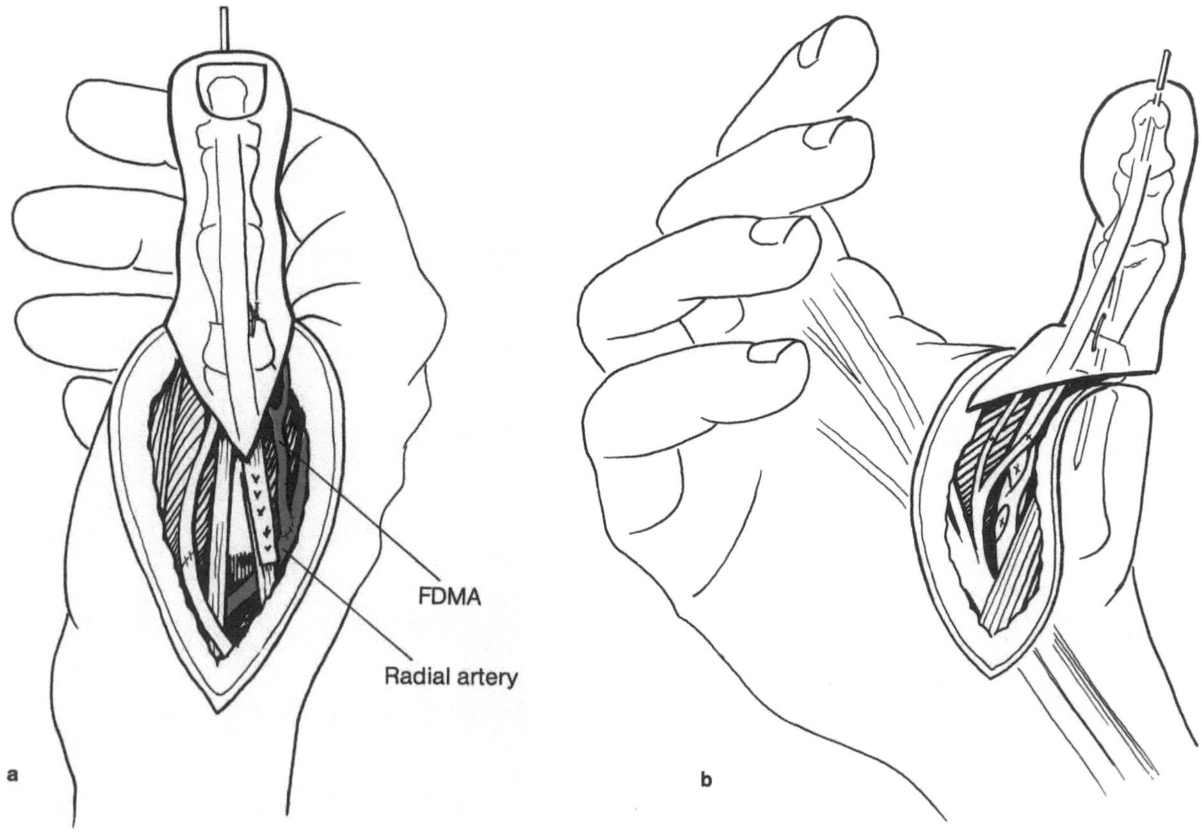

Fig. 20-9 a, b. The second toe in the proper position for opposition, with all dorsal and volar structures repaired

3. Do an end to end venous anastomosis. If the veins are smaller than the artery, do two venous anastomoses.

4. Do the arterial anastomoses without tension and with careful positioning of the pedicle, preferably as an end to side repair to the radial artery. Use 2 vessel loops on the radial artery - one proximal and one distal to the anastomosis to bring it out to the surface and to obstruct blood flow (Fig. 20-9a).

5. Suture the dorsal digital nerves of the toe to dorsal branches of the radial nerve.

6. Dorsal skin closure should be done as soon as the dorsal repairs are completed and before the volar structures are repaired. It is easy to obstruct with the artery or vein by compression or kinking during the skin closure. If this obstruction occurs, it may be necessary to apply a skin graft rather than do a direct closure. If the dorsal skin closure is too tight, the compromised circulation will become apparent while the volar repairs are being completed before the patient leaves the operating room.

7. Do the digital nerve repairs without tension using 9 or 10-0 microsutures. Be sure that the thumb digital nerves are undamaged at the site of the repair (Fig. 20-9 b).

8. On both sides of the base of the toe, it is frequently necessary to apply small skin grafts as local thumb stump flaps may not provide complete coverage.

9. Apply a well-padded splint which supports the wrist in a neutral position. The splint and dressing must not come in contact with the dorsum of the thumb reconstruction or there is chance of pressure on the pedicle.

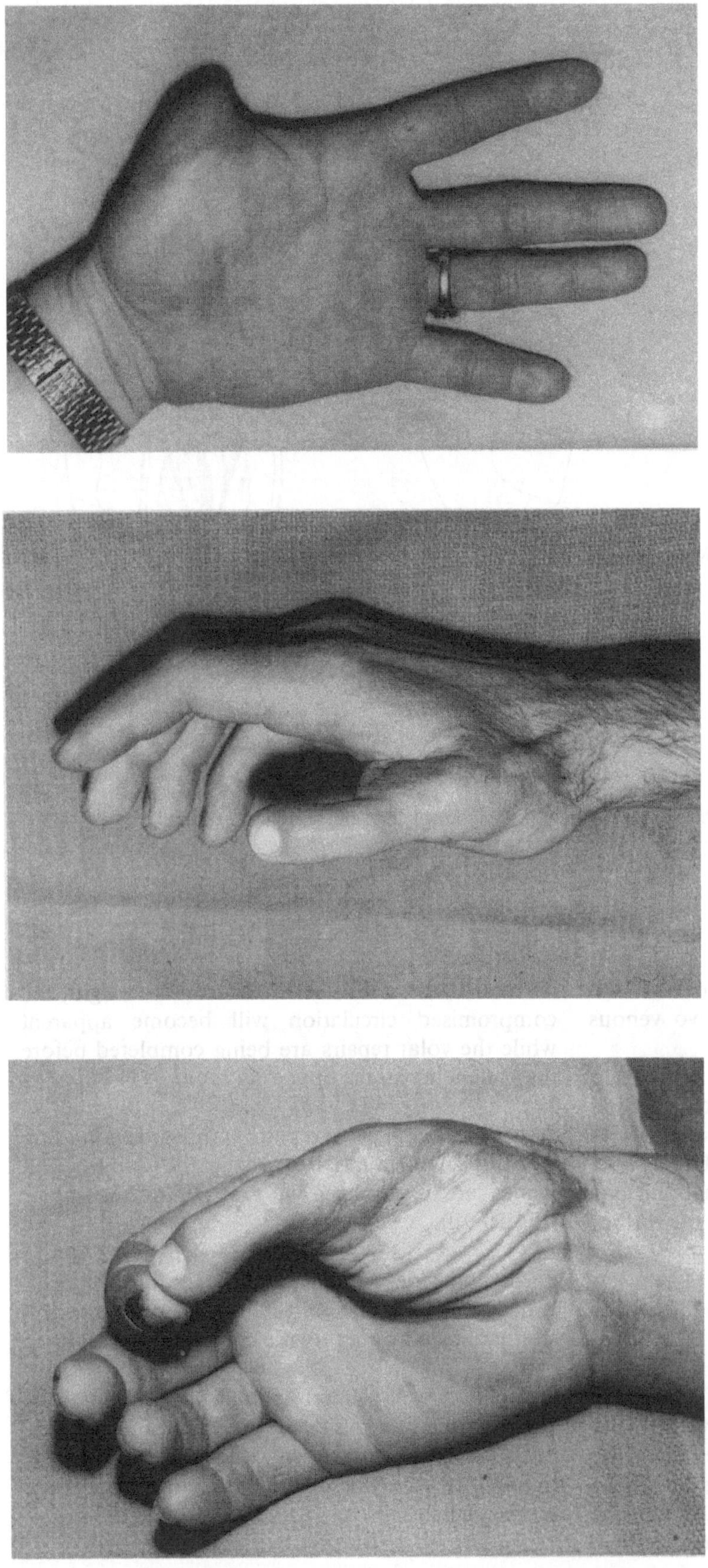

a

b

c

Fig. 20-10. a This carpenter sustained an avulsion of the thumb through the MP joint. **b, c** Following second toe transfer, the patient has good grip and pinch function and acceptable cosmesis. He returned to work as a carpenter

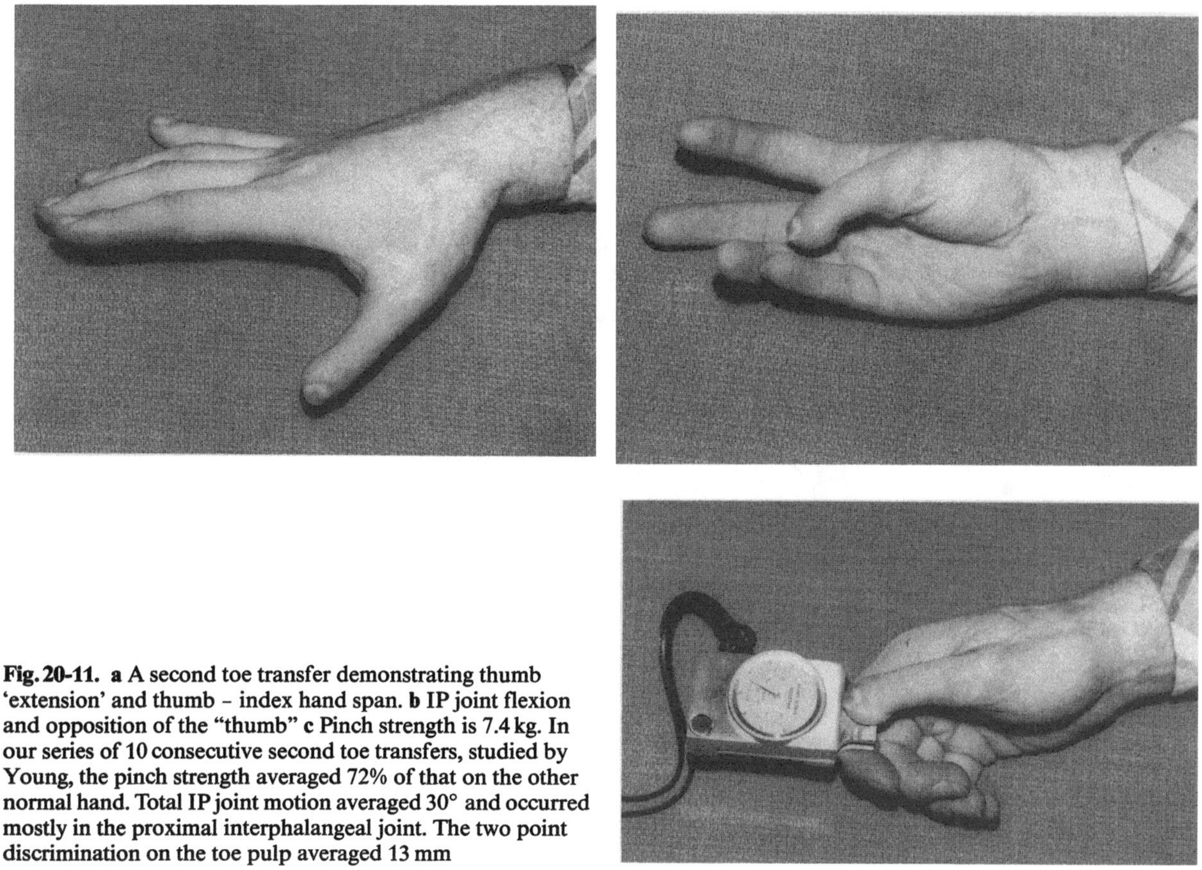

a b c

Fig. 20-11. a A second toe transfer demonstrating thumb 'extension' and thumb - index hand span. b IP joint flexion and opposition of the "thumb" c Pinch strength is 7.4 kg. In our series of 10 consecutive second toe transfers, studied by Young, the pinch strength averaged 72% of that on the other normal hand. Total IP joint motion averaged 30° and occurred mostly in the proximal interphalangeal joint. The two point discrimination on the toe pulp averaged 13 mm

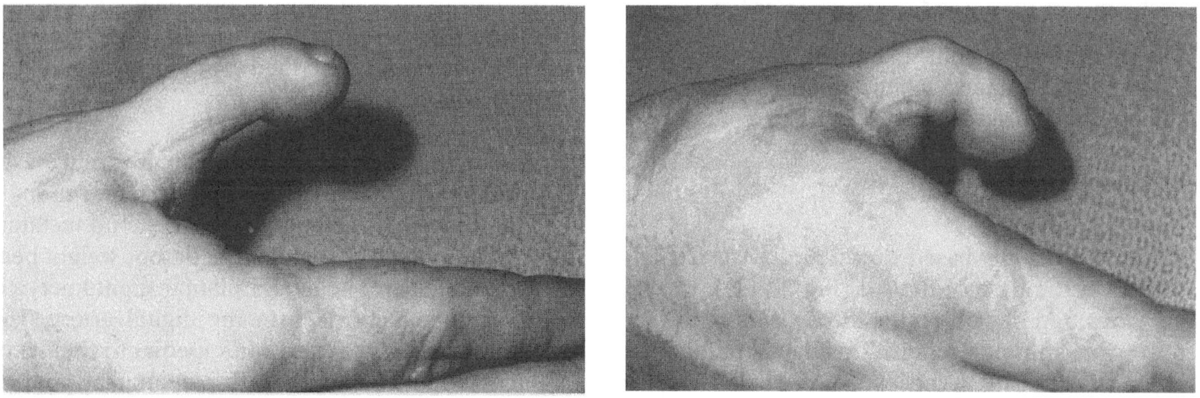

a b

Fig. 20-12 a, b. Second toe in extension (a) and in flexion (b). In some patients, such as this, although the second toe provides good function, it is too small to provide a good cosmetic reconstruction. Alternate techniques may be preferred

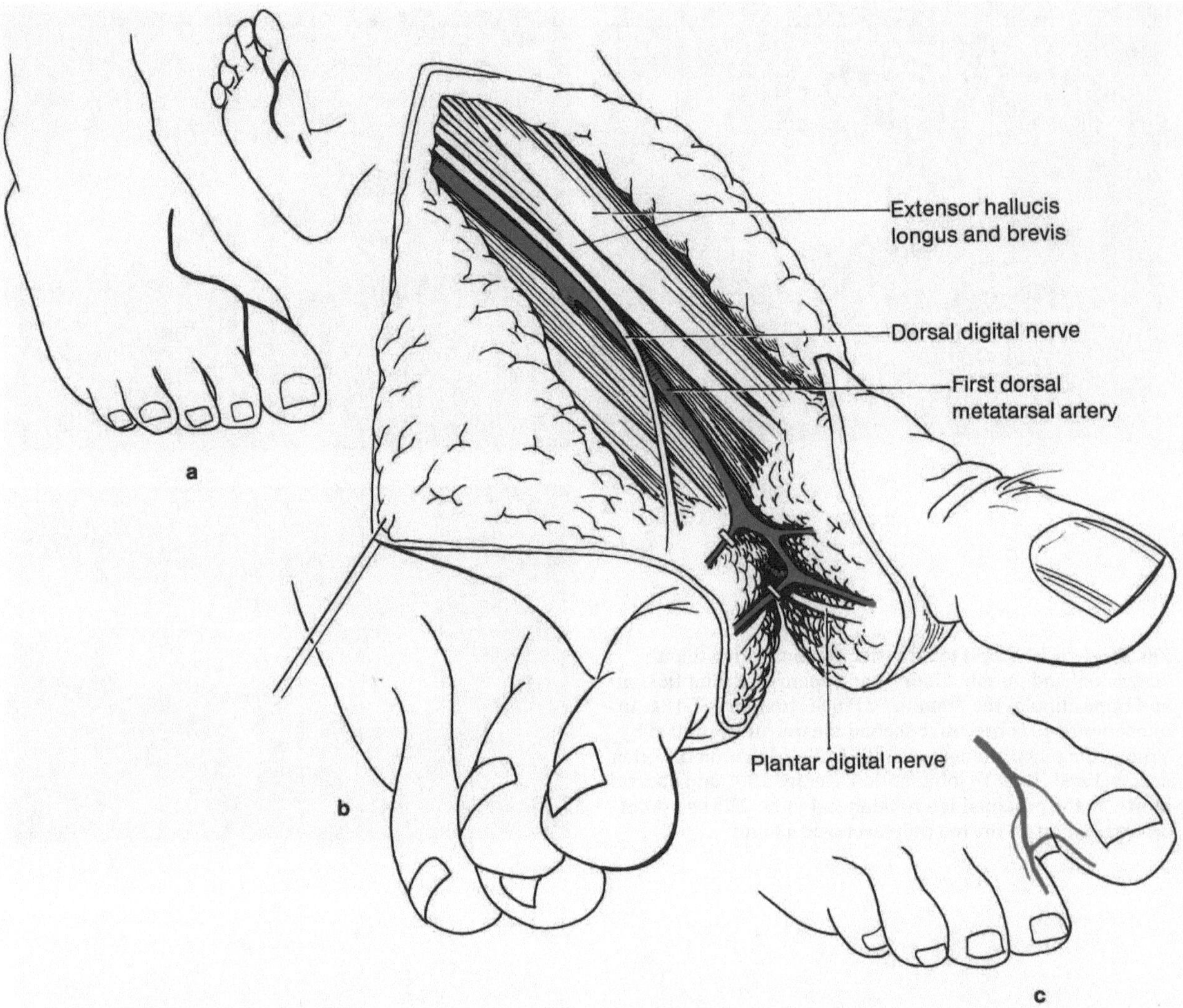

Fig. 20-13. **a** Flaps and incisions for removal of the first toe. **b** Pedicle preparation with application of clips to the dorsal and plantar digital arteries to the second toe. **c** A first dorsal metatarsal artery which deviates to the second toe may inadvertently be divided proximal to the plantar digital artery

Technique of First Toe to Thumb Transfer

Except for a few points, the technique of 1st toe transfer is the same as for the 2nd toe. These points will be emphasized in the discussion to follow.

I. Preparation of the First Toe

Surgical Technique

1. Outline distally-based dorsal and volar triangles of skin at the base of the toe (Fig. 20-13a). Leave a generous flap of skin on the medial side of the foot to provide stump coverage. This flap should extend at least 2 cm distal to the level of bone division. The toe will likely require a skin graft on its medial aspect after transfer to the hand.

2. Extend the dorsal incision proximally to provide exposure, and prepare the veins, artery and extensor tendons as was described for the second toe (Fig. 20-13b, c).

3. Extend the plantar skin incision in a curving fashion proximally from the apex of the plantar triangle into the space between the first and second metatarsal heads, so that the metatarsals do not weight bear on a plantar scar. The lateral plantar digital nerve is found immediately deep to the digital artery. The medial plantar digital nerve lies medial to the flexor hallucis longus, adjacent to the metatarsal phalangeal joint capsule.

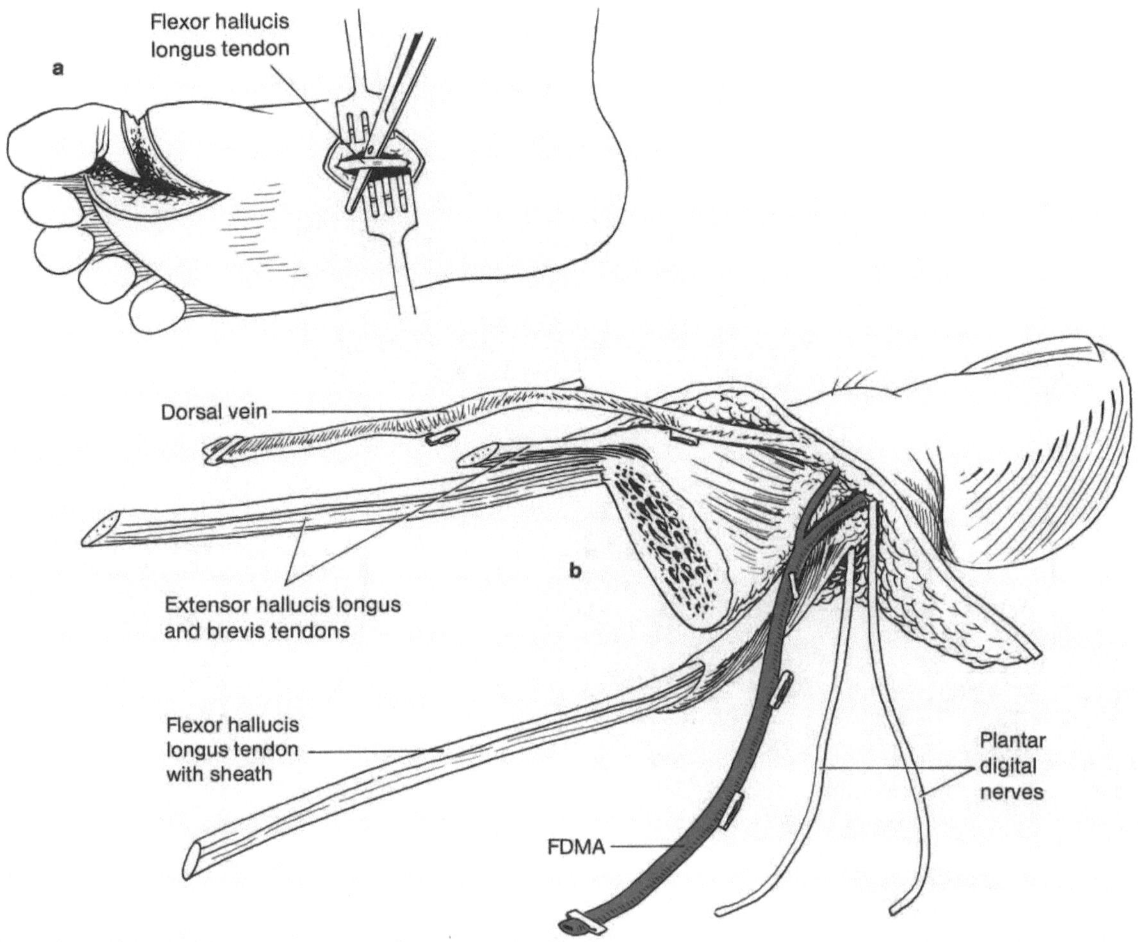

Fig. 20-14. **a** Medial plantar incision to identify the flexor hallucis tendon. **b** First toe removed through the head of the metatarsal with all structures prepared for transfer

4. To remove a long length of the flexor hallucis longus tendon, make a separate medial foot and medial malleolar incision. Carry the medial mid-foot incision dorsal to the abductor hallucis brevis and identify the tendon lateral to the medial digital nerve to the first toe (Fig. 20-14a). Through an incision behind the medial malleolus, identify the tendon posterior to the neurovascular bundle and divide it. Traction on the tendon at the medial foot incision and at the MT joint will deliver the tendon.

5. If the thumb is amputated proximal to the MP joint, take the toe MT joint to provide a thumb MP joint. If this joint is not required, disarticulate the first toe through the MT joint.

To remove a functioning MT joint and leave adequate plantar length on the first metatarsal, cut through the head of the metatarsal at 45° angled dorsally. Place the saw cut just proximal to the attachment of the collateral ligaments to the metatarsal head.

As May emphasized, cutting the metatarsal head at an angle and placing the oblique metatarsal osteotomy transversely on the metacarpal stump converts the hyperextending MT joint to a flexion MP joint. The oblique osteotomy leaves the plantar pushoff area of the first metatarsal intact and maintains foot function.

6. Leaving the pedicles intact, place the disarticulated toe back on the foot, wrap it in gauze and release the tourniquet. The toe must perfuse well on the foot prior to the division of the vascular pedicles and transfer to the hand (Fig. 20-14b).

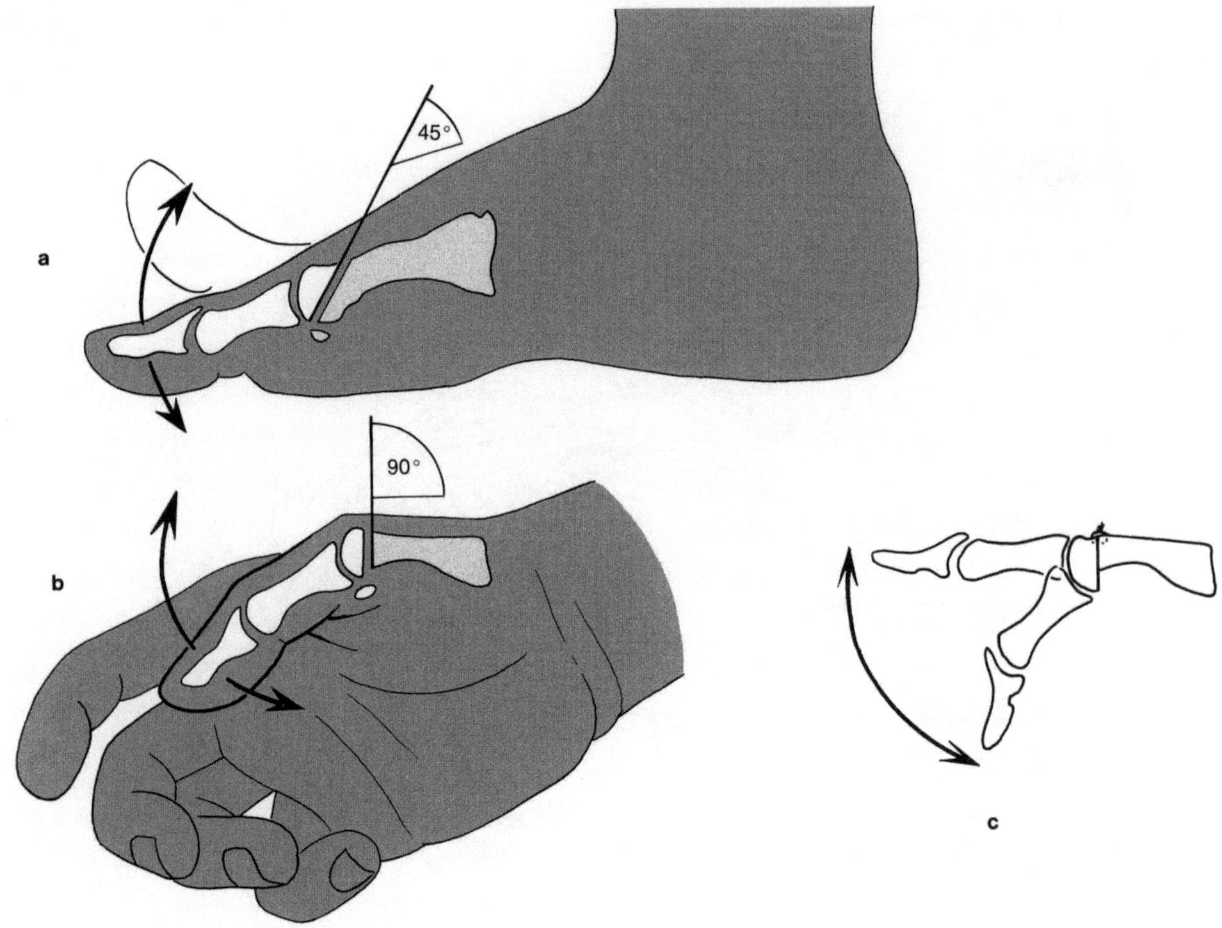

Fig. 20-15 a–c. Most of the range of motion of the first metatarsophalangeal joint is in hyperextension. In order that this joint provide a range of motion in flexion, the metacarpal head is cut obliquely on the foot (**a**) and applied transversely on the hand (**b**). This technique provides a good range of thumb flexion following transplantation (**c**)

7. Close the foot by bringing the medial flap over the end of the stump. The skin flap should not be tight or blistering and skin loss can be expected. Primary healing of the foot is an important goal in order to minimize the chance of tender scars.

II. Preparation of the Hand

All structures, except for the skin and flexor tendon, are prepared the same as for the second toe.

Surgical Technique

1. If the skin over the stump is suitable, raise it as a radially and palmar-based flap. Use this flap to cover the medial side of the transferred toe. If the skin is not suitable, use a straight line incision in the desired plane of flexion-extension of the toe transfer as used for the second toe transfer.

2. Identify the flexor pollicis tendon in the wrist. One of the advantages of the first toe is the long flexor hallucis longus tendon which is available. This allows the repair to be done in the wrist where adhesions are less likely.

III. Transplantation of the First Toe

Surgical Technique

1. If the amputation is at the base of the proximal phalanx, bone fixation is between this bone and the proximal phalanx of the first toe. Use two interosseous wire loops and supplement, if necessary, with an oblique k-wire. Also place a longitudinal k-wire to maintain the IP joint of the toe in full extension.

If the patient is a child, preserve the epiphysis at the proximal end of the phalanx by shaving only the articular cartilage from the base of the proximal

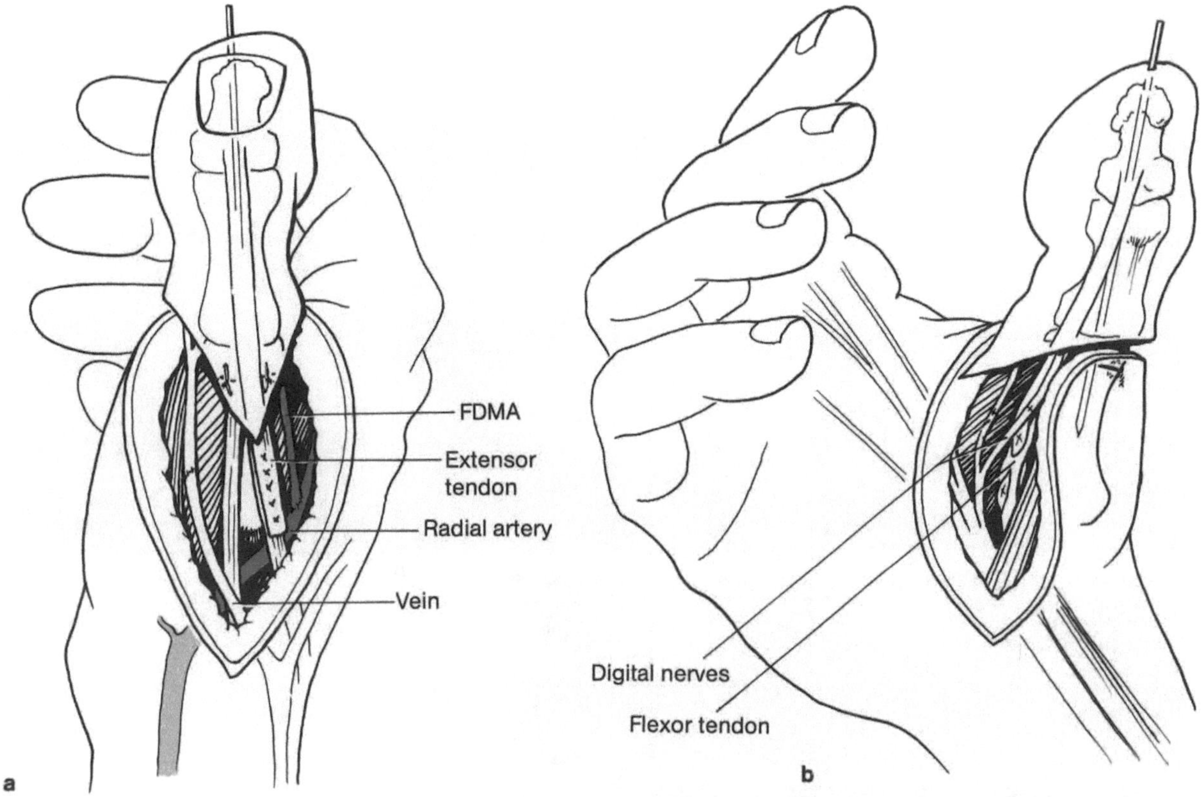

Fig. 20-16 a, b. The first toe fixed to the hand with the repair of all volar and dorsal structures

phalanx of the toe, and obtain bone fusion with longitudinal k-wires.

2. If the amputation passed through the metacarpal shaft, the transfer will include the metatarsophalangeal joint. Hold the toe on the stump in the desired position. While observing the cut surface of the metatarsal head which is held transversely on the stump, place a transverse osteotomy through the metacarpal in the appropriate plane (Fig. 20-15 a–c). In order that they not interfere with joint movement, place two interosseous wires through only the dorsal cortex of metacarpal and metatarsal and insert a longitudinal k-wire.

If the joint still tends to hyperextension, shorten the volar plate and tack it to the volar surface of the thumb metacarpal.

3. Suture the extensor tendon, vessels and nerves as described for the second toe transfer (Fig. 20-16 a). Suture the flexor hallucis longus tendon to the flexor pollicis longus tendon with an interweaving suture. The correct tension can be evaluated by palpating the tendon, and by flexing the wrist motion while observing the thumb motion at the carpalmetacarpal joint.

Postoperative Care

All of the usual postoperative considerations designed to maintain peripheral perfusion are particularly important in a toe transfer because of the susceptibility of peripheral vessels to reactive vasospasm. It is particularly important that postoperative hypovolemia, hypotension, body cooling and compression of the extremity are prevented.

Observe the toe half hourly for color, capillary return, and tissue turgor. Maintain temperature monitoring, using small probes placed on the tip of the toe. Use an adjacent finger as a control temperature. The temperature of the transfer is usually the same as in the adjacent digit but may be a degree higher or lower. A drop in the temperature of the transfer, while the control digit remains the same, indicates that there is a decrease in the volume of blood circulating through the toe. The cause of this decrease must be found immediately. Using the clinical signs

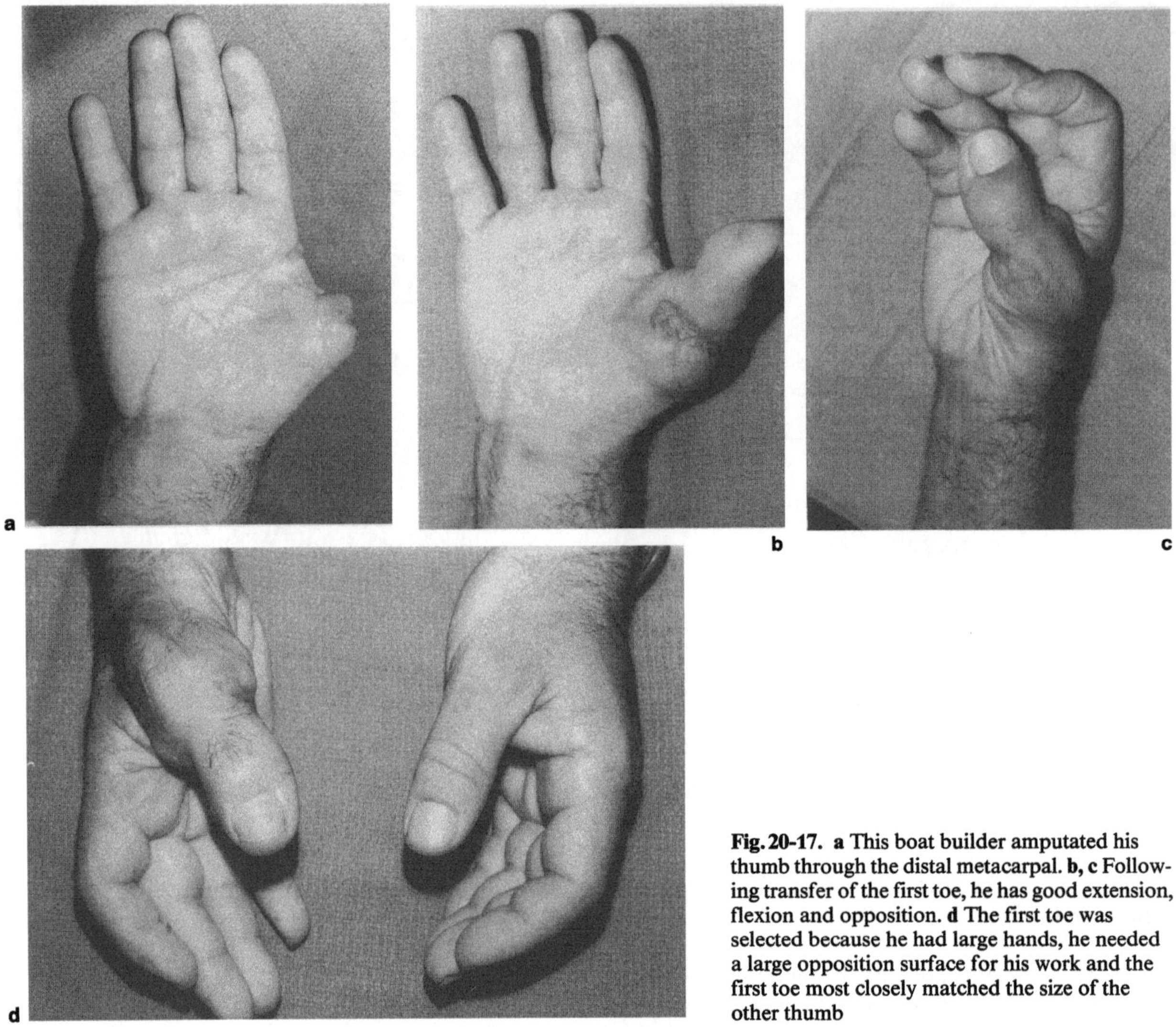

a b c d

Fig. 20-17. **a** This boat builder amputated his thumb through the distal metacarpal. **b, c** Following transfer of the first toe, he has good extension, flexion and opposition. **d** The first toe was selected because he had large hands, he needed a large opposition surface for his work and the first toe most closely matched the size of the other thumb

of color, capillary return and tissue turgor, it is usually possible to determine whether this is an arterial inflow problem or a venous obstruction problem. Appropriate conservative measures, such as elevating or lowering the arm, removing tight dressings or tight sutures, increasing the patient's blood volume, warming the patient, or administering antispasmotics or anticoagulents are all productive in overcoming decreasing circulation. The danger in not picking up these hemodynamic alterations early is that, with further progression, they may lead to anastomosis thrombosis.

Anticoagulation is not routinely used. However, if an anastomosis thrombosis occurs, full anticoagulation with intravenous heparin is given after revision of the anastomosis.

Change the dressing for a removable plastic splint prior to discharge from hospital. The splint supports the wrist and prevents pressure on the pedicle. Bed rest is required for at least five days to allow good foot healing.

The postoperative therapy program is important. It includes a program of active and passive motion which is begun at 3–4 weeks following the removal of the k-wire. The adequacy of bone fixation determines the vigor of the exercise program. This is followed by resisted exercises and a nerve relearning program when bone union and nerve regeneration have occurred. Activities of daily living are gradually incorporated.

References

1. Buncke HJ Jr, Buncke CM, Schultz WP (1966) Immediate Nicoladoni procedure in the Rhesus monkey or hallux-to-hand transplantation utilizing micro-miniature vascular anastomoses. Br J Plast Surg 19: 332
2. Bunnel S (1952) Digit transfer by neurovascular pedicle. J Bone Jt Surg 34A: 772
3. Cobbett JR (1969) Free digital transfer: report of a case of transfer of a great toe to replace an amputated thumb. J Bone Jt Surg 51B: 677-689
4. Frykman GK, O'Brien BMcC, Morrison WA, MacLeod A, Ciurleo A (1984) Long term functional value of toe to hand transfers. Presented at American Society for Surgery of the Hand, February 7, 1984, Atlanta, Ga
5. Gilbert A (1976) Composite tissue transfers from the foot: anatomic basis and surgical technique. In 'Symposium on Microsurgery' ed. Daniller A, Strauch B. CV Mosby, St. Louis
6. Gillies HD, Millard DR (1957) The Principles and Art of Plastic Surgery, 2: 486 Little Brown and Co, Toronto
7. Lister GD, Kalisman M, Tsai TM (1983) Reconstruction of the hand with free microneurovascular toe to hand transfer: experience with 54 toe transfers. Plast Reconstr Surg 71: 372
8. Matev I (1970) Thumb reconstruction after amputation at the metacarpo-phalangeal joint by bony lenthening. J Bone Jt Surg 52A: 957
9. May JW, Daniel RK (1978) Great toe to hand free tissue transfer. Clin Orthop 133: 140
10. Morrison WA, O'Brien BMcB, MacLeod AM (1980) Thumb reconstruction with a free neurovascular wrap around flap from the big toe. J Hand Surg 5: 575
11. Nicoladoni C (1897) Daumenplastic. Wien Klin Wochenshar 10: 663
12. Nicoladoni C (1900) Daumenplastic und organischer ersatz der Fingerspitze (Anticheiroplastik und Daktyloplastik). Arch Klin Chir 61: 606
13. Poppen NK, Norris TR, Buncke HJ Jr (1983) Evaluation of sensibility and function with microsurgical free tissue transfer of the great toe to the hand for thumb reconstruction. J Hand Surg 8: 516
14. Simonetta C (1979) Reconstruction of the thumb by tube pedicle, bone graft and island flap, In 'Mutilating Injuries of the Hand', ed Reid DAC, Gosset I. Churchill Livingstone, New York
15. Yoshimura M (1980) Toe to hand transfer. Plast Reconstr Surg 66: 74

Lower Extremity Reconstruction

Free tissue transfers have been particularly useful in reconstruction of the lower extremity. The most common applications have been soft tissue coverage of the tibia and the sole of the foot, and replacement of large bony defects of the leg. Prior to the advent of reconstructive microsurgery, patients with these problems required multi-staged operative procedures or amputation of the extremity.

Vascular Anatomoses in the Lower Extremity

In the early days of reconstructive microsurgery, free tissue transfers to the lower extremity had the highest incidence of flap failure of any area of the body. This problem has been partially solved by an appreciation of the need to maintain normal peripheral perfusion during the operation and postoperative period, by an appreciation of the importance of using undamaged vessels and by the use of new surgical techniques.

During the operation, blood pressure, blood volume and the patient's temperature must all be preserved at normal levels. If any of these are allowed to drop, the effect on blood flow is first felt in the peripheral circulation where the anastomosis is done. If the blood volume is not maintained, peripheral vasoconstriction will attempt to conserve the body's diminished blood supply, resulting in a decreased perfusion pressure to the peripherally-placed tissue transfer. If the patient becomes cooled, by the time that the core temperature has begun to drop, the peripheral temperature will usually be well down and the perfusion in the extremities significantly decreased.

Microvascular patients should be monitored by the anaesthetist in such a way that they are sure of the adequacy of their fluid replacement. In wounds which are open for a long time, there is often a slow but steady oozing of blood which results in a significant blood loss, the extent of which is often unappreciated by surgeon and anaesthetist. A tendency to overreplacement of fluids is indicated.

Torniquets, although useful for exposure of vessels, allow an extremity to become quite cool during their use. In addition, when the tourniquet is let down, if it has not been loosely applied, it may produce mild obstruction to venous return, which, when present for a long time, may significantly increase edema in the extremity.

For free tissue transfers to the lower leg, either the anterior tibial or posterior tibial vascular bundles are available for anastomoses. It is preferable to do the anastomoses near the ankle because the vessels are superficially located and more accessible. If anastomoses are done to the more deeply-placed vessels in the proximal leg, swelling of the leg musculature between which the pedicle must pass may cause compression and venous obstruction to the pedicle.

All subacute and chronic tissue defects are surrounded by a zone of tissue which has undergone an inflammatory and healing response. Vessels which are within this zone of injury, even when the healing response appears quiescent, are prone to develop spasm when dissected or divided. Vessels within this region do not have the normal pristine appearance of an artery and vein, but are fixed in place by a thin layer of fibrous tissue and appear a little more rigid than normal. When these arteries are divided, there is retraction and spasm of the vessel. The vessel will have a less than normal spurt of blood and, over a few minutes, the spurt will change to a dribble. An anastomosis to this vessel will always thrombose because of the low flow rate. Godina and Ikuta first brought to our attention the value of an end to side anastomosis in the lower leg. This has become a standard technique with lower extremity transfer. A useful aid to cutting the side hole is the Acland-Banis arteriotomy clamp which is used as a template to cut an accurate side hole in the vessel. As a side hole does not allow vessel retraction and shortening, there is less tendency to spasm and anastomoses are more likely to remain patent. The other advantage of an end to side anastomosis is that it allows a free tissue transfer to be done to a leg which has only one functioning artery.

If at all possible, both the arterial and venous anastomoses should be completely outside the zone of injury. However, end to side repairs may be successful within the zone of injury when an end to end repair would fail. Although the problem of spasm is most severe in arteries within the zone of injury, veins are also susceptible, particularly the superficial veins of the leg. For this reason, we prefer to use venae comitantes.

In the lower leg, which normally has relatively tight skin, the pedicle can easily be obstructed by a tight skin closure. This tightness is exacerbated by pre- and postoperative swelling in the leg. Although it may be possible to close the skin over the pedicle, it is often better to leave the skin open and apply a skin graft, often using a portion of the transfer to cover the pedicle.

When determining the pedicle length, it is easy to make it too short or too long. If the pedicle goes around a portion of the leg which undergoes postoperative swelling, and there is no allowance for stretching of the pedicle, it may be obstructed in the postoperative period. The surgeon's reluctance to adequately shorten a good pedicle may result in a redundant loop of vessel which is prone to obstruction by kinking.

Postoperative elevation is important to minimize additional swelling and pedicle compression. The usual duration of bed rest is 10–12 days following transfer, followed by a program of gradual ambulation with an elastic support bandage. On this program, we have had no problems with late postoperative vessel thrombosis.

References

1. Godina M (1979) Preferential use of end to side arterial anastomoses in free flap transfers. Plast Reconstr Surg 64: 673
2. Ikuta Y (1975) Free flap transfers by end to side arterial anastomosis. Br J Plast Surg 28: 1

Chapter 21. Lower Extremity Coverage

A soft tissue defect of the lower extremity may be covered with many different types of free tissue transfers. These include cutaneous, muscle only, myocutaneous, and fascial transfers. Each of these has particular merit which recommends it to certain situations. In general, a free tissue transfer should not be used unless it provides advantages over other coverage techniques, such as split thickness skin grafts and local flaps. Free tissue transfers should be used only when these two techniques are not available, or there is a clear advantage to using a free tissue transfer.

The skin only free tissue transfer has major advantages in cosmesis and the development of sensibility. A skin flap certainly provides the most acceptable surface, color, and consistency of any of the free tissue transfers. As an innervated skin transfer, the dorsal foot and forearm flaps provide durable, easily contoured and not too bulky skin cover which has protective sensibility and is particularly useful for the sole of the foot.

Muscle only transfers have the advantage that they are flexible and can readily be contoured to fit irregular shapes and cavities. The muscle will shrink to approximately one half of its pre-transplantation bulk and, with a skin graft applied, it develops a smooth, cosmetically acceptable contour. Although the skin graft does not look normal, it usually is quite acceptable and often preferable to the excess bulk which is present when a myocutaneous flap is transferred. There is less chance of infection developing when a muscle is placed in a contaminated bed than occurs when a skin flap is used.

When compared to skin transfers, a disadvantage of the muscle only transfer is the greater difficulty in postoperative monitoring of the muscle's circulation.

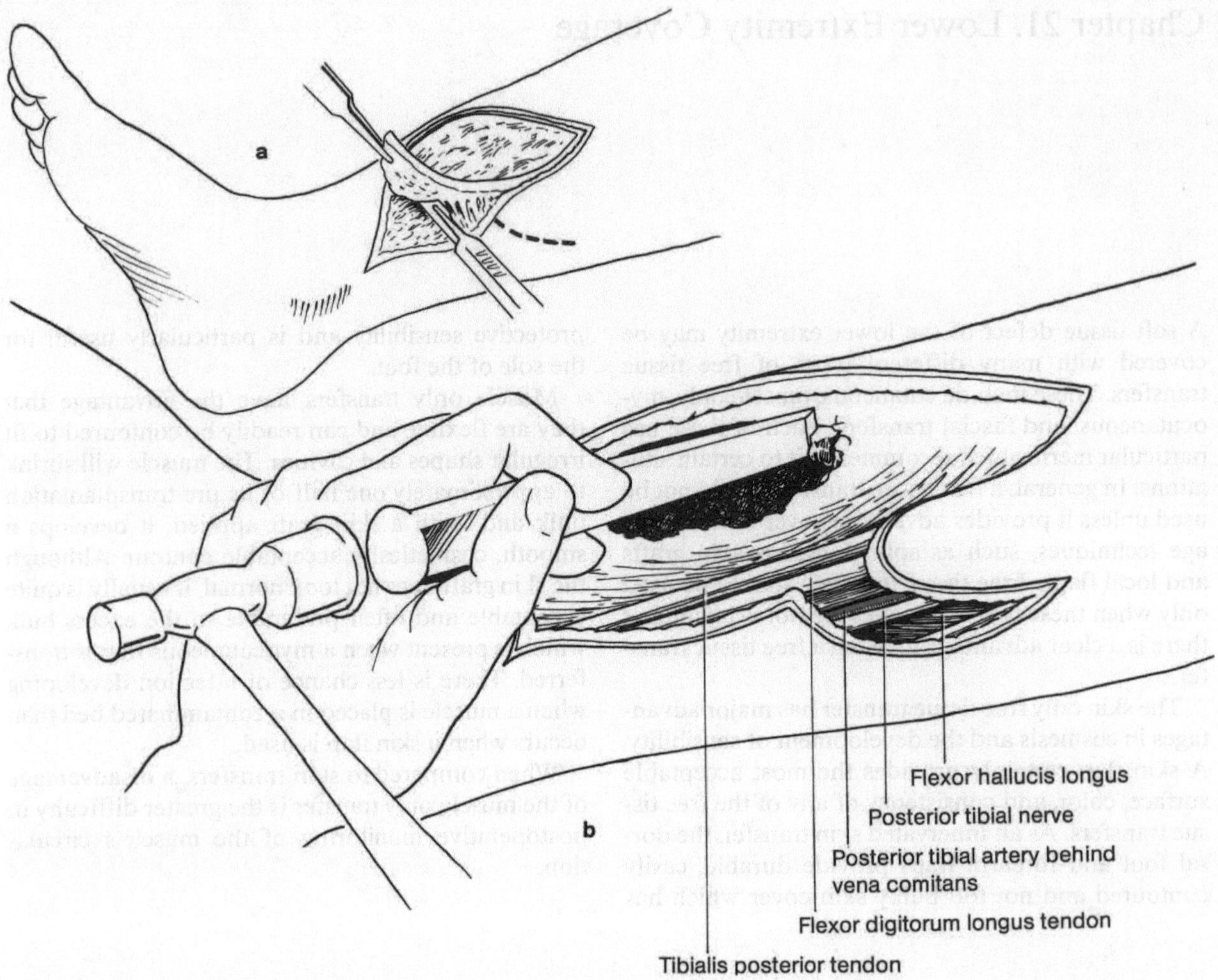

Fig. 21-1. **a** Treatment of osteomyelitis begins with a radical resection of all scar tissue about the area of osteomyelitis. **b** Bone is resected until healthy bleeding bone remains

Technique of Leg Coverage with a Muscle Transfer for Osteomyelitis of the Tibia

Preparation of the Leg

1. Outline on the leg the maximum size of the soft tissue defect which will be produced by the resection. The resection should include all of the previously infected and poorly-vascularized scar tissue about the osteomyelitis. Mark the site of the recipient vessels and the route which the pedicle will likely take to reach them (Fig. 21-1 a).

2. Make a pattern of these markings and transfer it to the muscle to be selected.

3. Do a radical excision of all the scar tissue about the area of osteomyelitis, and a radical sequestrectomy of bone, removing bone until only well-vascularized bone remains (Fig. 21-1 b).

4. Place an incision over the posterior tibial vessels and identify the posterior tibial neurovascular bundle (Fig. 21-2 a).

5. Separate the venae comitantes from the posterior tibial artery. There are usually 2 or 3 venae comitantes and they are often joined together by many cross connections which will need to be severed to allow exposure of the artery and the development of an adequate length of venous pedicle (Fig. 21-2 b). The artery should have a good pulsation and normal appearance.

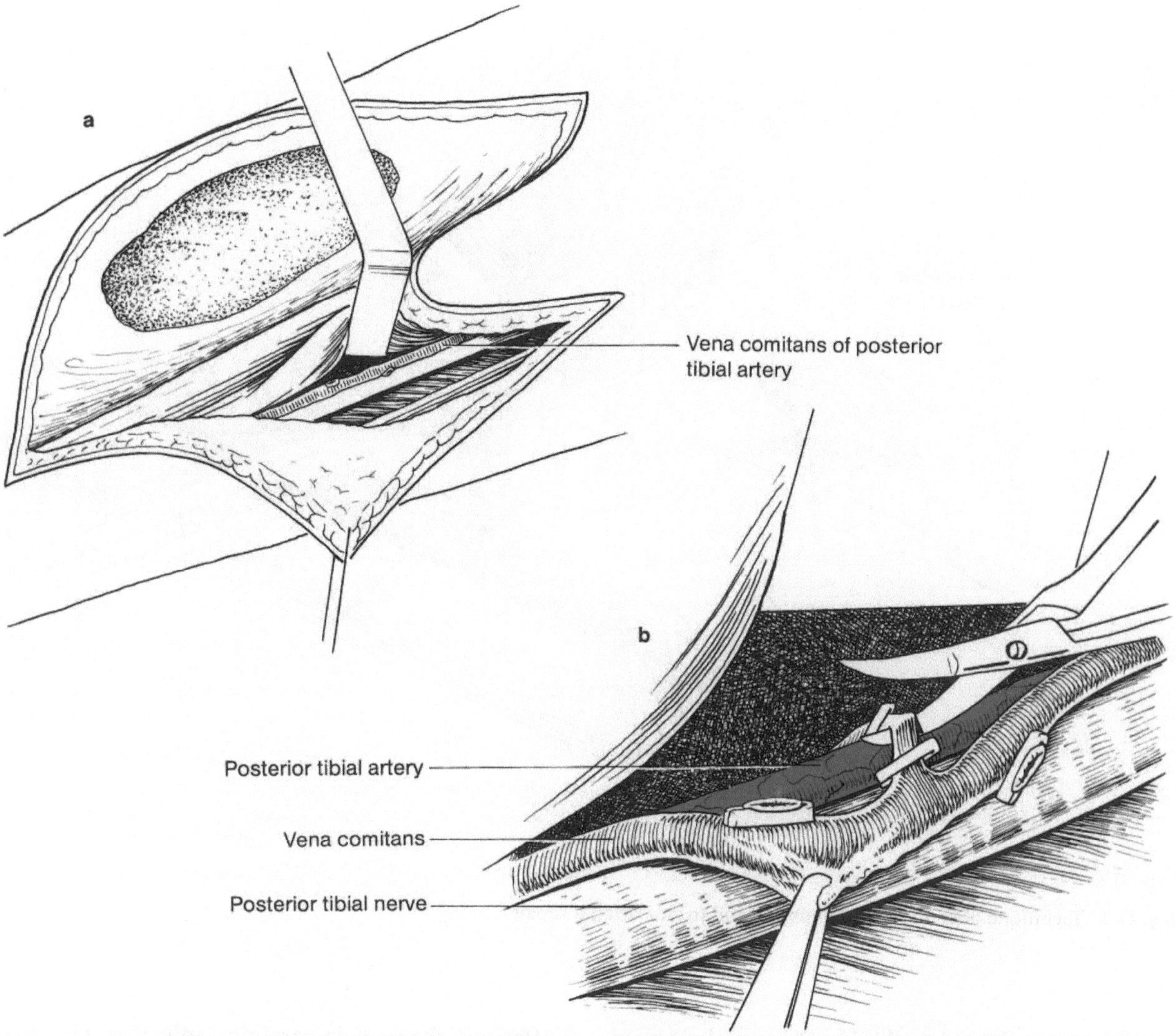

Fig. 21-2. **a** Identification of the recipient vessels, posterior to the tibialis posterior and flexor digitorum longus tendons. **b** Division of cross connections between venae comitantes after applying vessel clips

Preparation of the Muscle

The usual muscles for coverage of the lower extremity are the gracilis, rectus abdominis and latissimus dorsi. The gracilis is the smallest muscle of the three and all or a portion of it may be used. Its pedicle length, which is approximately 6 cm, is usually enough to reach the location of the planned vascular anastomoses. However, if this is not long enough, then the rectus or latissimus can be used. Both muscles have long pedicles which, by muscle excision, can be developed up to 10-12 cm in length. Sometimes, the diameter of these vessels is too large at the end for an end to side anastomosis to the anterior or posterior tibial vessels. Another disadvantage of the latissimus dorsi is that the vena comitans of the thoracodorsal artery may have a diameter of 5-6 mm, which is much larger than the 2.3 mm diameter of the venae comitantes of the distal posterior tibial and anterior tibial vessels.

The rectus abdominis muscle is particularly well suited to a long narrow defect as is sometimes present over the anterior tibia. For large wide defects, the latissimus dorsi muscle provides excellent coverage.

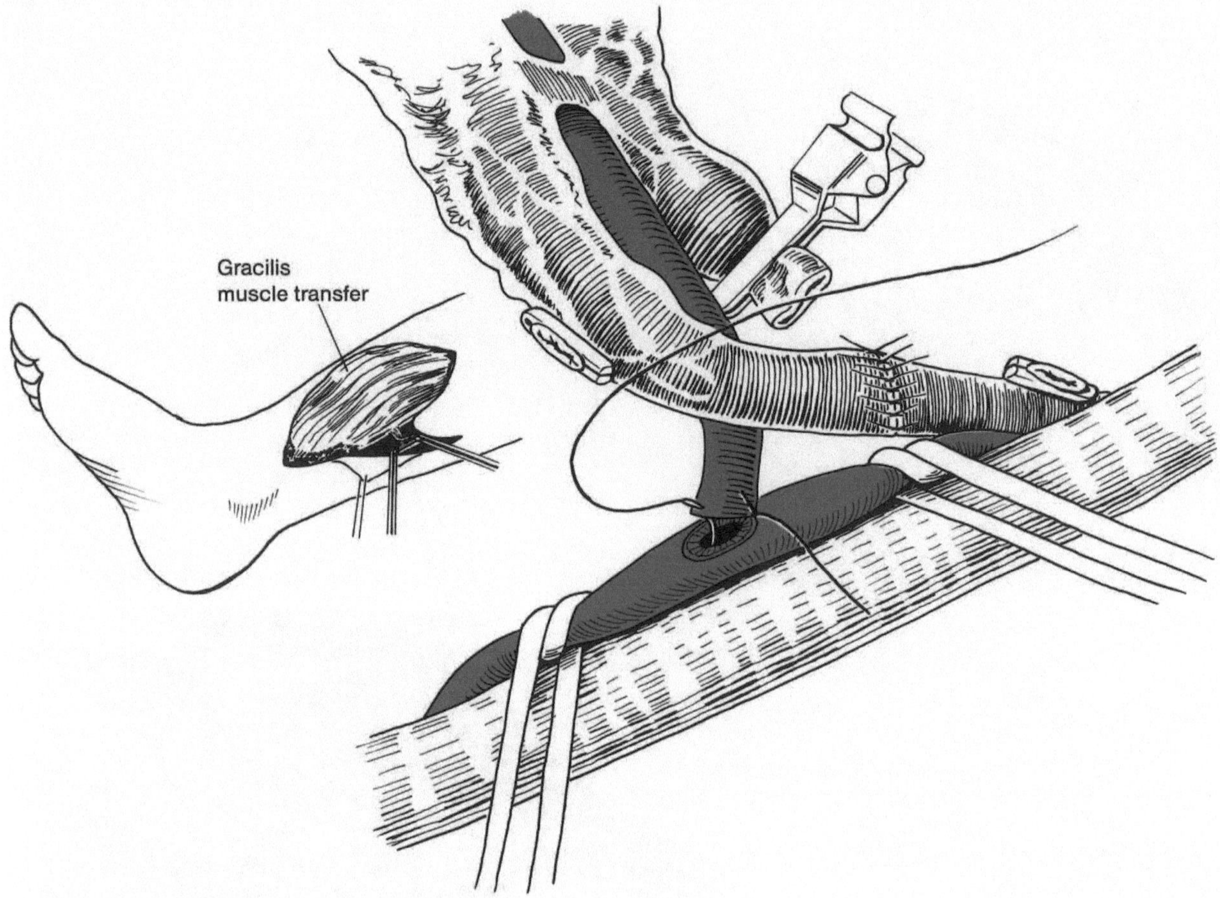

Fig. 21-3. Technique of end to end venous and end to side arterial repair

When transplanted to the leg, the muscle should be placed with its deep surface down, so that the pedicle will be covered and protected by the muscle. This positioning can be accomplished by selecting the muscle from the appropriate side of the body. There is evidence that, in some instances, a muscle may not pick up a vigorous blood supply from the surrounding tissues and may depend on the vascular pedicle permanently. Therefore, it is best that the pedicle be buried as deeply as possible so that it will be protected from subsequent trauma.

The technique of muscle elevation is described in Chapters 6, 7, and 8.

Transplantation of the Muscle to the Leg

1. Place the muscle in the defect, temporarily tack it about the margins so that it will not shift during the anastomosis, and cover it with damp gauze.

2. Position the pedicle carefully, adjusting it so that there is sufficient length to reach the recipient vessels but not enough length for kinking. Remember that when the vessels are distended, they will be longer than they appear when empty.

3. Do venous end to end anastomosis and arterial end to side anastomosis. When the arterial repair is being done, a useful technique to bring the recipient vessels up from the depths of the wound and also occlude the vessels is to use elastic vessel loops placed proximally and distally to the intended anastomosis (Fig. 21-3). When traction is placed on these elastics, the vessel is lifted into a more accessible position.

4. Following the anastomoses, give the muscle a chance to perfuse before suturing it into the defect. Observe the muscle's color for the adequacy of its circulation. Trim any muscle of questionable color back to bleeding muscle.

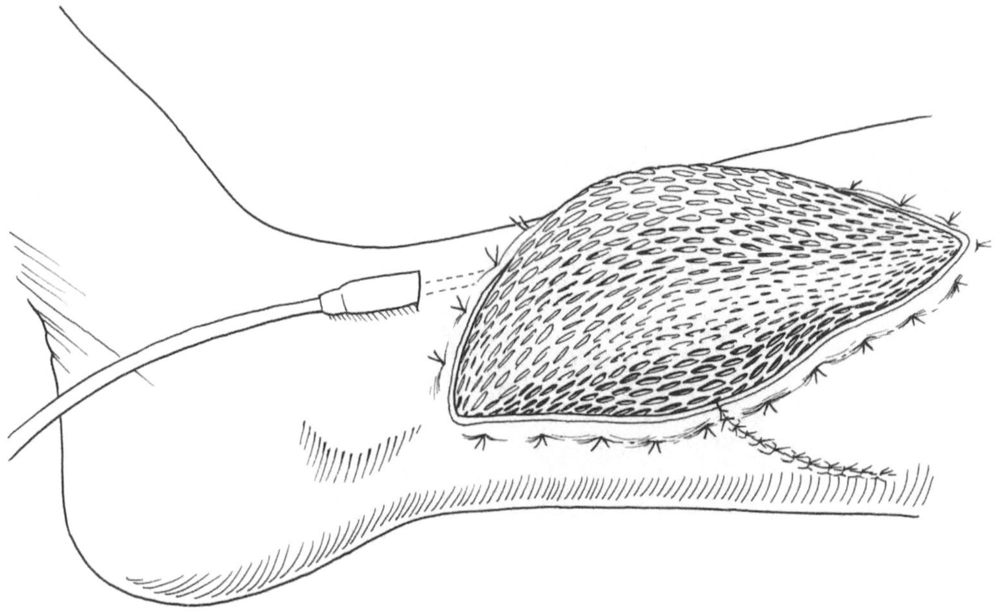

Fig. 21-4. Completed transfer with meshed split thickness skin graft in place and suction drain under muscle

5. Insert a suction drain under the muscle and multiple penrose drains about the margins. These must be placed with care so that they do not come in contact with the pedicle. Undermine the skin edges for 1 cm and insert the muscle under the skin edge, fixing it with multiple interrupted mattress sutures to provide a layered closure at the margins (Fig. 21-4).

6. Cover the pedicle by closing the skin incision with a portion of the muscle used for the transfer. The latter is a wise move if direct closure of the skin is tight.

7. Apply a skin graft to the exposed muscle, tacking it about the margins. A meshed, unexpanded graft allows blood which collects under the skin graft to escape (Fig. 21-4).

8. Dress the extremity from the knee to toes with a bulky gently-applied dressing, reinforced with a plaster back slab from the calf to toes. Be careful that the plaster slab does not place pressure in the area of the anastomoses.

Place an opening in the dressing over the muscle. A small flap of skin graft can be turned like the page of a book. This allows a 'window' on the muscle for frequent postoperative observations to assess the circulation.

When the anterior tibial vessels are used for an anastomosis, it is helpful to hold the foot in dorsi flexion to relax the extensor musculature and prevent compression of the pedicle where it passes between the muscles to the deeply placed recipient vessels.

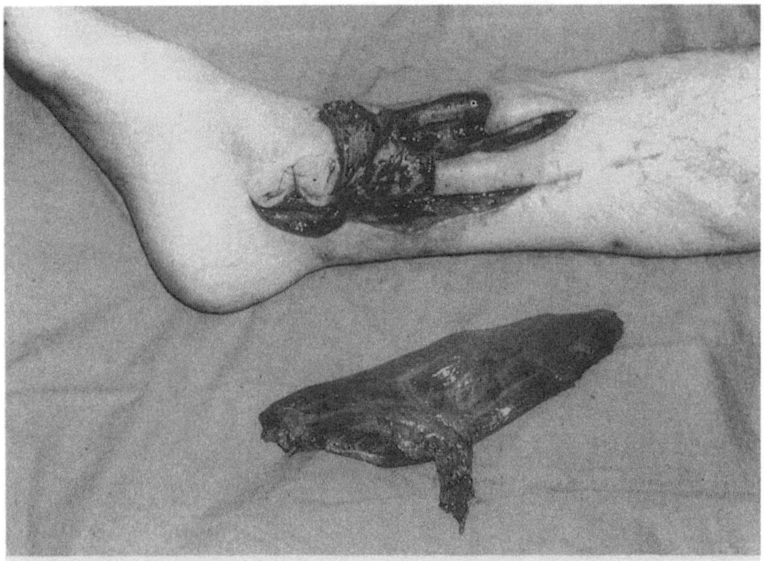

a **Fig. 21-5.** **a** Subsequent to a compound fracture, this patient had chronic osteomyelitis of the tibia for 9 years. Following each of his three previous sequestrectomies, his leg had been allowed to heal by secondary intention. He continued to have chronic drainage and pain. Surgical management included radical excision of his pretibial soft tissues and radical sequestrectomy. The gracilis muscle is seen below the prepared leg.

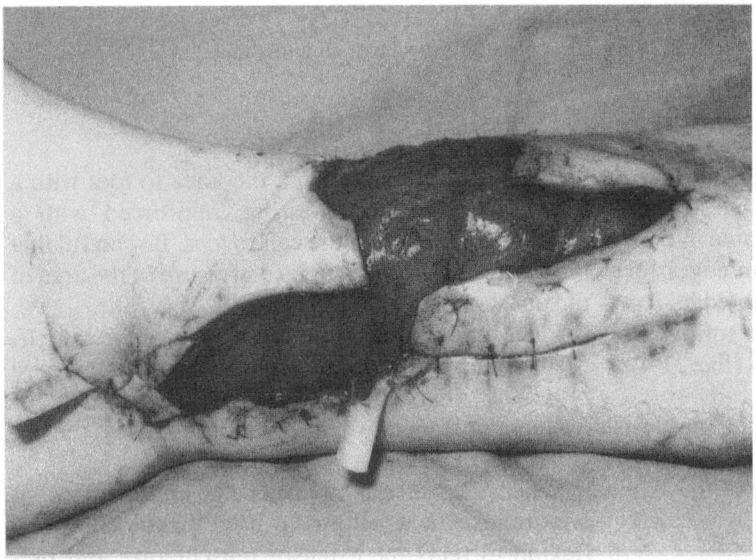

b

b Gracilis muscle has been fitted into the defect and the pedicle has been sutured to the posterior tibial artery and vena comitans. Muscle has been used to cover the pedicle which is just above the ankle, without attempting a too tight direct closure.

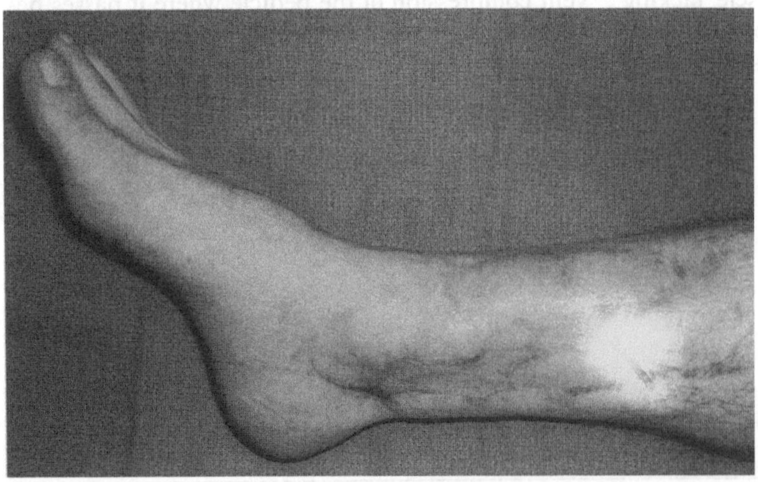

c

c Following a meshed split thickness skin graft, the appearance of the healed leg is quite acceptable, with good contour, color match, and a durable coverage

Fig. 21-6. **a** Medial aspect of right lower leg following a motor boat accident in which the patient sustained an extensive soft tissue and bony loss.

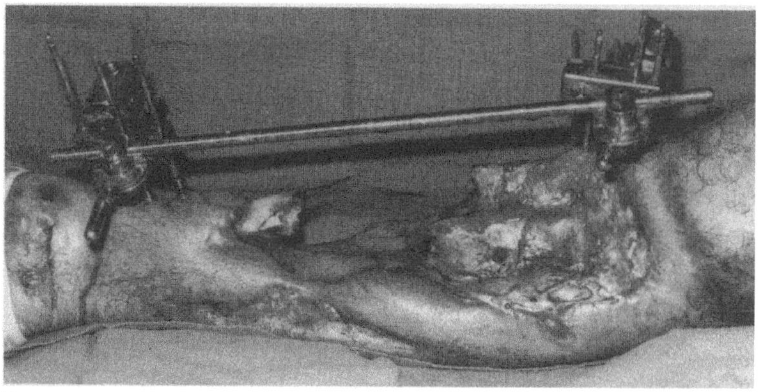

a

b Lateral aspect of leg following debridement and preparation of a 15 × 36 cm latissimus dorsi myocutaneous flap. Proximal anterior tibial artery and vena comitans are prepared for anastomosis.

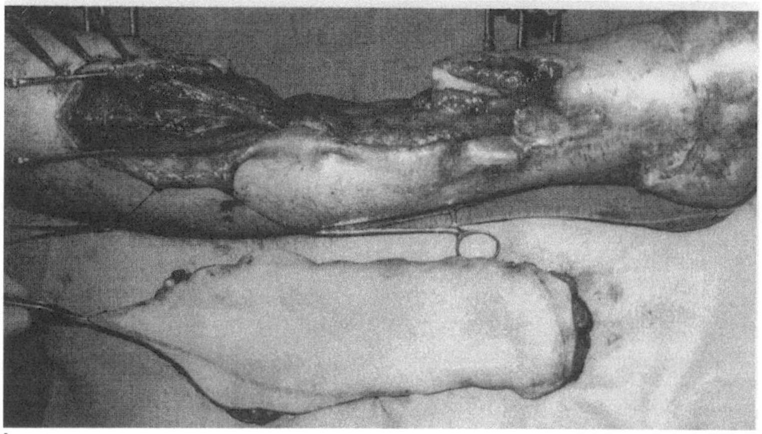

b

c Following transfer, this flap provided good cover with an acceptable appearance. At a second operation, a vascularized fibula was inserted into the tibial defect. **d** The donor area could not be closed directly and required split thickness skin grafting. This produced hyperpigmented scarring which the patient disliked

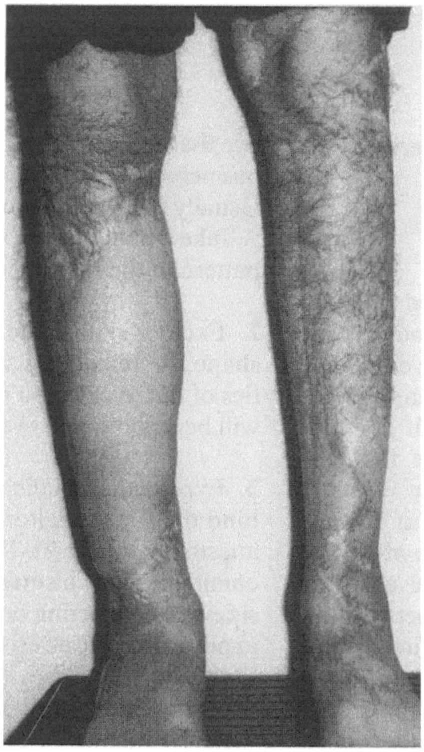

c

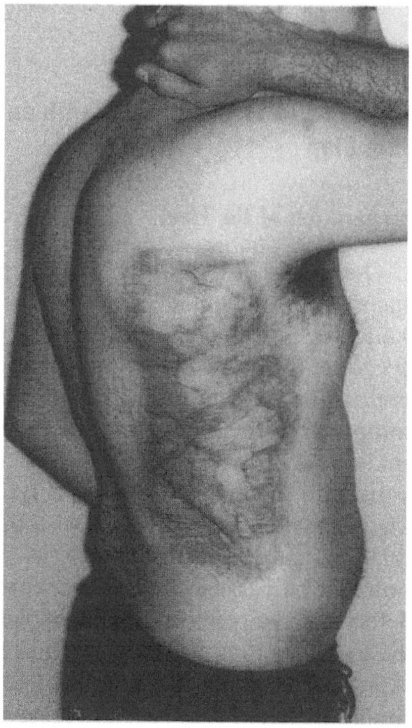

d

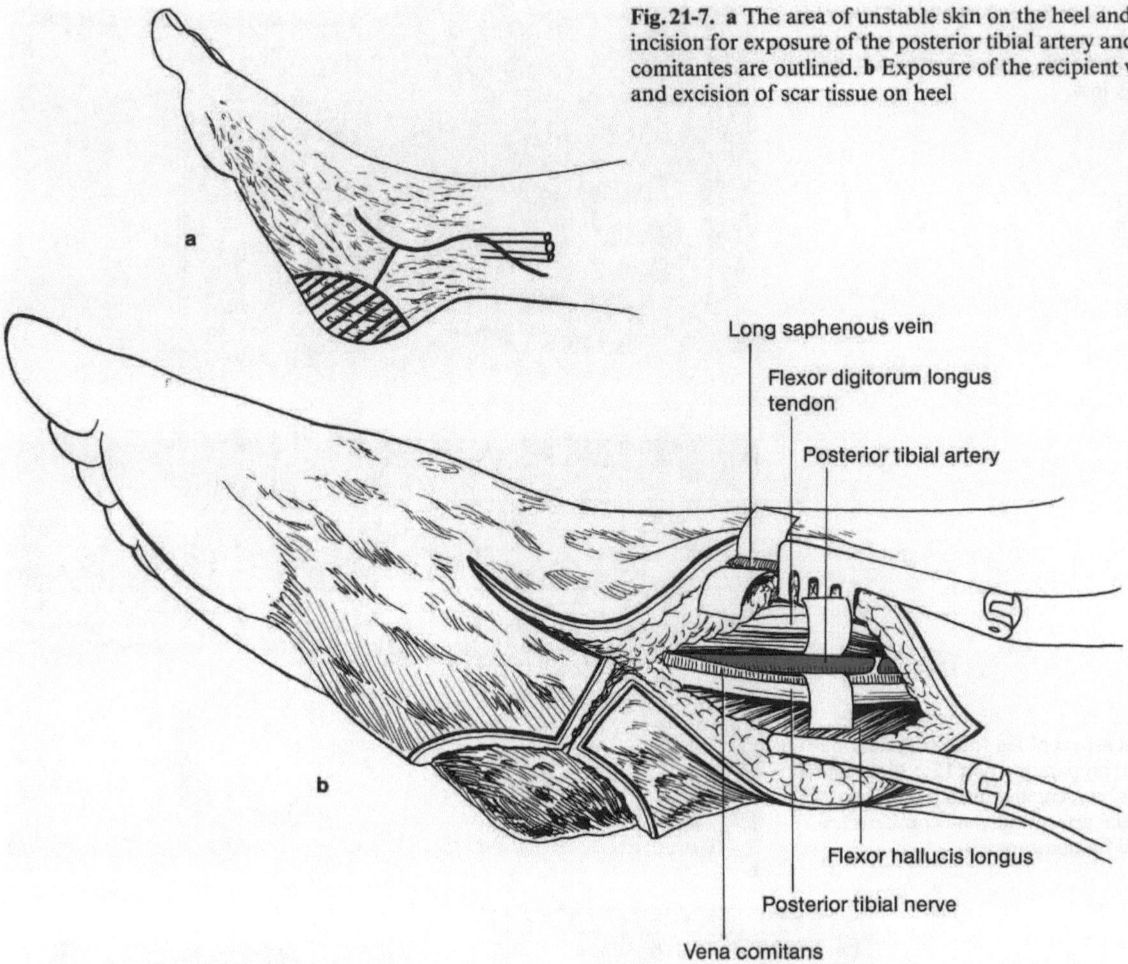

Fig. 21-7. a The area of unstable skin on the heel and the incision for exposure of the posterior tibial artery and venae comitantes are outlined. **b** Exposure of the recipient vessels and excision of scar tissue on heel

Technique of Heel Coverage with an Innervated Skin Flap

Preparation of the Heel

1. Outline the defect which will be created when the unstable epithelium over the heel is removed, and mark the expected site of the recipient vessels and the route of the pedicle. Plan the incision from the heel to the pedicle in such a way that it does not compromise the remaining skin on the foot and ankle, and provides a non-kinked route from the transfer to the recipient vessels (Fig. 21-7a). It is unwise to tunnel the pedicle under a bridge of scarred skin and subcutaneous tissues, as vessel compression can be expected. Use an incision between the defect and recipient vessels and close it directly after the transfer or apply a skin graft on the pedicle. If a skin graft is going to be applied to the pedicle, it should be taken with an extra layer of fatty connective tissue. Mark the expected location of the cutaneous nerve which will be used for innervating the flap. Usually this will be the sural.

Take a pattern from the markings and transfer this pattern to the flap donor site.

2. Excise the unstable epithelium over the heel and shape the remaining scar tissue and any irregularities of the os calcis so that the surface under the flap will be smooth and even.

3. Expose the tibialis posterior vascular bundle behind the flexor digitorum longus and prepare it for anastomosis (Fig. 21-7b). Dissect free the 2–3 venae comitantes which surround the artery and divide the side and connecting branches sufficiently to provide exposure for the arterial and venous anastomoses.

4. Expose the sural nerve and examine it under magnification to be sure that it is undamaged.

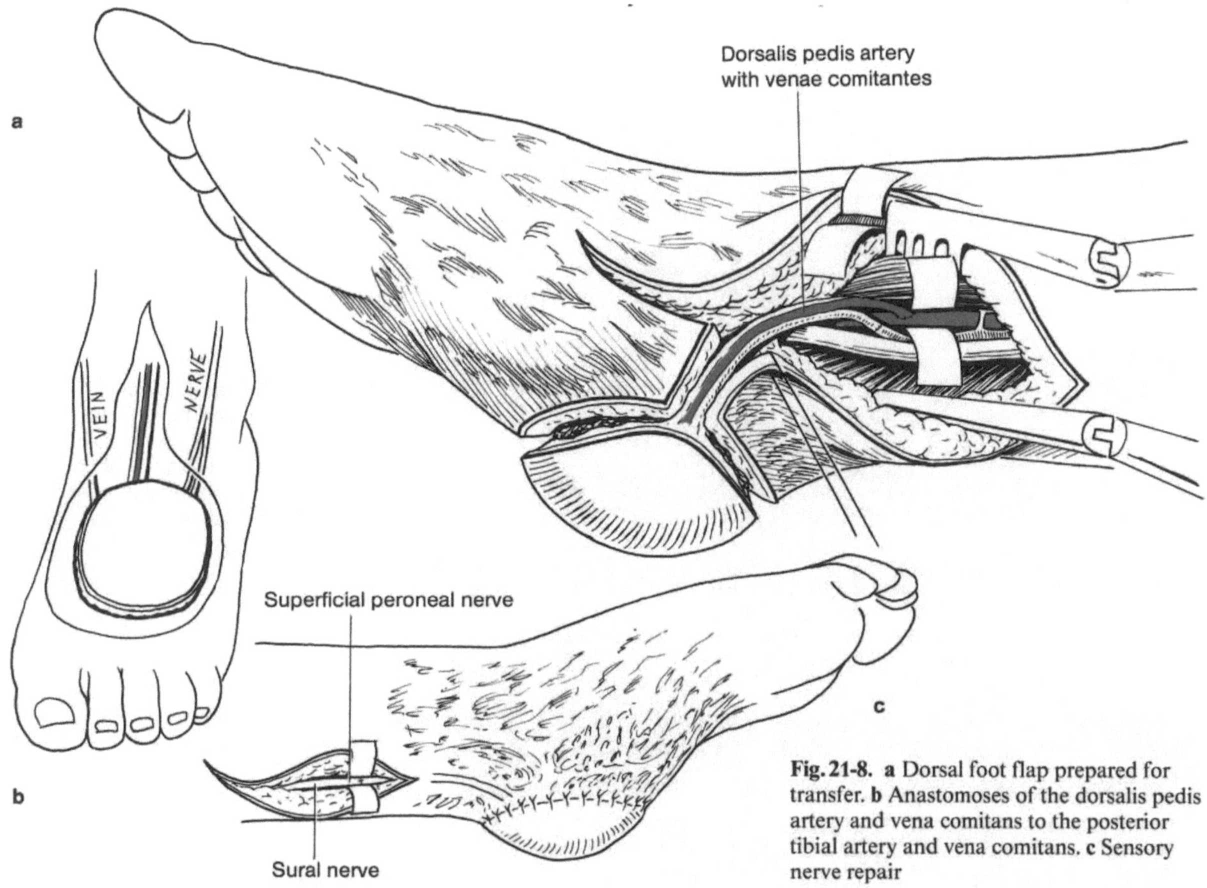

Fig. 21-8. a Dorsal foot flap prepared for transfer. b Anastomoses of the dorsalis pedis artery and vena comitans to the posterior tibial artery and vena comitans. c Sensory nerve repair

Preparation of the Skin Flap

The transfer is taken as described in Chapter 3. The size of the transfer should be slightly larger than the pattern which has been taken from the defect to allow for postoperative swelling (Fig. 21-8 a).

Transplantation of the Skin Flap to the Heel

1. Place the flap on the heel and temporarily tack it in place.

2. Carefully position the pedicle from the flap to the recipient vessels with sufficient length to allow an easy repair, but not excess redundancy which might produce kinking of the pedicle.

3. Do a venous end to end and an arterial end to side anastomosis (Fig. 21-8 b). Use vessel loops to retract the artery.

4. Suture the skin flap edges and insert multiple small penrose drains about the margins to allow escape of blood.

5. Take care in closing the incision over the pedicle. If it is tight, leave it open and apply a skin graft directly on the pedicle.

6. Do a microsurgical nerve repair between the sural nerve on the foot and the superficial peroneal nerve on the flap (Fig. 21-8 c).

Postoperative Care

Following a flap to the heel, the best position of the patient is lying face down. Alternate with periods on both sides. In this way, the flap can be left open and exposed with the foot resting on a pillow.

If the patient insists on lying supine, a back slab is placed on the distal sole of the foot and posterior calf, but not allowed to produce pressure to the heel. This technique runs the risk that inadvertent pressure may be applied to the pedicle or flap in the postoperative period.

Whichever technique is used should allow exposure of a portion of the flap so that it can be monitored for capillary return, color and swelling.

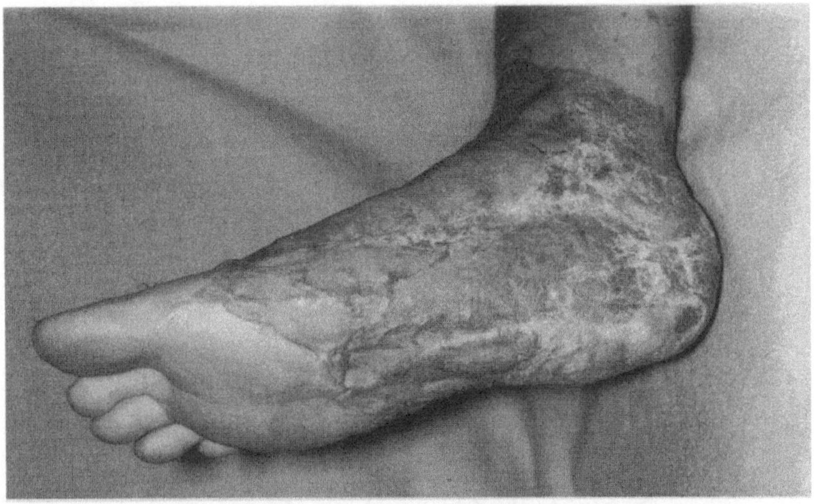

a

Fig. 21-9 a. Patient sustained a degloving injury of the foot in a motor vehicle accident. She was unable to bear weight on her heel because of an unstable split thickness skin graft applied directly to the os calcis

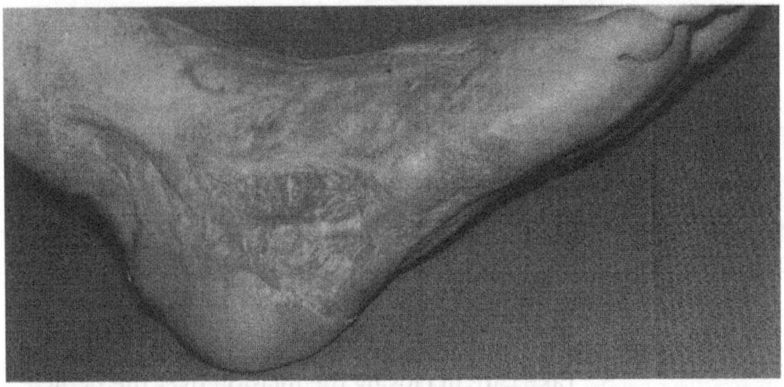

b

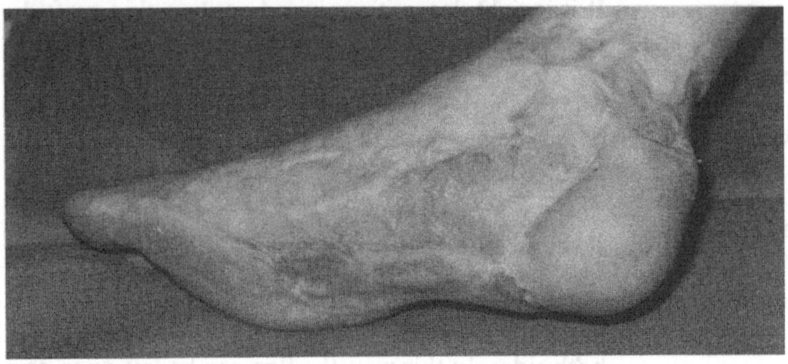

c

Fig. 21-9 a–c. Appearance of heel one year postoperative. Flap has protective sensation and allows full weight bearing without skin breakdown

Chapter 22. Bone Reconstruction

The development of vascularized bone grafts has provided a solution to the management of large bony defects. In small conventional bone grafts, some osteocytes may survive in well-vascularized beds. However, in large grafts, the osteocytes do not survive and the bone is replaced by a process of creeping substitution [1, 2]. During this process, which takes 6-12 months, the graft actually becomes weaker before it becomes stronger. It is susceptible to fractures and non union and, in the presence of contamination, readily becomes infected and lost.

In the vascularized bone graft which is transferred with microvascular anastomoses, the osteocytes survive. Survival and normal function are indicated by the results of tetracycline labelled bone biopsies, positive bone scans following transfer, and rapid healing between the graft and recipient bone.

The indication for a vascularized bone graft is a large bony defect which cannot be adequately reconstructed with a non-vascularized graft. Many surgeons favour a vascularized bone graft for any bony defect greater then 6-8 cm in length. However, the likelihood of survival of conventional cancellous bone grafts depends not only upon the size of the defect but also the vascularity and sterility of the bone graft bed. Some surgeons have had success grafting very large bony defects with cancellous bone chips. The key to this success is the radical resection of contaminated scar tissue and bone, and the application of a vascularized muscle transfer as the first stage of a two-stage procedure. Others have had success with massive homografts for replacement of large bone defects. However, these grafts will not survive in the post traumatic bed which is usually contaminated, and their incorporation time is often a few years [3]. Many large bone defects result from trauma, particularly compound fractures from motor car and motor cycle accidents. These accidents can produce devastating injuries to the lower leg with extensive tibial and soft tissue destruction. As vascularized bone grafts tolerate contamination, they are particularly suitable for post traumatic reconstruction. Vascularized bone grafts often allow severely damaged extremities, which would otherwise require an amputation, to be salvaged. The surgeon must reserve the vascularized bone graft for salvage of legs which have a useful functional potential.

Selection of Bone Graft for Extremity Reconstruction

Taylor is credited with introducing both the fibula and the iliac crest, the most useful grafts for long bone reconstruction.

In our experience with 97 vascularized bone grafts, 53 have been used for mandibular reconstruction and 39 for extremity reconstruction. This experience includes 14 fibular grafts, and 23 iliac crest grafts used for lower extremity reconstruction. Of these lower extremity grafts, three iliac crests and one fibula did not survive. Two cases required additional cancellous bone grafting at one end of the graft. Stress fractures occurred in 2 patients and healed uneventfully. All of these grafts were used to manage defects which were too large for conventional grafting. The three iliac crest failures resulted from use of damaged recipient vessels and occurred in our early experience with this transfer.

Fibula

The fibula provides a long straight and strong cortical bone which can be removed in lengths up to 25 cm. This bone is most useful for extremity reconstruction for medium to long bony defects when soft tissue coverage is not required (Fig. 22-1). However, very small soft tissue defects associated with fibular transfer can be covered with a split thickness skin graft placed over a muscle sleeve which is taken with the fibula. This muscle sleeve can be augmented by leaving a large portion of the flexor hallucis longus or the soleus attached to the fibula and applying a skin graft to the muscle. However, the patient may not wish to lose flexor hallucis longus function. It is

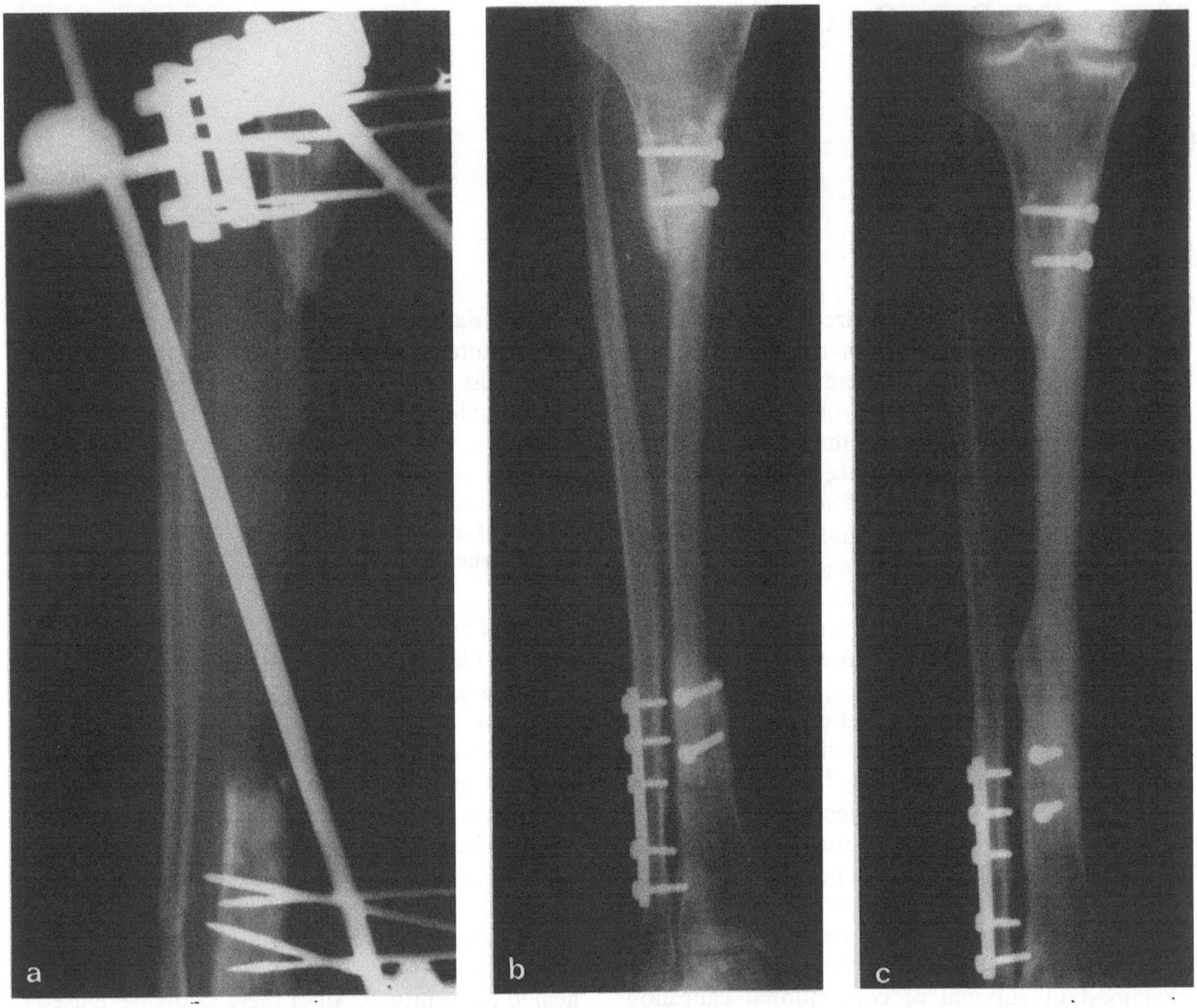

Fig. 22-1. **a** A 20 cm long post-traumatic defect of the tibia. **b** Appearance 6 months following fibular transfer. The fibula has united to the tibia but hypertrophy has not begun. **c** Hypertrophy of the fibula 3 years following transfer. A stress fracture occurred at the lower end of the fibula one year postoperatively and healed with a generous callous

also possible to carry a small skin flap based on the fasciocutaneous perforators which lie on the posterior crural intermuscular septum. This flap is useful for small skin defects of up to 5 to 6 cm in width. For wider defects, the benefits of a wide flap are likely to be outweighed by the disadvantage of an unsightly donor site which will have to be skin grafted. If a long bony defect requires a large soft tissue coverage, usually a preliminary skin, muscle or myocutaneous flap is done, or an iliac crest osteocutaneous transfer is used.

Iliac Crest

The iliac crest transfer is a curved piece of cortical and cancellous bone which is particularly well-vascularized. The advantages of using the crest are the rapid union which occurs between the bone graft and the remaining bone of the extremity, and the large vascularized skin flap that may be carried with the transfer. By utilizing the relatively straight anterior portion of the crest, the surgeon can reconstruct bony defects of 6–9 cm (Fig. 22-2). The iliac crest is the preferred graft for short bony defects of this length, both with and without soft tissue defects. Beyond this length, the bone curvature becomes a problem and requires a straightening osteotomy. With an osteotomy, a straight 12–15 cm graft is avail-

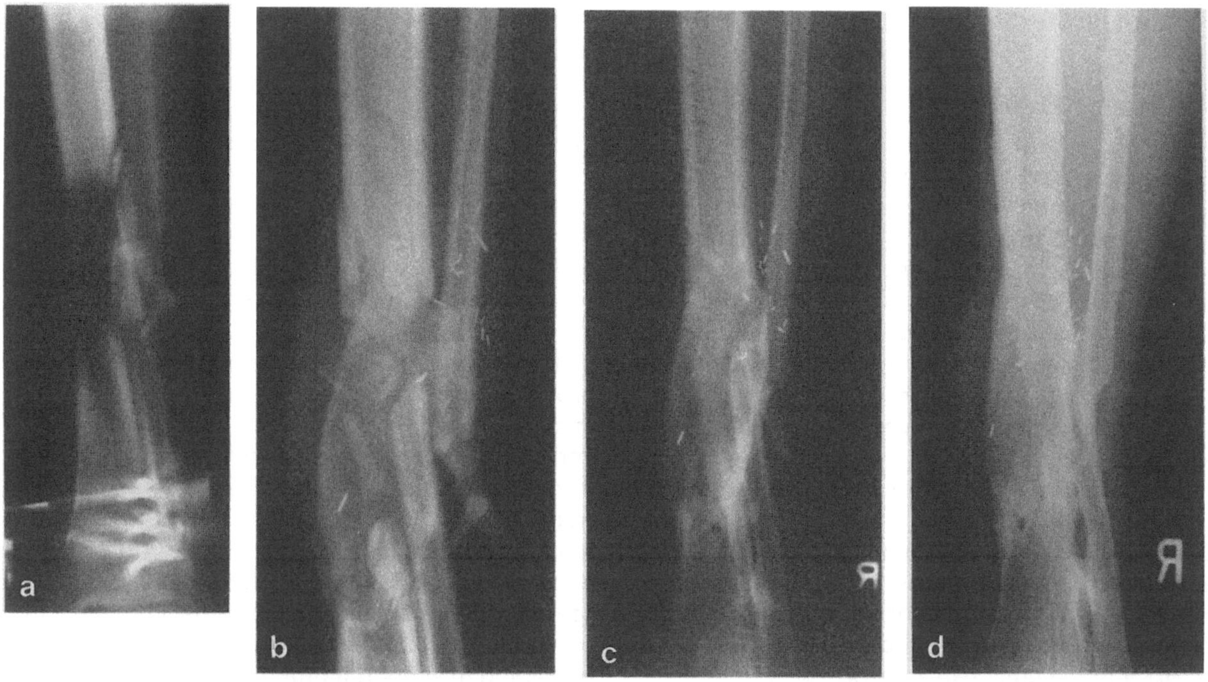

Fig. 22-2. **a** Following a compound fracture of the tibia and fibula in a motor vehicle accident, there was an 8 cm defect in the lower third of the tibia. **b** Appearance immediately following iliac crest transfer. **c** Six months following transfer, union has occurred between graft and tibia. **d** Two years following the iliac crest reconstruction, there is solid union, bone hypertrophy, and bony remodelling

able. It is used for large defects only if there is an associated large soft tissue defect.

The disadvantages of this transfer are that the bone is curved and of limited size, and the skin flap is frequently bulky. The bone is also bulky, and can, with the thick skin flap, produce a bulge which may be a cosmetic concern.

Principles of Bone Fixation

Large bony defects are difficult to manage. Good techniques of osteosynthesis are required. The graft must come into good apposition and be securely fixed to the recipient bone by means of butt, step, or mortice and tenon joints. Any bone defects at the junction of the bone graft and recipient bone must be packed with cancellous bone chips. The graft must be firmly fixed to the recipient bone without disturbing the graft's circulation. In order to maintain this circulation, there should be minimal periosteal stripping and minimal hardware placed in the graft. One or two screws are adequate for graft to recipient bone fixation. The proximal and distal ends of the injured bone are stabilized with an external fixator or a long AO plate which spans the graft. Care must be taken that the bone graft is placed in the defect so that the vascular pedicle which runs along the bone is not compressed or obstructed.

Fibula Transfer to the Tibia

Preoperative Planning

Using x-rays and clinical evaluation, make an estimate of the amount of bone required. Often this is a greater length than initially supposed because of non viable fragments of bone at the tibial ends and the obliquity of the fracture fragments. Although this reconstruction is done as a two team procedure with simultaneous preparation of the transfer and recipient site, the fibula is not usually cut until the damaged bone ends are prepared and the required length of graft determined.

An arteriogram is done for both legs. The arteriogram in the injured leg will show the presence, condition and location of potential recipient vessels and any altered vascular patterns. The arteriogram of the donor leg will indicate the location and length of the peroneal artery and rule out developmental absence of either of the other two arteries.

Technique of Tibial Reconstruction with the Fibula

Preparation of the Recipient Leg

1. Draw the likely location of the bone graft and its pedicle on the injured leg and mark the incision for exposure of the recipient vessel.

Although it is possible to tunnel the pedicle to the recipient vessels, it is preferable, particularly about the ankle, to make a direct incision. Not only does this allow good visualization for the anastomosis, but it allows observation of the pedicle and a gentle closure without compression of the pedicle. Gentle closure is facilitated by inserting the pedicle under one margin of the incision, which is left open and skin grafted. Alternatively, the flap may be defatted where the pedicle is located and direct closure obtained.

2. Place an incision at both the upper and lower ends of the bone defect. Expose the entire defect between the two ends of the tibial segment, or create a tunnel if the bed was previously prepared with a skin flap. Excise scar tissue which lies in the intervening bed between the bone ends.

3. Remove non viable fragments of cortical bone. Excise the ends of the tibia until bleeding is obtained and the bone appears healthy. Do not do the final shaping of the tibia until the fibula is available to allow precise insetting of the graft ends. Measure the maximum length of bone which will be required so that the surgeon removing the fibula can proceed.

4. Dissect the recipient vessels and prepare the artery and the venae comitantes for anastomosis.

5. If a Hoffmann fixator is used for fixation of the proximal and distal bone ends, it may be applied at this time. Align the foot, bring the leg out to length and apply the fixator using whichever configuration is most suitable, usually transfixion pins and double frame fixation. The bars on the side of the vascular repair can be removed for access to do the anastomosis and then replaced at the termination of the procedure. The fixator is useful at the end of the operation to suspend the leg from an orthopaedic bed frame and to support a drop foot splint.

Preparing the Fibula Bone Transfer

The fibula is prepared as described in Chapter 9.

Transfer of Fibula to Tibia

1. Fit the fibula into the defect. Be sure that the peroneal artery which runs parallel to the fibula lies in a position where it will not be compressed. The pedicle should lead directly to the recipient vessels without tension, kinking or compression. Strip back the periosteum at the ends of the fibula, leaving it attached to the fibula and in contact with the tibia. Fit the fibula into the tibia with either a modified mortice and tenon or step joint. Sometimes the size of the bones will allow the fibula to be telescoped into the medullary cavity of the tibia. Fasten the fibula to the tibia with one or two screws. If there are defects between the fibula and the adjacent tibia, fill them with iliac crest cancellous bone chips. Petelage of adjacent surfaces of the fibula and tibia may stimulate osteogenesis.

2. If fixation of the proximal and distal tibial bone fragments is obtained with an AO plate, it is important that the plate not compress the peroneal artery. Apply the plate first and obtain normal leg length and alignment, and then insert the fibula.

3. Do an end to side repair with the recipient artery and an end to end venous repair with a vena comitans (Fig. 22-3). If there is a major vessel defect in the leg, it is possible to use the peroneal artery as a vessel graft to span the defect, suturing the distal end of the peroneal artery to the distal end of the divided leg vessel.

4. Close the skin over the pedicle and bone, leaving the distal bone exposed, and observe the distal end of the peroneal artery to see if pulsations are still present after skin closure. Since the circulation to the fibula cannot be monitored after closure, particular care is required to prevent vascular obstruction.

Do a bone scan within the first 5 days following transfer. A 'hot scan' is good evidence that the bone is vascularized and the anastomosis is patent. If the scan is done after one week, a 'hot scan' may be produced by neovascularization about the margins of a non-vascularized graft.

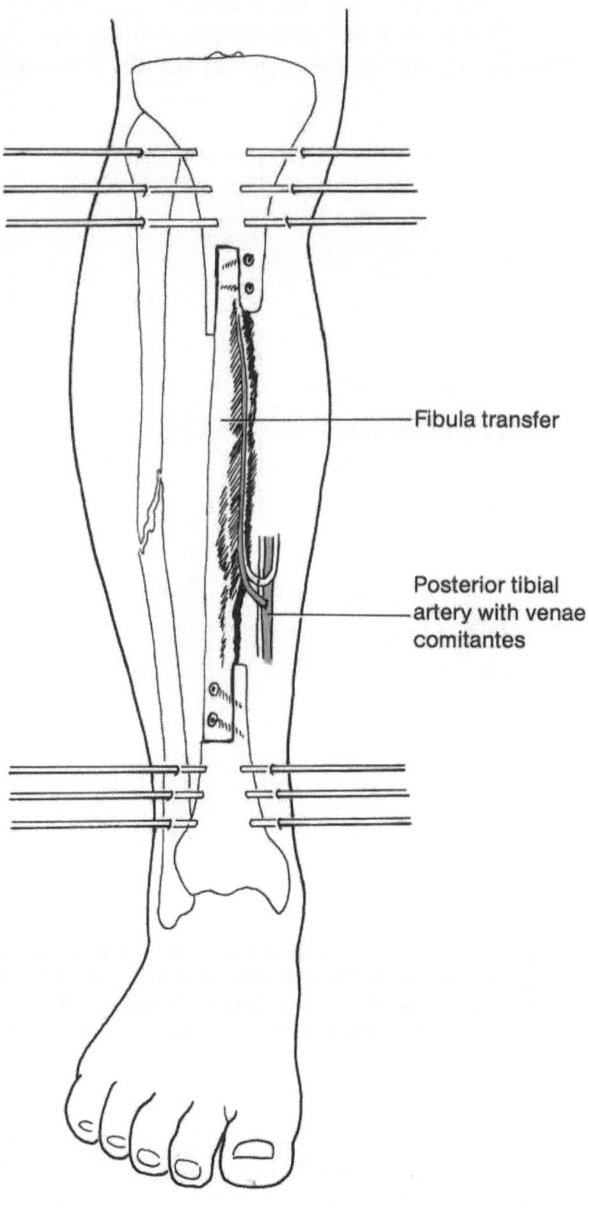

Fig. 22-3. The fibula transfer completed. A 4-bar external fixator maintains the relative positions of the proximal and distal tibial segments. The fibula is dowelled into the lower end and morticed into the upper end of the tibia with one screw in each location. The peroneal artery and vena comitans are sutured to the posterior tibial artery and vena comitans near the ankle

Iliac Crest Reconstruction of the Tibia

Preoperative Planning

There are three individual tissues which must be considered in planning each transfer. These are the bone, with its compound curves; the iliacus muscle which carries the vascular pedicle; and the skin flap attached to the abdominal musculature, which is attached to the superior margin of the crest.

It is helpful to have a model of both the right and left iliac crest which can be placed on the injured leg to assist in the visualization of the location of the various structures. The bone and skin on the transfer must fit the bone and skin defect, and the pedicle must lie adjacent to the recipient vessels. The deep circumflex iliac artery enters the anterior end of the transfer and lies on the medial aspect of the iliacus. The transfer must be positioned so that the pedicle is not compressed, and leads directly into the recipient vessels.

There are four possible longitudinal orientations of the iliac crest in each leg. The crest may be positioned in the leg so that the pedicle and the anterior superior spine are either proximal or distal, and the bone may be rotated so that the superior margin of the crest faces anteriorly or so that the iliacus musculature faces anteriorly. Either position of rotation usually allows the pedicle to be positioned so that it will not be compressed. The most common orientation which fits the requirements of bone reconstruction is to have the superior margin of the crest facing anteriorly. In this position, the iliacus and

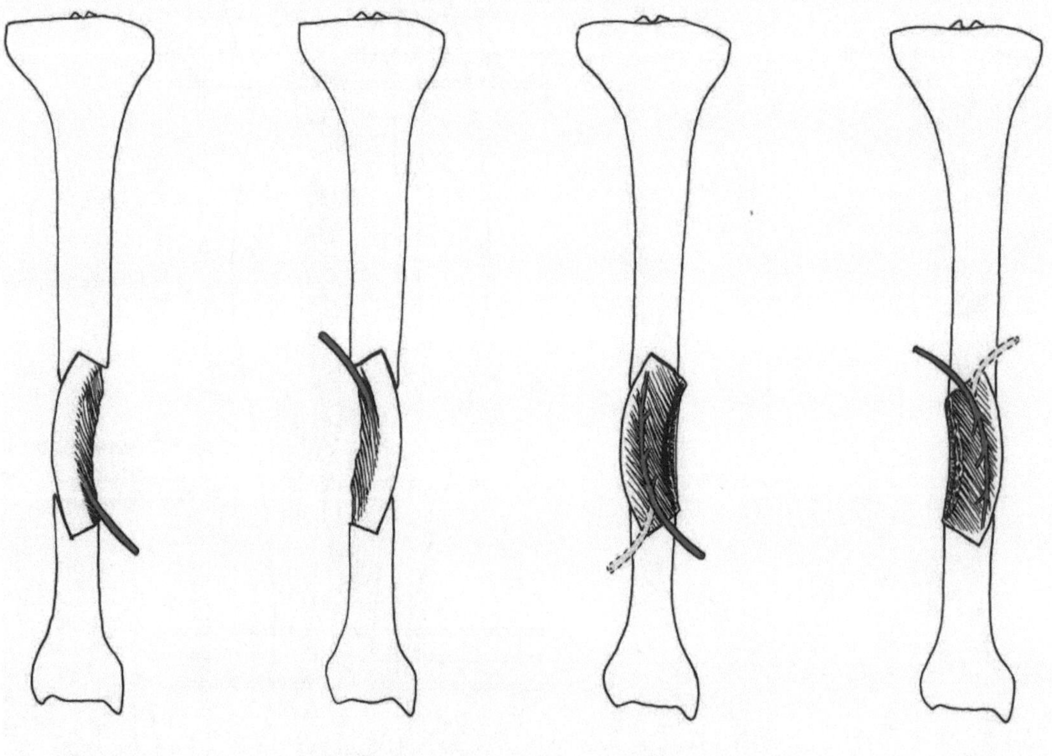

Fig. 22-4 a–d. There are 4 different positions which are possible for each iliac crest. The right iliac crest is illustrated. Each position places the pedicle in a different location and determines the choice of recipient vessels. Lying on the iliacus, the DCIA must not be compressed when placed in the leg defect. If either the superior surface of the crest (**a, b**) or the iliacus (**c, d**) faces anteriorly, the DCIA will usually be unharmed

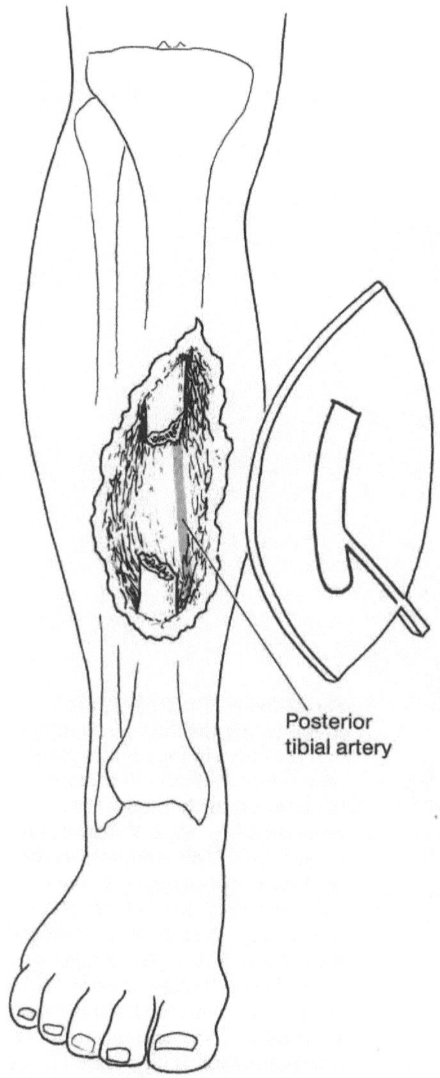

Fig. 22-5. A pattern is made of the bone and soft tissue defect. The anticipated recipient vessels are the posterior tibial. This pattern is then used to plan a transfer which, in this case, will be from the right hip.

pedicle will lie on either the medial or lateral side of the leg and the recipient vessels must be on this side (Fig. 22-4a, b). However, if the bone is placed with the iliacus facing anteriorly, the pedicle can be led to either side (Fig. 22-4c, d). The side of the pelvis chosen for the donor site will depend upon the location of the preferred recipient vessels, and the shape of the bony defect.

Technique of Tibial Reconstruction with the Iliac Crest

Preparation of the Leg

The preparation of the leg is the same as for a fibular transfer.

Outline the area on the leg which will require soft tissue coverage, the area of the bone defect and the expected location of the pedicle and recipient vessels. Take a pattern of this plan and transfer it to the appropriate iliac crest (Fig. 22-5).

Preparation of the Iliac Crest Transfer

The technique of taking the iliac crest is described in Chapter 10.

If a short length of bone is required, it will be taken from the anterior portion of the crest. If a longer length is required, with an anticipated straightening osteotomy, bone can be removed to as far back as a few centimeters from the sacroiliac joint. Anticipate the extra length of crest which will be required to fit the graft into the tibial ends and to allow for shortening at the time of the straightening osteotomy.

If an osteocutaneous transfer is used, because of the bulk of the transfer the skin flap needs to be wider than might be anticipated.

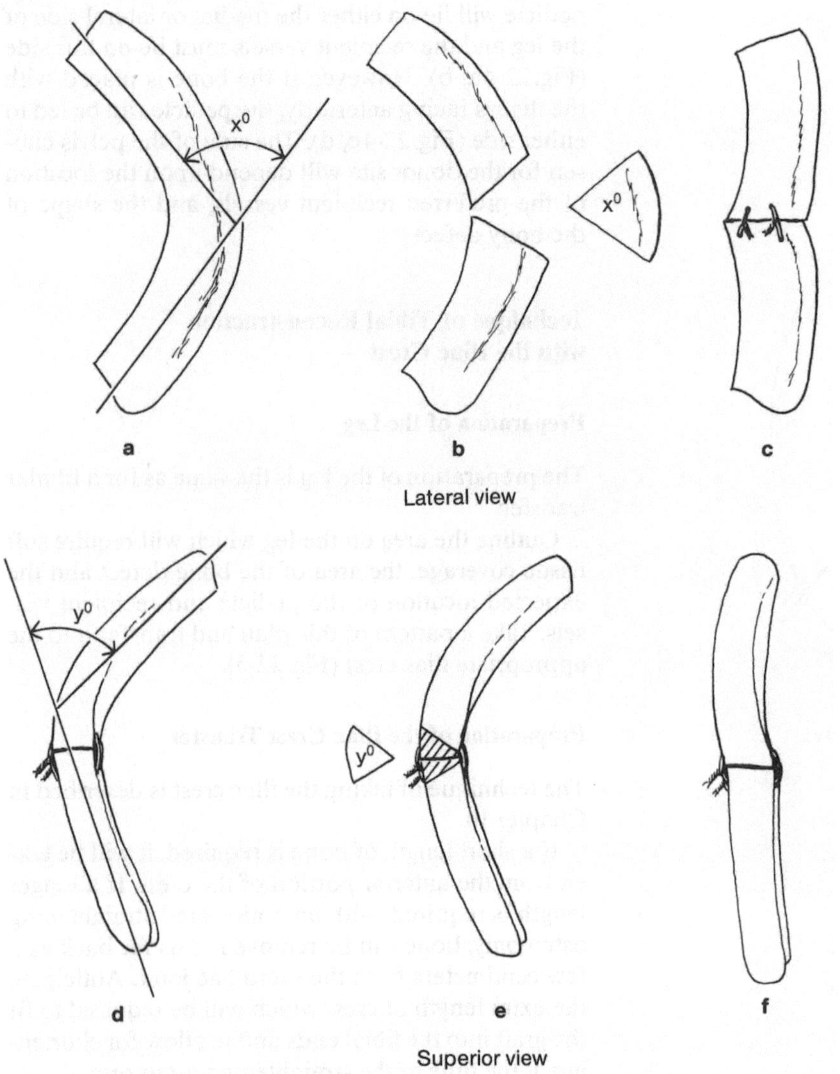

Fig. 22-6a–f. The technique of straightening the iliac crest requires that the curve in the sagittal plane, represented by angle X degrees and the curve in the horizontal plane, represented by angle Y degrees, be straightened. This straightening can be done in two steps. A wedge of bone angled X degrees is first removed from the side of the crest and the two pieces are placed together (**a–c**). Then, a wedge of bone angled Y degrees is removed from the superior surface (**d–f**), and this produces a straight piece of iliac crest

Transfer of Iliac Crest to Tibia

1. Use the osteotomy technique to straighten the crest if a large defect is being reconstructed.

Set up a sterile sculpture table with measuring and bone cutting instruments. The crest is curved in both the horizontal and sagittal plane and both of these curves must be removed to provide a straight bone transfer.

Study the shape of the iliac crest. Two separate bone wedges can be removed at the same site, one in each plane (Fig. 22-6a–f), or a single wedge can be planned which is angled in both planes to effect the straightening of the crest (Fig. 22-7a–c). Every crest has an individual shape in both of the curves. In planning the straightening osteotomies, it is useful to think of the iliac crest as being angled at the tubercle rather than curved. The technique of straightening will be to remove a wedge of bone at the tubercle of the iliac crest to correct both angles. Place a straight line along the axis of both the anterior and posterior portions of the iliac crest, in both the sagittal and horizontal planes of the pelvis. Measure the angles between these lines and outline the angles on the top and side of the crest. Expose the bone by elevating the abdominal musculature, iliacus and periosteum adjacent to these angles.

Use a sharp oscillating saw and remove a precise triangle or triangles of bone, maintaining an intact bridge of periosteum and iliacus. Check the correction and, if not adequate, remove further bone.

Fix the two fragments of bone with two asymmetric interosseous wire loops.

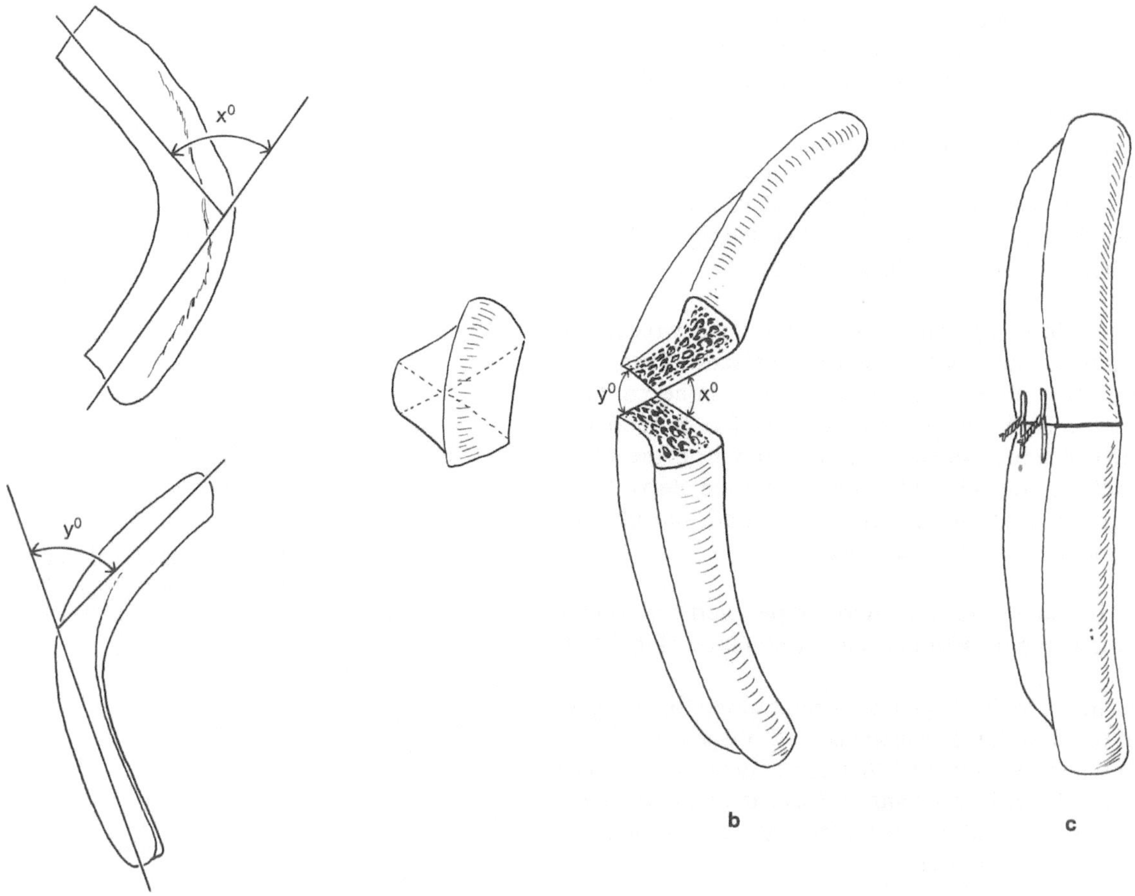

Fig. 22-7 a–c. Instead of removing the wedge in two steps, it may be removed in one. A wedge is removed with angles X degrees and Y degrees in the sagittal and horizontal planes respectively. The periosteum and iliacus are preserved between the two fragments of bone to maintain the blood supply to each.

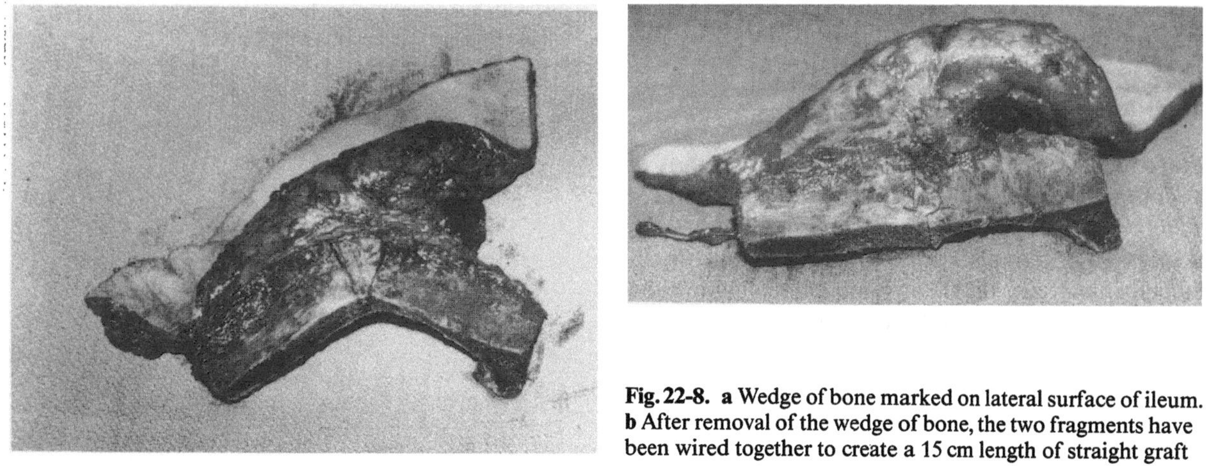

a b

Fig. 22-8. **a** Wedge of bone marked on lateral surface of ileum. **b** After removal of the wedge of bone, the two fragments have been wired together to create a 15 cm length of straight graft

This technique provides good straightening and solid bone fixation but does shorten the length of the crest. Taylor has described another straightening technique which involves a sagittal split of the crest with the split packed with cancellous bone. This technique does not allow as firm a bone fixation and has a projecting plate of internal iliac crest. However, it does not produce bony shortening and has resulted in good union in his hands.

2. Fit the straightened iliac crest into the two ends of the tibia, shaping the adjacent surfaces of the tibia and crest to provide good bone to bone contact. Scrape back the periosteum from the crest in the area of bony contact and lag screw it to the tibia. Pack any defects with cancellous bone chips. Petelage the adjacent surfaces of the graft and tibia to stimulate osteogenic activity.

3. Do an end to side arterial repair and end to end venous repair with the venae comitantes (Fig. 22-9).

4. Insert multiple penrose drains along the margins of the skin flap and insert at least one suction drain. Position all drains so that the pedicle is not compressed. With this transfer, there is often considerable postoperative oozing from the cut surfaces of the bone and muscle.

5. Use the Hoffmann external fixator and elevate the leg by suspending the fixator from an orthopaedic bed frame to decrease venous pressure, oozing and swelling in the transfer.

6. Monitoring. The cutaneous flap provides a good indication of the circulation to the bone transfer. However, as the cutaneous flap represents the terminal branches of the vascular tree, it is possible to have it die when the bone graft and underlying musculature are well perfused.

Modifications of Surgical Technique

For coverage of a small soft tissue defect, a cuff of abdominal musculature may be used instead of a skin flap. This musculature provides a good bed for skin grafts and is preferable to trying to take an attached small skin flap. For bone defects with good skin cover, the transfer is taken without any abdominal musculature.

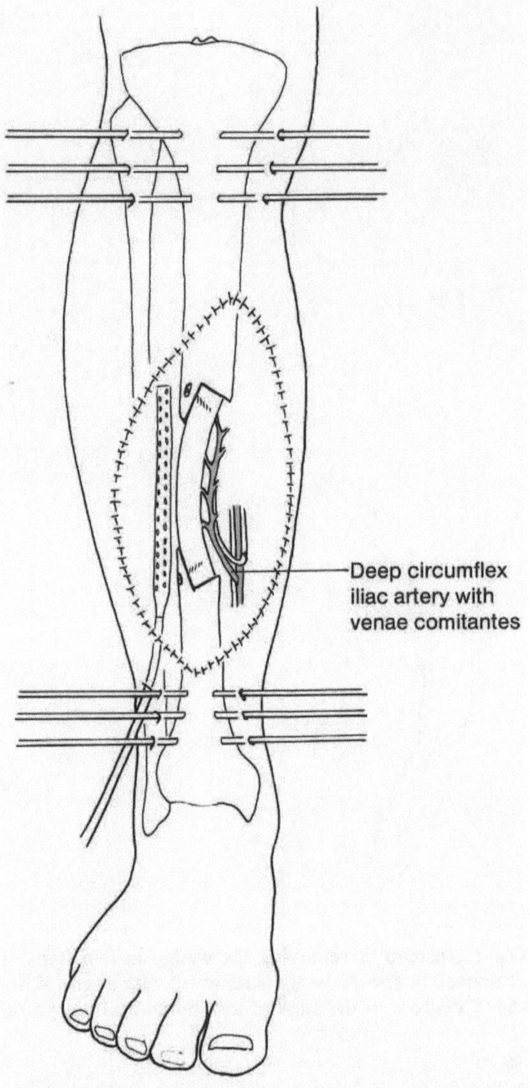

Fig. 22-9. The iliac crest can be used without osteotomy to reconstruct a 10 cm defect in a tibia. A 4-bar external fixator maintains the relative positions of the proximal and distal tibial segments, while the crest is firmly fixed to the tibial fragments with a lag screw at each end

Postoperative Care

The patient is confined to bed with the leg elevated for 10-14 days to establish the inital soft tissue healing and allow the anastomosis to stabilize. Following periods of increasing dependency, the patient is ambulated non-weight bearing in the external fixator for 8-12 weeks. When this is removed, a patellar tendon bearing cast is applied and worn for 16 to 20 weeks until there is evidence of good radiological union and early bone hypertrophy. When the PTB cast is removed, a Saramiento brace is fitted and worn for approximately 6 months. For hypertrophy to occur, the graft must be stressed by a program of increasing and protected weight bearing.

Although the iliac crest and fibula will heal promptly to the adjacent bone, the graft does not have sufficient strength to function as a tibia or a femur until graft hypertrophy has taken place. Following bone union, the graft will tolerate compression stresses well, but is prone to fracture with rotational or angular stresses. However, these fractures are accompanied by a voluminous callous, have no long term ill effects and may even be a stimulus to graft hypertrophy.

The fibula will continue to enlarge in response to stress for at least 2 years. Although the diameter of the fibula may not become as large as a tibia, the width of the cortex often becomes thicker than the normal tibia (Fig. 22-1).

An iliac crest reconstruction will develop thickening along the cortices as well as within the cancellous part of the graft (Fig. 22-2).

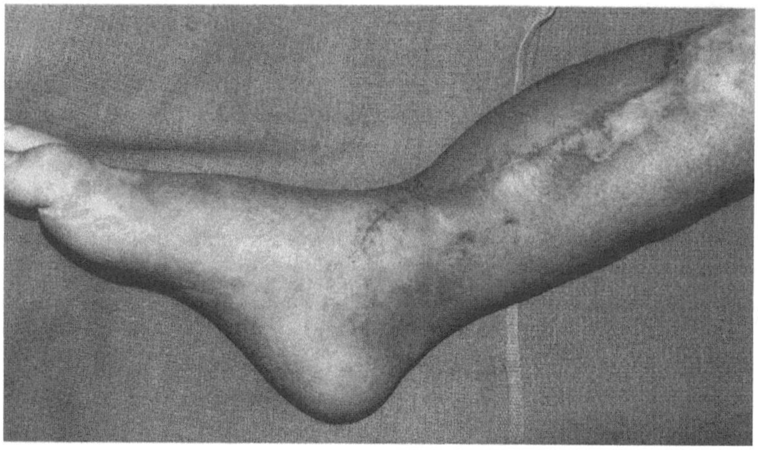

Fig. 22-10. Typical prominent appearance of the leg following an iliac crest osteocutaneous reconstruction

References

1. Albrektesson T (1980) The healing of autogenous bone grafts after varying degrees of surgical trauma. J Bone Joint Surg (Br) 62: 403
2. Berggren A, Weiland A, Dorfman H (1982) Free vascularized bone grafts: factors affecting their survival and ability to heal recipient bone defects. Plast Reconstr Surg 69: 219
3. Gross AE, McKee NH, Langer F, Pritzker KPH (1983) 'Surgical techniques and clinical experience with articular allografts at the knee'. In: Osteochondral Allografts: Biology, Banking and Clinical Applications. ed Friedlaender GE, Mankin HJ, Sell KW, Little Brown & Co, Massachusetts, Chapter 28, 289
4. Taylor GI (1975) The free vascularized bone graft. Plast Reconstr Surg 55: 553
5. Taylor GI (1977) Microvascular free bone transfer. A clinical technique. Orthop Clin N Am 8 (2): 425
6. Taylor GI (1978) One stage repair of compound leg defects with free, revascularized flaps of groin and iliac bone. Plast Reconstr Surg 61: 494
7. Taylor GI (1983) The current status of free vascularized bone grafts. Clin Plast Surg 10 (1): 1985

Chapter 23. Paediatrics

Ronald M. Zuker

Reconstructive microsurgery offers new hope for difficult and complex problems that previously defied adequate surgical management. The reconstructive paediatric surgeon must not only deal with acquired traumatic deformities but also address difficult congenital anomalies. Many conditions which were fraught with surgical failure and disappointment may now be served better through the use of microsurgery.

Preoperative

The preoperative assessment of the child requires a relaxed rapport between the child and the examiner. Frequently the child cannot readily demonstrate activities that the examiner wishes to see. Certain tasks may require encouragement, particularly in hand surgery. Appropriate games and toys in the examining room are helpful as well as the co-operation and understanding of the parents. The clinical examination may have to be repeated in order to gain adequate information regarding the abilities of the child. Radiological assessment is often helpful to assess bony age and perhaps predict limb growth. Angiography is difficult to carry out under local anaesthesia in young children and, in most instances, is best done under general anaesthesia which eliminates the problem of vascular spasm and pain. Once a surgical course has been outlined, it is imperative that the parents and child understand the nature of the surgery and the specific environmental changes that the child will undergo.

At the time of operation, several technical factors must be taken into consideration. The most obvious is the vessel size. Blood vessels in children are surprisingly large when one compares total body weight to that of the adult. A review of our cases has revealed the following average sizes of vessels for 2–3 year old children:

Posterior tibial artery	1.0–2.0 mm
Vena comitans of posterior tibial	1.0–2.0 mm
Peroneal artery	1.2–1.5 mm
Vena comitans of peroneal artery	1.0–2.0 mm

Intraoperative

During the microsurgical transfer itself, as with adults, it is critical to maintain warmth, hydration and a normocarbic state. The physiological response of children to prolonged anaesthetic is much the same as that of an adult, although their metabolic requirements are slightly higher. Thus, ventilation must be more rapid and fluid requirements slightly increased.

Anaesthetics: The anaesthetic agents used usually consist of a narcotic infusion, diazepam or droperidol, nitrous oxide and oxygen, a muscle relaxant where this is not contraindicated by the surgical procedure, and isoflurane which allows quick awakening and involves minimal metabolism. The latter is also somewhat greater in its vasodilatory capacity than the others. An endotracheal tube is used which should have a leak if the intubation is to be prolonged. A too snug fit may predispose to postoperative laryngeal edema or endothelial necrosis.

Monitoring: With children, the margin of error is smaller, and consequently careful monitoring is imperative. An arterial line is mandatory for constant blood pressure monitoring and for ease of blood sampling. This is supplemented with a blood pressure cuff and Doppler. A reliable large bore intravenous line is used for fluid replacement. A central venous line is helpful to assess intravascular volume and catheterization is useful for measuring hourly urine output. The temperature is measured either rectally or through the esophagus, and expired carbon dioxide monitored with an endotracheal carbon dioxide monitor.

Supportive Measures: It is imperative to sustain an adequate temperature, and so warming blankets are used on the upper surface of the child. A ripple mattress is used beneath the child to prevent pressure sores. All fluids are warmed and the ventilation system includes a heated humidifier.

Co-operation and discussion between the surgeon and anaesthetist are imperative so that each understands the other's problems and needs.

Postoperative

The postoperative monitoring of microvascular flaps in children is much the same as in adults. The transfer may require added protection as the child may not understand the need for co-operation. Extra care is required for dressings such as hand dressings which are placed above the elbow in order to prevent them from slipping. During the postoperative phase, it is mandatory to keep the parents and the child well informed as to the various manoeuvres and manipulations that are necessary to monitor the flap. Understanding is a major step towards cooperation. Parents are encouraged to stay with the child and help with the child's care and positioning. The child himself is stimulated as much as his level of growth and development allows with suitable play equipment. It is often helpful to have a favourite toy or animal bandaged and have the child look after his 'patient'. Once the trust and co-operation of the child has been obtained, everything else seems to fall into place.

Intra-Abdominal Testis

The management of the intra-abdominal testis continues to challenge the surgeon. A strong case can be made for orchiectomy in unilateral cases in postpubertal patients. Orchiopexy with preservation of the vessels of the vas deferens and transection of the testicular vessels has met with only limited success. Similarly, staged orchiopexy, bringing the testis to the scrotum in two stages, has not improved testicular survival. Testis relocation with revascularization of the testicular vessels using microvascular anastomoses was first described by Silber and Kelly in 1976. The procedure proved difficult because of the size of the testicular vessels (0.5-0.7 mm). However, the initial results appear encouraging. Testicular size was maintained by this technique, suggesting survival and function of the relocated testes. However, the effect of the procedure on fertility and hormone production is still unknown.

I feel that microvascular autotransplantation of the testis is indicated in bilateral nonpalpable testis and probably in prepubertal unilateral nonpalpable testis, where the potential for fertility is high. Both testes are transplanted in bilateral cases, usually at two separate operations. It is probable that even with repositioning of the abdominal testis, the significantly increased risk of testicular cancer is not affected. However, having the testis in the scrotum facilitates examination for malignant change. The preferred age for the procedure is 4-5 years.

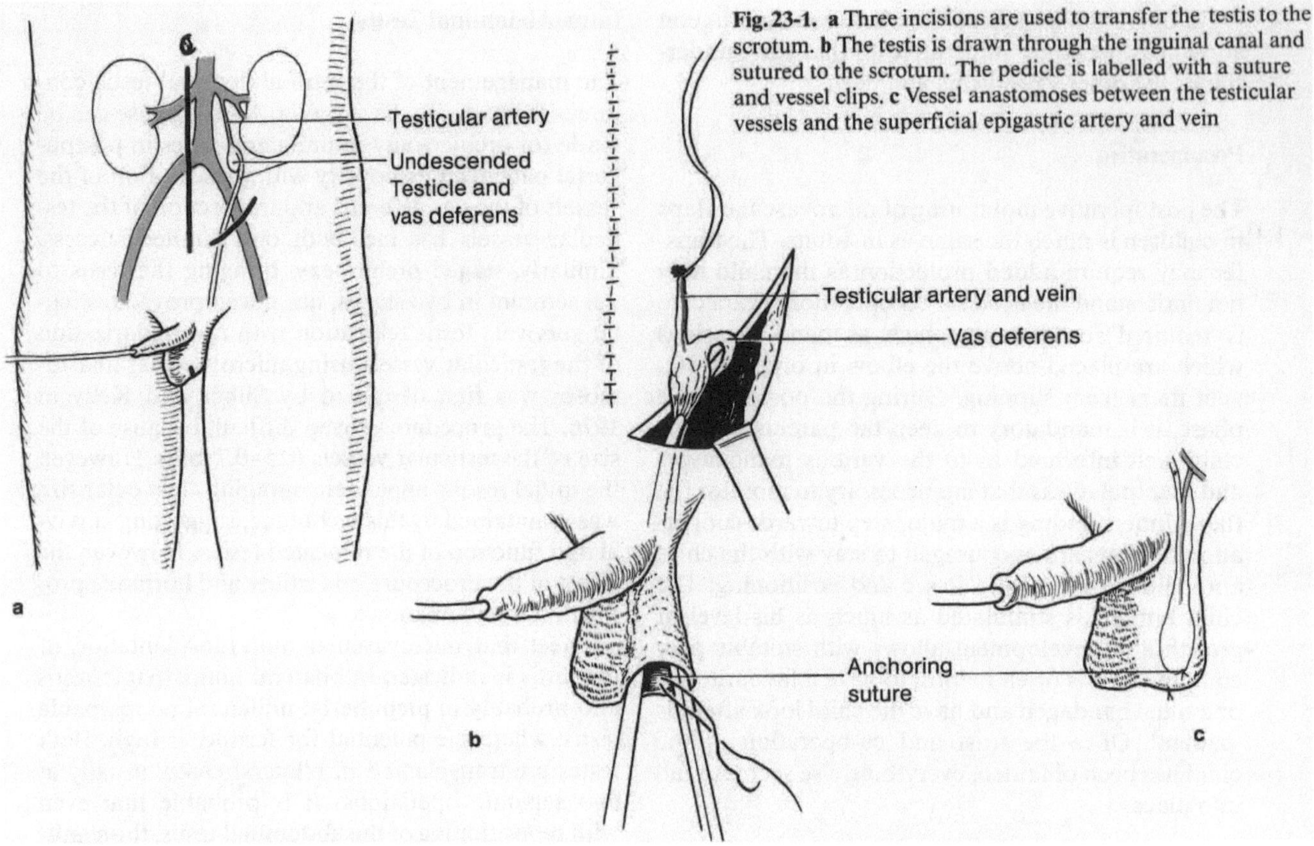

Fig. 23-1. a Three incisions are used to transfer the testis to the scrotum. **b** The testis is drawn through the inguinal canal and sutured to the scrotum. The pedicle is labelled with a suture and vessel clips. **c** Vessel anastomoses between the testicular vessels and the superficial epigastric artery and vein

Technique of Transplantation of the Abdominal Testis to the Scrotum

The surgical procedure consists of moving the intra-abdominal testis to the scrotum. The vas and its vessels are kept intact, and the testicular vessels are anastomosed to vessels in the groin.

1. Through a midline infra-umbilical incision, identify the testis in its retroperitoneal position (Fig. 23-1 a). Dissect free the testicular artery and vein and mobilize the testis. Free the vas deferens while protecting its vessels. Clip the testicular vessels as close as possible to their origin from the renal artery and vein (aorta and inferior vena cava on right). Use two clips for the artery and one clip for the vein to facilitate later identification.

2. Make a transverse lower abdominal incision. Expose the inguinal canal by opening the external oblique aponeurosis. If a hernia sac is present, it should be obliterated. Bring the testis through the internal ring into the canal and down into the scrotum, using a low scrotal incision. Suture the testis to the scrotal sac (Fig. 23-1 b).

3. The testicular vessels are left in the inguinal canal. Through the transverse abdominal incision, identify and prepare the superficial epigastric artery and vein for anastomosis. Do an end to end venous anastomosis with 11-0 nylon. In a 5 year old child, the testicular vein is approximately 0.8 mm and the inferior epigastric vein is 1.5 mm in diameter. Do an end to side arterial anastomosis. The superficial inferior epigastric artery may require mobilization to bring it to a more advantagenous position for anastomosis. The difference in size between the 0.5 mm testicular artery and the 1.2 mm inferior epigastric artery suggests the use of an end to side anastomosis (Fig. 23-1 c).

4. Upon completion of the anastomosis, observe the venous outflow to confirm revascularization of the testis. Close the wounds in layers.

5. A morphine infusion is a useful means of providing postoperative analgesia for the first night. The patient remains in bed for 5 days postoperatively. Caffeine restriction is maintained for one month.

Congenital Pseudarthrosis of the Tibia

Historically, the management of tibial pseudarthrosis has been fraught with repeated failures. Inadequate resection of the diseased segment, lack of osteogenic stimulus and poor bony fixation account for these failures, which may eventually lead to limb amputation. Vascularized bone transplantation with the contralateral fibula is now our preferred treatment. The procedure involves a radical resection of the diseased bone, and its replacement with a vascularized bone graft. The objective of the procedure is to place a vascularized bone graft in contact with healthy tibia in order to effect bony union. Leg length discrepancy and malalignment are easily corrected. The disadvantages of the procedure are the difficult bony fixation and the small vessel microanastomoses [2].

Technique of Tibial Pseudarthrosis Reconstruction with a Vascularized Fibula

1. Make a recipient site incision which allows exposure of the diseased bony segment as well as the posterior tibial vessels (Fig. 23-2a, b). Resect the diseased bone segment, removing bone until normal appearing bone is encountered. Prepare the recipient vessels just proximal to the medial malleolus.

2. Remove the fibula as described in Chapter 9. If surgery occurs prior to epiphyseal closure, securely join the distal fibular segment on the donor leg to the tibia to avoid a progressive valgus ankle deformity. Place a screw through the residual distal fibular metaphysis into tibia, taking care not to involve the epiphyseal plate.

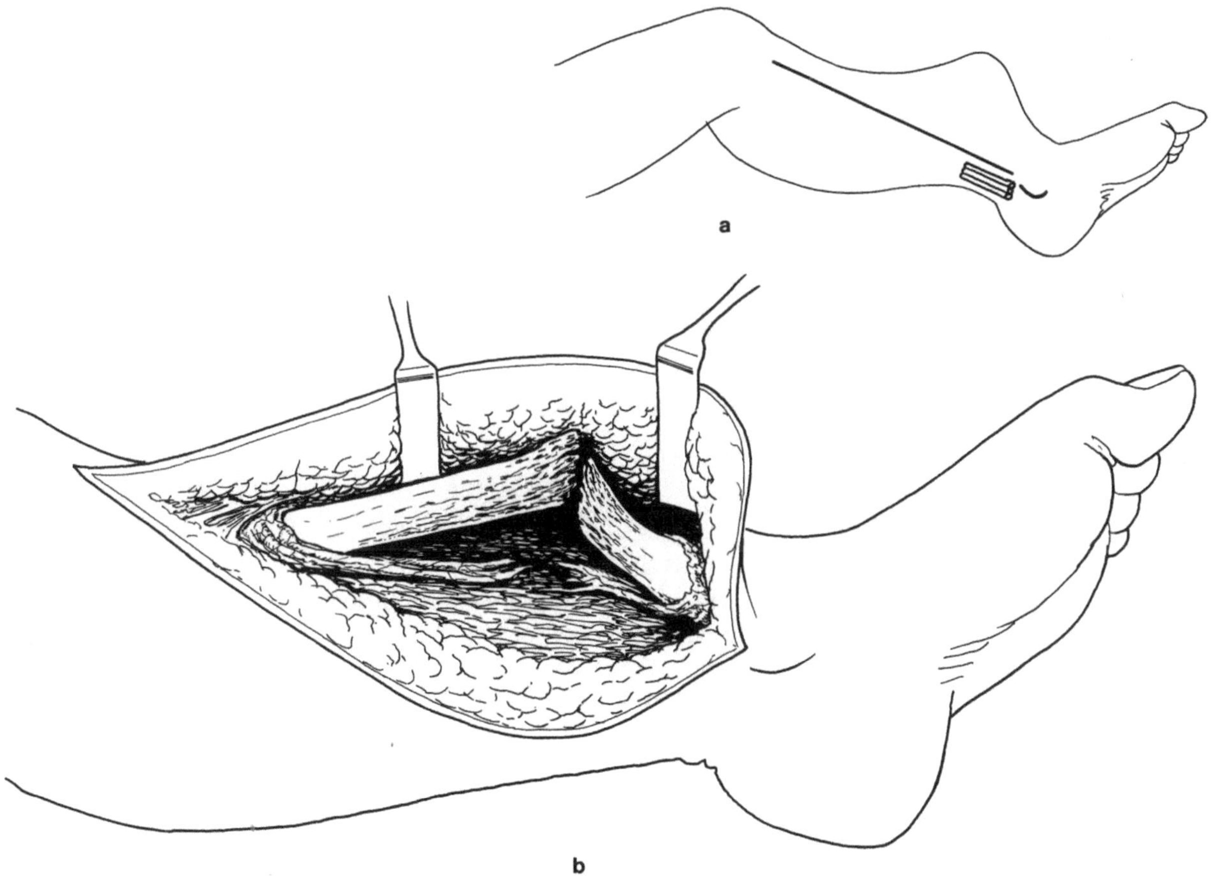

Fig. 23-2. a Incision for the exposure of the pseudarthrosis and posterior tibial vessels. **b** Exposed pseudarthrosis

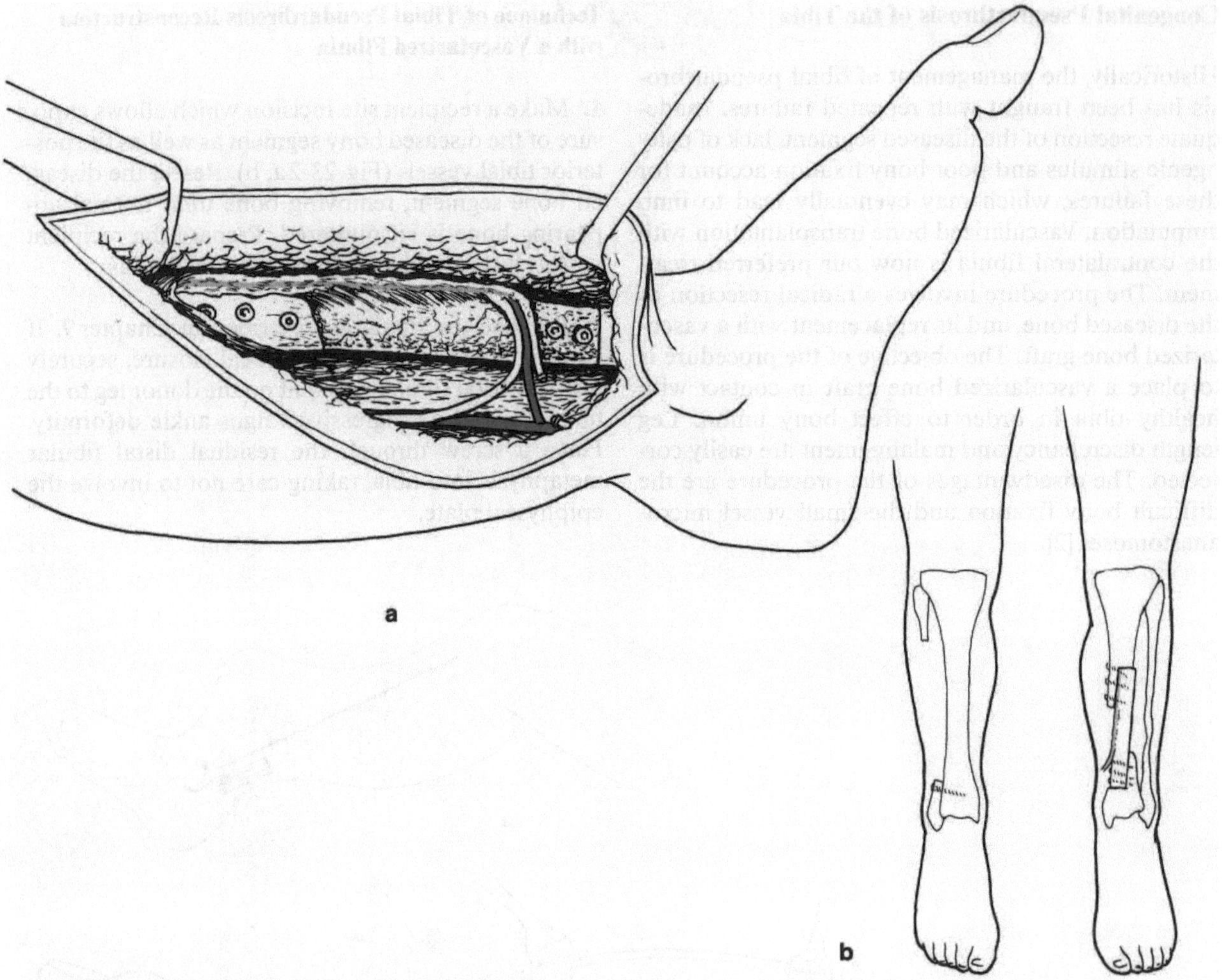

Fig. 23-3a, b. Following resection of the pseudarthrosis. The fibula has been fixed to the proximal and distal bony segments. Anastomoses are between the peroneal artery and posterior tibial artery and between their respective venae comitantes

3. Fit the fibula into the tibial defect. Place the proximal fibula into the distal tibial defect so that the fibular pedicle is close to the recipient vessels in the ankle. Rotate the fibula so that the peroneal vessels drape easily toward the posterior tibial vessels. In this position, the peroneal vessels attached to the fibula are not compressed. Bring the leg out to correct alignment and fix it into position with mini plates or screws. Plate fixation to the small distal bone fragment may be awkward. Do an end to end anastomosis between the peroneal vena comitans and a posterior tibial vena comitans, and an end to side anastomosis between the peroneal artery and the posterior tibial artery (Fig. 23-3). Assess the perfusion by observing venous outflow as well as bone and muscle cuff oozing.

4. Close all wounds in layers with suction drains in each extremity. Apply above the knee plaster splints on both legs.

Postoperative Care

Protect the pseudarthrosis limb by splinting and non-weight bearing until bony union is evident radiologically. The donor leg should be protected similarly if a tibial fibular synostosis is desired. Allow gradual weight bearing and follow fibular remodelling.

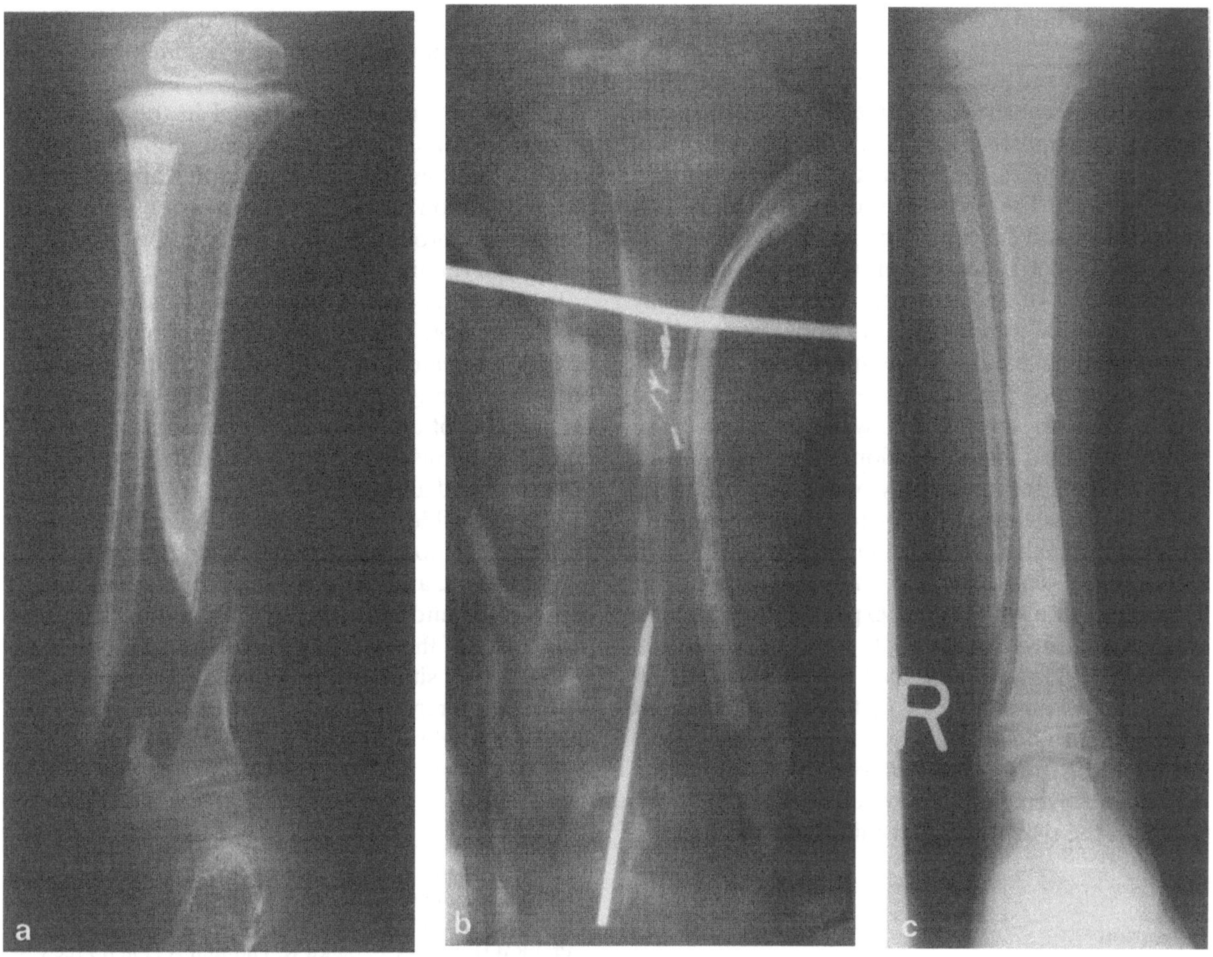

Fig. 23-4. **a** Tibial pseudarthrosis in 1½ year old child. **b** Radiological appearance of leg immediately after fibular transfer for tibial pseudarthrosis. Longitudinal insertion of k-wire through os calcis into end of fibula. Distal fragment of tibia was too small to accept a plate. **c** Appearance of leg 3 years postoperative showing bone union, hypertrophy, and remodelling of the graft

Congenital Hand Anomalies

Congenital hand anomalies remain a major challenge to the reconstructive surgeon. Where digits are lacking, toe transfers are a new avenue of reconstruction providing an alternative to conventional techniques [3]. The prime purpose of toe transfer is to increase hand function. The potential for achieving grip or pinch function can substantially upgrade the usefulness of an extremity. Although there may be a substantial improvement in appearance with a toe transfer, the hand will not appear normal. However, toes are not fingers, nor are they thumbs, and to expect them to substitute fully is unrealistic. The transfer can be a major functional asset but the lack of hand-like appearance may be a disappointment.

The major advantages of toe transfers for congenital hand anomalies are that the toe provides a digit with motion, sensibility, and an appearance similar to a digit. Growth can be expected to match its anticipated growth on the foot.

The major disadvantages are the donor defect on the foot, the possibility of systemic complications during the prolonged transfer procedure, the potential need for further revisionary surgery to achieve increased movement or more appropriate toe position, and the risk of vascular failure with loss of the toe.

Indication

Currently, toe to hand transfer is most useful in congenital amputations and in amniotic band syndromes. In severe repressive anomalies, toe transfer can upgrade power grip and pinch functions. Occasionally, the radial ray anomaly is suitable for a toe transfer.

Gilbert of Paris has pioneered in the use of the second toe transfer for congenital amputations. As vestigial tendon and nerve structures are present at the amputation stump, the toe transfer has the potential for reproducing most functions, especially in congenital thumb amputations.

In severe repressive anomalies, usually only one digit is present. The transfer of a toe, which is almost always anomalous as well, can provide gross grip and significantly improve overall hand function. As the position of the toe usually necessitates its amputation to allow shoe fitting, its transfer improves both the hand and foot.

When feasible, congenital radial ray anomaly may be treated by toe transfer. When the thumb is vestigial or absent, and there is a functional carpal-metacarpal joint, and some thenar musculature is present for control of the transplant, a toe transfer would be helpful. This situation, however, is unusual. Index pollicization remains the procedure most often indicated in radial ray anomaly.

References

1. Silber SJ, Kelly J (1976) Successful autotransplantation of an intra-abdominal testes to the scrotum by microvascular technique. J Urol 115: 452
2. Pho RWH, Levack B, Satku K, Patradul A (1985) Free vascularized fibular graft in the treatment of congenital pseudarthrosis of the tibia. J Bone Jt Surg 67B: 64
3. Gilbert A (1982) Toe transfers for congenital hand defects. J Hand Surg 7: 118

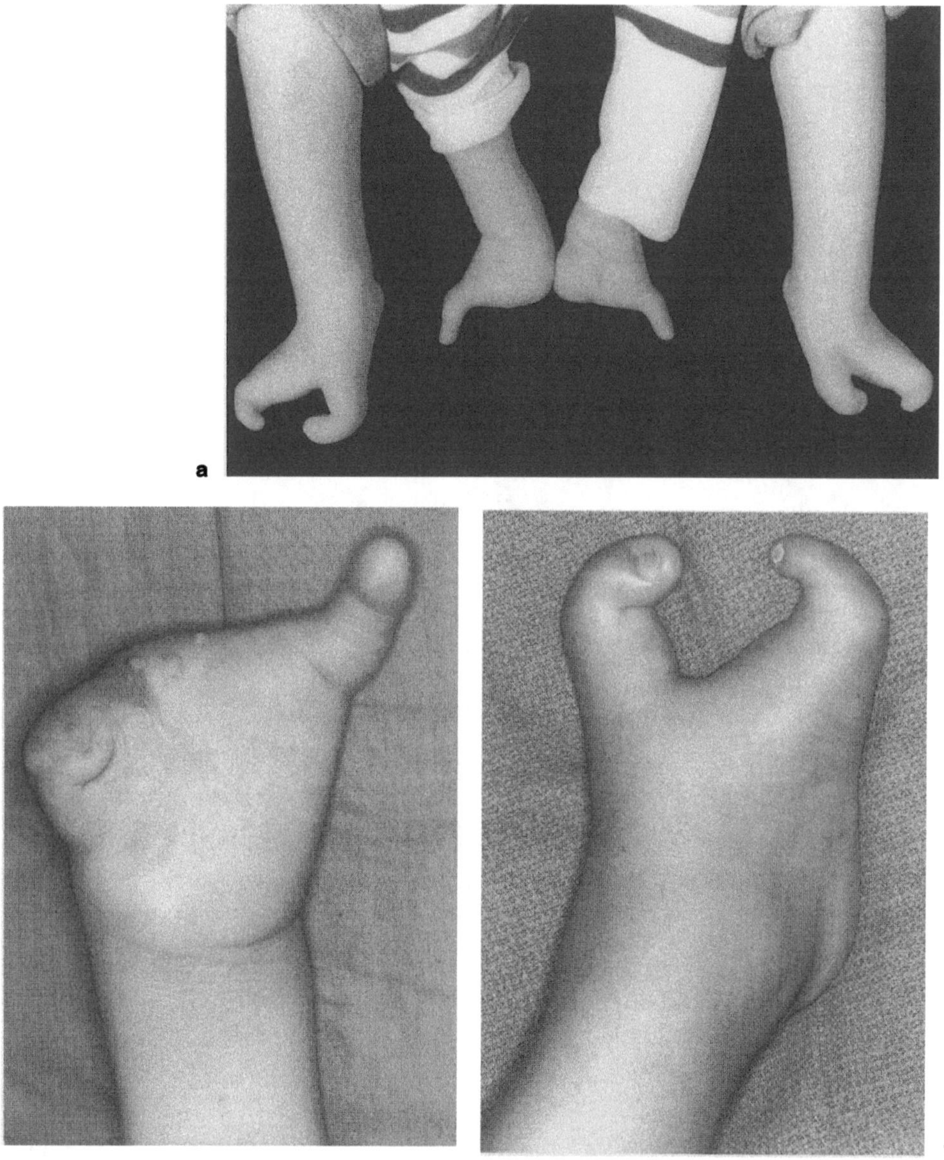

a b c

Fig. 23-5. **a** A three and a half year old boy had severe bilateral recessive anomalies of both hands and both feet. **b** Each hand had only a single ulnar digit. **c** Each foot had two toes forming a lobster claw deformity. The operative plan was to transfer the right great toe to create a right thumb. In planning the incisions, care was taken to prepare for skin flap coverage on the future foot stump and for the vessel and tendon repairs in the hand. Digital models proved extremely valuable in this regard.

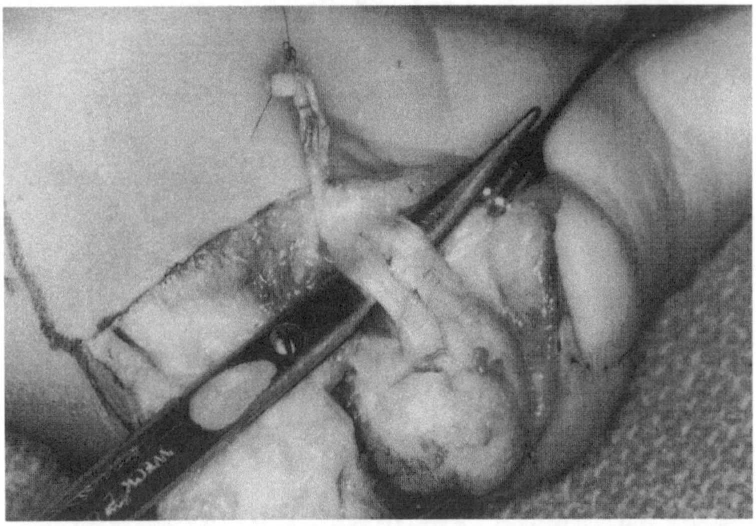

d

Fig. 23-5. d In the hand, the radial artery, superficial dorsal vein, palmar digital nerves, and tendons were prepared. Both flexor and extensor tendons were found fused to each other over the stump of the second metacarpal as seen in the photo

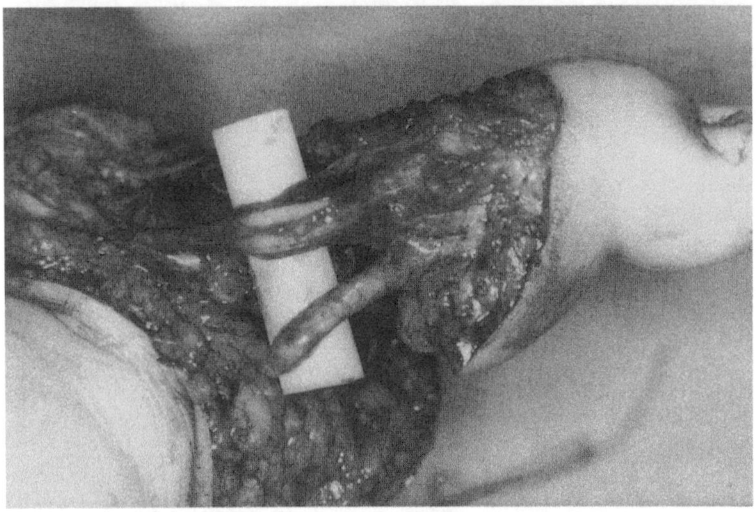

e

Fig. 23-5. e The second team prepared the toe and isolated the posterior tibial artery, a dorsal foot vein, volar digital nerve (single) and flexor and extensor tendons. Both the tendons were found on the lateral side of the toe as seen in the photo. Despite separation and attempted dorsal and plantar repositioning, on traction each tendon produced a lateral deviation of the toe. The bone was prepared for transection 1 cm proximal to the metatarsal phalangeal joint. Prior to division of the vessels, perfusion was assessed on the posterior tibial artery and dorsal vein of the foot and found to be adequate

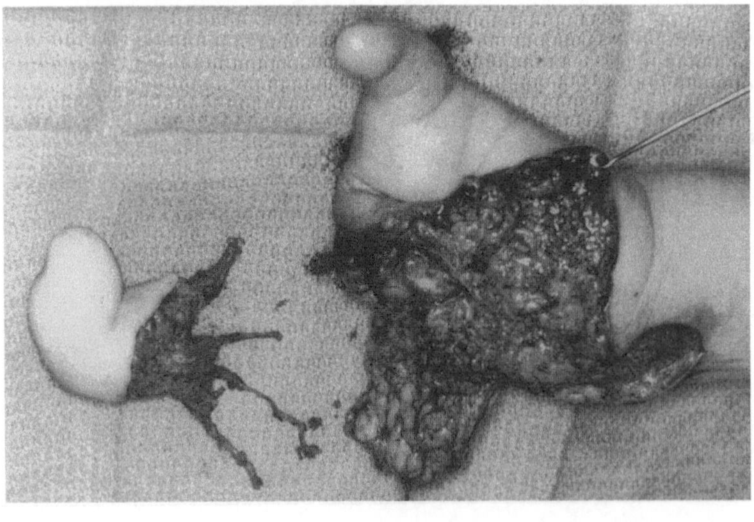

f

Fig. 23-5. f With division of the vessels on the foot, the digit was transferred to the hand. Osteosynthesis was achieved with two K-wires between the second metacarpal and the metatarsal. The toe was positioned with a radial and palmar angulation in order to provide pinch and grasp function with the little finger. Tendons, nerves and vessels were connected between the toe and hand

Fig. 23-5. g Appearance of the hand 6 months after surgery.

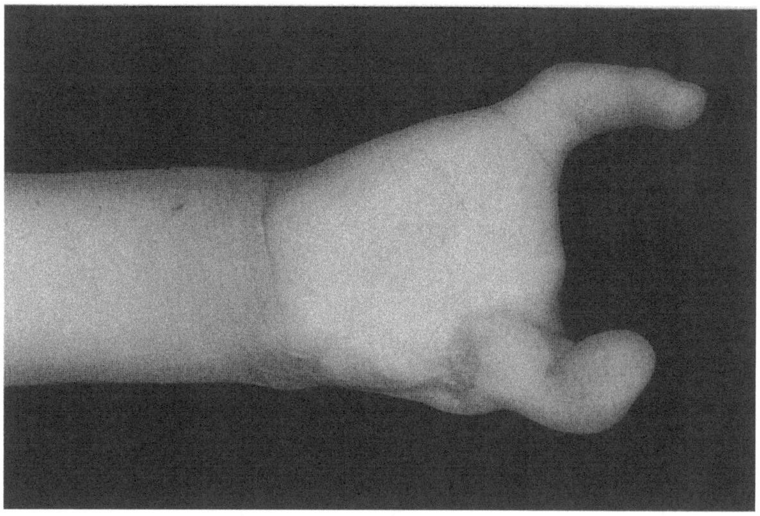

g

Fig. 23-5. h The reconstruction provided good pinch function.

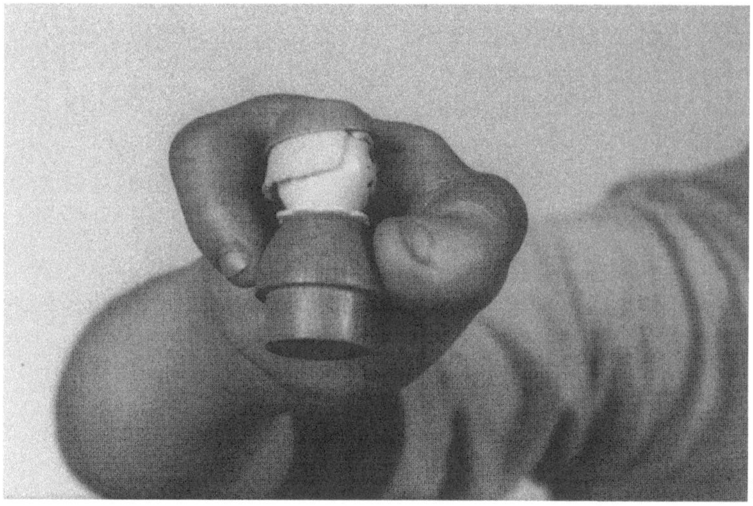

h

Fig. 23-5. i Useful grasp function is provided for large objects. It is well accepted now that successful vascularization of the epiphyseal plates will maintain function of the growth plate. Radiologically, these plates remain open following transfer and growth of the toe seems to proceed at the normal rate for a toe

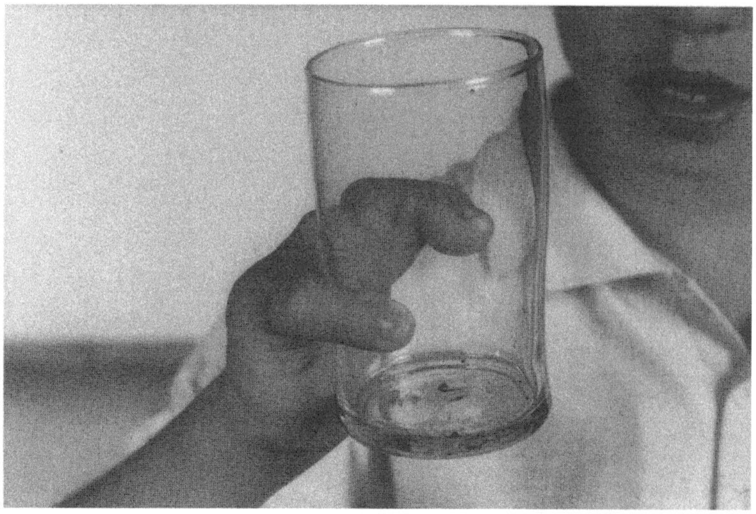

i

Subject Index

The Greater Omentum

Anatomy, Physiology, Pathology, Surgery
With an Historical Survey

Editors: **D. Liebermann-Meffert, H. White**
Consulting Editor for Section of Surgery: E. Vaubel
With a Foreword by Sir A. Parks

1983. 262 figures, some in color. XIX, 369 pages
ISBN 3-540-11882-9

Contents: Anatomy and Functional Anatomy. - Physiology and Functions. - Clinical Aspects. - Pathological Conditions, Specific Investigations, and Therapy. - Experimental Basis for Reconstructive Surgery Using the Omentum. - Historical Review.

This is the first comprehensive review and updating of the anatomy and physiology of the greater omentum and its uses in various surgical techniques. Recent advances have shown that far from being the Cinderella of the abdomen this organ is of increasing importance in reconstructive surgery. With the development of microvascular techniques the omentum will have even greater applications. It has been used in vivo studies of immunological and microcirculatory questions and has been found to be an excellent matrix for grafts. In this book the anatomy of the omentum in man and laboratory animals is described, the embryology and physiology of the omentum are presented, and details of animal experiments of clinical value are given. The section on pathology compiles the rare tumors of the omentum for the first time. A historical review is also provided.
Although omental surgery is undertaken in numerous centers, its application is still somewhat neglected. This book will help surgeons establish techniques with the omentum more widely and will serve as a foundation for future developments.

Springer-Verlag
Berlin Heidelberg
New York Tokyo

Springer

MIX
Papier aus verantwortungsvollen Quellen
Paper from responsible sources
FSC® C105338

If you have any concerns about our products,
you can contact us on
ProductSafety@springernature.com

In case Publisher is established outside the EU,
the EU authorized representative is:
Springer Nature Customer Service Center GmbH
Europaplatz 3, 69115 Heidelberg, Germany

Printed by Libri Plureos GmbH
in Hamburg, Germany